The Inevitable

DISPATCHES ON THE RIGHT TO DIE

Katie Engelhart

Atlantic Books
London

First published in the United States in 2021 by St. Martin's Press,
an imprint of St. Martin's Publishing Group.

First published in hardback in Great Britain in 2021 by Atlantic Books,
an imprint of Atlantic Books Ltd.

This paperback edition published in 2022.

10 9 8 7 6 5 4 3 2 1

A CIP catalogue record for this book is available from the British Library.

Paperback ISBN: 978-1-78649-566-2
E-book ISBN: 978-1-78649-565-5

Printed in Great Britain

Atlantic Books
An imprint of Atlantic Books Ltd
Ormond House
26–27 Boswell Street
London
WC1N 3JZ

www.atlantic-books.co.uk

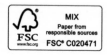

MIX
Paper from
responsible sources
FSC® C020471

For my parents

CONTENTS

If suicide is allowed then everything is allowed. If anything is not allowed, then suicide is not allowed.

—Ludwig Wittgenstein, *Notebooks, 1914–1916*

How can reason not reasonably detest and fear the end of reason?

—Julian Barnes, *Nothing to Be Frightened Of*, 2008

A NOTE ON SOURCES

Where indicated with an asterisk, I have used a pseudonym and sometimes changed several identifying details to protect the privacy of the person concerned. Otherwise, all names and details are real.

The
Inevitable

Introduction

Betty* said that she would go to Mexico herself. "I'm going to do it," she told the others. Lots of people went to Tijuana, but Betty chose Tecate, a small city off Federal Highway 2 surrounded by mountains. She had read in her online suicide manual about Mexican pet stores where in-the-know foreigners could buy lethal poison. All you had to do was tell the employee at the register that your dog was very sick and needed to be put to sleep—and that you were there to buy the sleeping agent. "I'm on the case," Betty texted her friends from outside a local shop. She was a little bit scared, but not too scared. She didn't think the police would seriously target a woman in her seventies. "They're not going to go after a little old lady," she said. "And I could pull the little-old-lady cover if I had to. I could sit and cry if I had to. No problem."

Back in Manhattan, before she left for Mexico, Betty had bought a handful of expensive-looking cosmetics bottles and printed labels to stick on the front of them: FOR SENSITIVE SKIN ONLY. The idea was that she would transfer the pet-store poison into the decoy containers before driving back over the border into California and flying home. The drugs would belong jointly to her and her two best friends. They would hold on to them quietly, in their respective Upper West Side apartments, until someone got sick. "We have a pact," Betty said. "The first one who gets Alzheimer's gets the Nembutal." The fast-acting barbiturate would put the drinker to sleep quickly, but not suddenly. Once she was asleep, her breathing would likely slow over the course of fifteen or twenty minutes, before it stopped.

Betty told me this shortly after we met. It was at a wedding. I was a friend of the bride. She was the mother of the groom. We first spoke outside, on the lawn, beside an old canoe filled with melting ice and bottles of white wine. Later, we talked at her apartment, which had chandeliers in the hallways and a rheumatic wood-paneled elevator. Betty's reading glasses hung from a cord around her neck, and she put them on and took them off and put them on again, again and again, as we spoke. I hadn't been looking for her—we met by chance—but when I told Betty about the book I was writing, she laughed and said that she had a story for me. By the time I heard it, I had interviewed enough people to know that all across America, sick and elderly men and women are meticulously planning their final hours: sometimes with bottles from Mexican pet stores or powders from drug dealers in China or gas canisters from the Internet or help from strangers. I also knew that while most reporting about the so-called right to die ends at the margins of the law, there are other stories playing out beyond them. Away from medical offices, legislative chambers, hospital ethics committees, and polite conversation. I knew that this was where I wanted my book to begin.

It had recently occurred to Betty that she had no interest in growing very old or dying very slowly. An old friend was in his nineties and it depressed her to see him still "hanging around." It depressed him, too. He was brittle and bored, and all his friends were dead already. And still he drifted, almost passively, almost without meaning to, from treatment to treatment. The end of life was strange that way. Betty blamed his doctors, and in turn all doctors. "Their whole education is 'Save a life! Save a life! Save a life!' Sometimes they forget what terrible shape people are in." She believed that it was better to cede to the limits of medicine than to fight them.

Her own husband had died quickly enough. Seventy-five years old. Cancer. Still, he suffered. Sometimes he cried. In his final days, Betty imagined taking firm hold of a pillow and smothering him, partly because she thought that's what he would have wanted, but also because she couldn't bear to see him that way. In the end, he grew so agitated that doctors gave him enough painkillers to knock him out. He spent three days in a morphine-induced languor and then died. Betty and her friends agreed that they would never let themselves get to that place and also that they would never rely on a physician to help them, because who knew where the bounds of a doctor's mercy lay?

Betty had learned about the Mexican drug from an online suicide manual, *The Peaceful Pill Handbook*, which was published by a fringe right-to-die group called Exit International. "You're only going to die once," its author said. "Why settle for anything but the best?" The handbook taught Betty that there was an alternative path. She could kill herself when she wanted to, only it wasn't as straightforward as most people assumed, if the end goal was a death that was foolproof and quick and painless. Reading through the text, Betty learned that many people try to end their lives and fail, on the weakness of their resolution, or by the foibles of their chosen poison, weapon, severed artery, or high-rise window. Or they take a handful of painkillers and die in writhing agony. Older methods of life ending had also been rendered impractical by advances in medicine and technology, which generally made the world safer, but also made it harder to achieve an easy death. Environmental regulations on the automobile industry had lowered permissible carbon monoxide emission levels, which made it more difficult to end a life by asphyxiation in the old way: running a car in a closed garage and funneling exhaust gas in through the window. Coal gas ovens had been replaced by less lethal natural gas equivalents. First-generation sleeping pills had been phased out and replaced with medicines that weren't as easy to overdose on. Even sympathetic doctors would have a hard time prescribing lethal pills to sick and dying patients like they used to: discreetly and quietly and with important things left off the patient's medical charts. Betty's book advised readers to acquire one of several drugs to hold for safekeeping and to use when the time was right.

Betty warned her friends that they would have to be careful in their planning, because even though suicide is legal, it is against the law to help someone else do it. Besides, if the wrong person found out, the women could find themselves under lockdown psychiatric watch, stripped of their belts and shoelaces and privacy, for hours or days. Interrogated and observed and accused. Betty had never broken the law before, and she didn't particularly want to. She would have preferred to do things properly: to wait until she was just about ready to die and then ask her doctors to make it so. But physician-assisted death is not legal in New York State. And anyway, even in the US states where it is legal, for terminally ill patients, a person can't qualify to die just because she is old and tired of living in an elderly body that she no longer wants or relates to.

As it was, she was feeling OK. She went to Pilates every week. She went to the theater. She saw interesting friends and read complicated books. But one day, all of that would end. When it did, Betty hoped that she could summon enough resolve to kill herself. Sometimes, she thought she should just pick an age and promise herself that she would not live beyond it. "There are two types of people in the world," Betty told me, "those who want to deal with death and get some control over it, and those who don't want to think about it. . . . I can't not think about it."

THE PUSH TO wrest bodily control, at the end of natural life, from the behemoth powers of Big Medicine and the state has been defined by individual stories: generally of white women whose personal end-of-life tragedies became family dramas, and then viral national dramas—and then talking points and turning points in a larger political crusade for "patient autonomy." In the US, this modern history begins in 1975, when twenty-one-year-old Karen Ann Quinlan went to a party at a bar in New Jersey, where she reportedly chased Valium with a few gin and tonics and then passed out. At the hospital, doctors attached the young woman to a mechanical respirator, but it was too late. Karen Ann's brain had been without oxygen for so long that it was damaged beyond repair. She was not dead, strictly speaking, but she had entered a "persistent vegetative state." Her weight dropped from 115 pounds to less than 70. Her eyes opened and shut and moved, but not in the same direction or in tandem. She seemed to grimace, though doctors assured her family that this was nothing more than a mindless muscle spasm. Several weeks later, Joseph and Julia Quinlan asked doctors to turn off their daughter's respirator, and the doctors refused. Hospital administrators said that removing the machine would lead to Karen Ann's death and thus would be murder.

The Quinlans filed suit in September 1975. When they did, the fight over young Karen Ann mutated into the nationally televised Quinlan affair. Dozens of journalists packed into the crowded Morristown courtroom and held vigil outside the Quinlan family home, flooding the front door in a wash of paparazzi flashbulbs whenever anyone came or went. The body of the voiceless, featherweight girl seemed to cry out for protection, and soon a cast of would-be saviors appeared. Politicians and priests spoke of rescuing her. Self-described faith healers and prophets arrived in New Jersey, some of them promising miracles—if only they could rest their hands on the "sleeping beauty." In daily news broadcasts, Karen Ann's inscrutable sleep assumed the form of a fairy tale or a morality play. In court, lawyers for the family said that Karen Ann deserved to die "with grace and dignity." On the other side, lawyers representing the hospital doctors compared the Quinlans' petition to Nazi atrocities during the Holocaust, "like turning on the gas chamber."

In November 1975, the Quinlans lost their case but quickly appealed

to the New Jersey Supreme Court, which reversed the lower-court decision. Justices ruled that Karen Ann's individual liberty interests were
greater than the state's interest in preserving her life, since doctors saw
"no reasonable possibility" that she would get better. By the court's logic,
when doctors turned off Karen Ann's life support, they would not be
murdering her, but instead allowing her "expiration from existing natural causes." The New Jersey justices referred to this act as "judicious
neglect," though others would call it "passive euthanasia." Later, at Karen
Ann's funeral, a parish priest named Monsignor Thomas Trapasso gave
an anguished homily. He said he prayed that the young woman's drawn-
out end would not "erode society's concern for the worth of human
life. . . . Only time will tell the full impact that Karen Ann's life and death
will have on future ethical practices."

In 1983, twenty-five-year-old Nancy Cruzan lost control of her car in
Carthage, Missouri, while driving home from her job at a nearby cheese
factory. She was found facedown in a ditch, not breathing. Again, doctors
declared the patient to be in a persistent vegetative state and put her
on life support. Again, the woman's parents insisted that their daughter would have preferred death to a vegetative life, and they asked for
her feeding tube to be removed. Again, hospital administrators refused.
And once again, the young woman lay in her hospital bed for days and
months and then years: her hands and feet contorted inward at unholy
angles and her body still, save for the occasional eye flutter or seizure or
round of vomiting. This time, the patient's fate was decided by the US
Supreme Court, which in 1990 issued its first-ever ruling in a right-to-die
case. In a 5–4 split, justices decided that any competent individual had the
right to refuse any medical treatment, regardless of her prognosis or how
effective a treatment might be. A patient could, for example, turn down
medicine that would save her life. Also, family members and healthcare
proxies could refuse treatment on behalf of an incompetent patient, as
long as she had left clear evidence of her wishes. Some right-to-die advocates celebrated the decision, but for many Americans there was a creepy

element to the court's ruling; judges had established a right that many people assumed they already had and always had.

When Nancy's feeding tube was finally withdrawn, she took twelve days to die. It was reported that her lips blistered and cracked and began to protrude. Her tongue swelled and her eyelids dried shut. Americans following her story were left to wonder whether withdrawing a machine and letting a person die of dehydration was so different from letting a doctor give a lethal injection to quickly end a patient's life, and which was better. "Even a dog in Missouri cannot be legally starved to death," said one reverend who traveled from Atlanta to stand outside the hospital as Nancy's body gave way. That same year, a twenty-six-year-old named Terri Schiavo went into cardiac arrest at her Florida home and inspired yet another right-to-die battle: this one pitting the woman's husband against her parents, with both sides claiming to speak for the unspeaking Terri, who had not left behind a legal will. Over the course of fifteen years, Terri's feeding tube would be inserted, then withdrawn, then reinserted (on the orders of a judge), then withdrawn again, then reinserted again (on the orders of then Florida governor Jeb Bush), before finally being removed forever in 2005.

Through these women's stories, a debate over the limits of lawful medical care transformed into a more aching conversation about fundamental rights and eventually into a campaign to take the patient autonomy movement even further. In 1994, Oregon residents passed Measure 16, making the state the first place in the world to legalize, by vote, what was then called assisted suicide, but which now, in the vocabulary of political lobbyists and patients who struggle to distance their cause from the laden s-word, is often called medical aid in dying (MAID) or physician-assisted death (PAD). After a string of legal challenges and a repeal campaign backed by nearly $2 million of Roman Catholic Church funding, the law went into effect in 1997. The Oregon Death with Dignity Act became a historic and moral turning point for the country and the world: a tilt toward utopia, or dystopia, depending on your view of things.

A year later, in 1998, an eighty-four-year-old Portland woman with metastatic breast cancer became the first person in the United States to legally die with her doctor's help. The woman was known to the public as Helen, and when she first told her doctor that she wanted to die, he said he didn't want to be involved. A second doctor advised her to enroll in hospice care and wrote in his notes that Helen was probably depressed. Helen found a third doctor. At her first appointment, she arrived in a wheelchair, attached to an oxygen tank. She explained that she had enjoyed living, but that each day was now worse than the day before it. Dr. Peter Reagan sent Helen to a psychiatrist, who spent ninety minutes evaluating her mood and competency before determining that in fact she showed no signs of depression. Reagan, in turn, wrote the woman three prescriptions: two for anti-nausea drugs, and the other for a barbiturate called secobarbital.

Before the Oregon law passed, Reagan told me, he had been "in enough situations where patients asked me for aid in dying. I turned it down because it wasn't legal. I knew there was a demand and I felt sick from that demand. I felt sick that I couldn't help people." But other doctors, Reagan knew, had helped their patients anyway, in the hospital shadows. In a 1996 survey in Washington State, 12 percent of doctors said they had received "one or more explicit requests for physician-assisted suicide" and 4 percent had received "one or more requests for euthanasia." A quarter of patients who made those requests were given lethal prescriptions. In a separate 1995 study of Michigan oncologists, 22 percent admitted to having participated in "assisted suicide" or "active euthanasia." And of course, there was Dr. Jack Kevorkian, who had become his own national scandal in 1990 after he helped a fifty-four-year-old Oregon woman take her life in the back of his beat-up Volkswagen van.

The Oregon law required patients to self-administer their lethal medications, so it was Helen who raised the glass of barbiturate to her lips. It took about twenty seconds for her to swallow all the liquid. She was at home with her two children, in the evening. When it was over, she asked for some brandy, but because she wasn't used to alcohol, she choked a little on the drink. Her daughter Beth rubbed her feet. Dr. Reagan took her small hand in his larger hand and asked how she was doing and Helen's response to him was the last thing she said. "Tired."

It was an inauspicious first. "It just happened," Dr. Reagan told me. He had been a workaday family doctor in Portland. When he agreed to help Helen, he didn't have any idea that her death would be the first. Then Helen's story hit the papers. "While doctors, religious leaders and politicians continue to debate the ethics of allowing physicians to help terminally ill patients kill themselves," wrote *New York Times* reporter Timothy Egan, "the issue took a sharp turn from the abstract today." Afterward, Reagan's name was leaked to reporters and he wondered what would happen to him. Would people throw rocks through his windows? Would they do worse—like they did to abortion doctors? But they did neither. Reagan continued to write prescriptions.

From the start, those opposed to physician-assisted death worried that any right to die would evolve, by tiny and coercive steps, into a duty to die—for the old, the enfeebled, and the disabled. A professor at the Oregon Health and Science University described it more bluntly: "There was a lot of fear that the elderly would be lined up in their R.V.'s at the Oregon border." But on the other side, advocates argued that a constitutional *right to life* had been perverted by the exigencies of modern medicine: that it had become, for most Americans, even ones who wanted to end their lives, an enforceable duty to live.

Under the Oregon Death with Dignity Act, an eligible patient has to be terminally ill, with a prognosis of six months or less to live. Prognostication is a fuzzy science, notoriously imprecise, and so two independent physicians must be in agreement. The patient must be over eighteen years old, a resident of the state, and mentally capable at the time of her request. If her doctor suspects that her judgment is impaired, for instance, by a psychological disorder, she should be sent for a mental health evaluation. The patient also has to make two oral requests to die, separated by at least fifteen days, and provide a written request to her attending physician, signed in the presence of two witnesses. Under the law, the patient's doctor is obliged to explain alternatives to assisted death, like pain management and hospice care, and also to request that she not end her life in a public place. The doctor will recommend that the patient notify her family members but cannot require it. At the heart of the law is the self-administration requirement; the patient needs to take the medication herself, since only assisted dying (where a patient self-administers lethal drugs, usually by drinking a powder solution) and not euthanasia (where a doctor administers the drugs, usually intravenously) is allowed.

When the Death with Dignity Act went into effect, advocates hoped that Oregon would give other states the moral impetus they needed to pass their own equivalent laws. Some proponents saw their movement as the logical continuation of other grand progressive battles: for the abolition of slavery, for women's suffrage, for racial desegregation. Baby boomers, the theory went, had seen their parents die ugly, protracted hospital deaths and wanted another way. But the post-Oregon elation did not quite play out. In 1995, the Vatican called assisted death a "violation of the divine law." The American Medical Association also declared itself opposed, on the grounds that "physician-assisted suicide is fundamentally incompatible with the physician's role as a healer" and his solemn pledge to do no harm. Healing, the thinking went, precluded killing. In the years following, dozens of states debated and rejected their own Oregon-style statutes. Doctors in Portland came to assume, as one said later, that assisted death would remain "one of those quirky Oregon things."

In 1997—the year that scientists in Scotland unveiled a cloned sheep named Dolly and Comet Hale-Bopp flew by earth—the US Supreme Court ruled on two assisted-death cases, from Washington and New York. In both cases, justices unanimously decided not to overrule state-level bans on physician assistance in death. In doing so, they concluded that physician aid in dying was not a protected right under the US Constitution. In other words, there was no right to die, or right to die with dignity—or even, in the words of Justice Sandra Day O'Connor, a "generalized right to 'commit suicide.'" Instead, the Supreme Court sent the issue back to the "laboratory of the states." In his principal opinion, Chief Justice William Rehnquist emphasized the state's interest "in protecting vulnerable groups—including the poor, the elderly, and disabled persons—from abuse, neglect and mistakes." He also alluded to the slippery-slope argument that had become a backbone of opposition thinking around the world. The theory went that once a limited right to die was granted, it would be impossible to rein it in; the law would inexorably expand and expand to include ever more categories of patients. The sick but not dying. The mentally but not physically ill. The old. The paralyzed. The weak. The disabled. Eventually, critics warned, there would be abuse. Of the poor. The unwilling. The compromised. The scared. The sixteen-year-old boy with a scorching case of unrequited love. Any given principle, US Supreme Court justice Benjamin Cardozo once observed, had a "tendency . . . to expand itself to the limit of its logic."

Elsewhere, though, legislators had different ideas about sanctity. In 1995, the Northern Territory of Australia legalized euthanasia. While the law was rescinded by the federal government just two years later, the global landscape was slowly shifting. In 1998, "suicide tourists" from around the world started dying in Switzerland, where assisted death had been decriminalized and where a new clinic, near Zurich, began accepting foreign patients. Then in 2002, both the Netherlands and Belgium legalized euthanasia. Later, they were joined by Luxembourg, making the tiny Benelux region the global hub of physician-mediated death.

Around the same time, a legal challenge in Britain failed to overturn the country's ban on assisted dying. The case was brought by Diane Pretty, a 43-year-old from Luton with motor neurone disease. Diane said she wanted to end her life, but that she couldn't, because she was paralyzed from the neck down. In this way, she said, her physical inability to suicide, as was her legal right, was depriving her of her human right to die with dignity. Diane, in turn, wanted her husband to kill her – and she wanted to be sure that when he did, he would not be jailed for murder. She brought her claim before a British court, and then the European Court of Human Rights in Strasbourg. On the day she lost her final appeal, in April 2002, Diane addressed a cluster of reporters in London, through a voice simulator. "The law has taken all my rights away," she said. A month later, she died, after days in terrible pain. She died "in the way she always feared," the *Telegraph* reported.

Back in the US, it wasn't until 2008 that Washington followed Oregon's lead. Then came Montana (by judicial ruling, rather than legislation); Vermont; Colorado; California; Washington, DC; Hawaii; Maine; and New Jersey. The laws had different names, which made use of different euphemisms: End of Life Options Act (California), Our Care, Our Choice Act (Hawaii), Patient Choice and Control at the End of Life Act (Vermont). According to a 2017 Gallup survey, 73 percent of US adults believe that a doctor should be allowed to end a patient's life "by some painless means," if the patient wants it and "has a disease that cannot be cured." That show of support, however, drops to 67 percent when people are instead asked whether doctors should be allowed to help a patient "commit suicide if the patient requests it." Language both reflects and shapes opinion, and the s-word still carries its weight.

In Oregon, where the movement started, the numbers have remained small: around 3 out of every 1,000 deaths. In 2019, 290 patients got a lethal prescription and 188 died by ingesting lethal drugs. The vast majority have cancer, while others have heart disease, lung disease, and neurological illnesses like amyotrophic lateral sclerosis (ALS, or Lou Gehrig's disease). The patients are, more often than not, white and over sixty-five and middle class, married or widowed, with some college education. They score low on measures of spirituality. Almost all have health insurance, and most are already enrolled in hospice care. They have the time and the temperament and the capital to figure out what they want and then get it. Other researchers have offered additional theories. They note that African Americans are generally less likely to access end-of-life care, including palliative and hospice care, and speculate that these same disparities and discriminations extend to aid in dying. They observe that lethal medications are expensive and aren't always covered by insurance and so are sometimes unaffordable. They insist that certain demographic groups take better care of their elderly than others, and so presumably have fewer older people wanting to kill themselves. They chalk it all up to differences in religiosity and communal belongingness and moral values.

We do know something about what motivates patients to choose early death, in the places where aid in dying is legal. What surprised me most, looking through Oregon Health Authority data, was that most people who ask to die are reportedly not in terrible pain, or even afraid of future pain. The vast majority cite "losing autonomy" as their primary end-of-life concern. Others worry about "loss of dignity," loss of the ability to engage in enjoyable activities, and "losing control of bodily functions." Where pain enters the equation, it is a fear of future pain, or a wish to fend off forthcoming pain—or sometimes the here-and-now psychic pain of not knowing how much more pain will come. Will it be a good death or a bad death? The uncertainty is what lends the question its urgency. In the end, patients choose to die for more existential reasons: in response to suffering that falls outside the established borders of modern medicine.

THIS BOOK INCORPORATES medicine, law, history, and philosophy, but it is not a book of argument and it is not a comprehensive accounting of the right-to-die movement. Primarily, it is a collection of stories and conversations and ideas. My work began in London in 2015, when I was working as a journalist at VICE News. That year, the British Parliament voted on whether to legalize physician-assisted death in the country. I did some reporting on the subject and worked with a few colleagues on a documentary film. I followed the national debate, which was both vehement and predictable. Proponents spoke of "personal autonomy" and told wrenching stories about sick and dying people who were driven to end their lives, in hideous ways, because of their pain. Opponents spoke of "the sanctity of life" and warned of a lack of safeguards to protect vulnerable people. On the day of the vote, protesters gathered outside the Parliament building to scream in each other's faces, purple-faced and bug-eyed. GIVE ME CHOICE OVER MY DEATH, read posters on the one side. BEWARE THE SLIPPERY SLOPE, DO NO HARM, read posters on the other. Later, after Parliament voted down the bill, I continued my own research, first across Britain and then in countries where assisted dying is legal: Canada, Belgium, the Netherlands, and the United States. I wanted to know what it meant to legislate a whole new kind of dying into being. It seemed so fundamental to how we understand the meaning of our lives and the social contracts we feel bound to.

When I turned my attention to reporting, I was surprised to find much less data than I had expected. In Belgium and the Netherlands, euthanasia oversight councils publish annual reports, but they reveal little about the individual people who make use of the laws. In the American states where aid in dying is legal, health departments release even less. In these places, physicians are required to turn in some amount of paperwork on each completed death, but these forms are filled out by doctors rather than by dying patients, whose self-reported thoughts and expressions are never captured by the medical system. Not every state collects much data at all, and not all of the collected data is published, because of confidentiality concerns. This leaves some researchers to mourn for all that is never known about these unusual patients—their specific geographic locations, their mental health histories, the nature of their family relationships, the size of their bank accounts. Across the world, systematic research on physician-assisted death is also scant. "There are reasons for that," Dr. Ganzini, who has published more on the subject than almost anyone else in America, told me. "It's hard to get it funded. It is the kind of research that, for example, the National Institutes of Health would be wary of." I knew that if I wanted to understand these patients, I needed to find them, and then to follow them through the brief slivers of time when they were planning their deaths.

But that wasn't all. As I learned more about US death with dignity laws – the kind that are considered, from time to time, in countries like the UK – they no longer seemed that philosophically radical. The laws, after all, apply only to dying patients who are going to die soon anyway. They speed up an inevitable process, but not by much. And they don't change its course. As the months and years passed, I started meeting other kinds of patients: men and women who didn't meet the criteria for physician-assisted death, even where it is legal, but who still wanted to die—for absolutely rational reasons, they said. Because they were chronically ill. Or in pain. Or old and tired, or becoming demented. Or because they didn't want to live as long and as sick as their parents had. These people were very different from one another, but they seemed to share a common vocabulary. In our conversations they spoke of "rational suicide," a kind of life ending that is, at least in theory, not impulsive or inspired by mental illness (what is sometimes called "despair suicide," which is most suicides) but instead by the ostensibly cooler and more sober mathematics of cost-benefit analysis. Given everything: to die or to live?

Many people told me stories about coming up against the limits of the law and then looking for solutions outside them. And finding them. Sometimes, help came in the form of loved ones. Other times, people found relief on the Internet: in small but often highly organized clandestine groups, which some activists refer to as the "euthanasia underground." When I first learned about these networks, I was amazed by them. But then—well, of course. Hadn't I read about underground women's groups that offered abortions in the years before they were legal? Didn't I know that whenever the law falls short, people find a way? I decided to make these people the focus of my reporting and the protagonists of this book.

Over the course of four years, I spoke with hundreds of people, all over the world, who are, in various ways, involved in assisted death, both within and outside the law. I interviewed patients, doctors, nurses, researchers, dogged advocates, stalwart opponents, a tormented mother, an indignant father, and a grandmother who locked herself in the basement when I arrived to ask questions about her grandson. I connected with a shaman in the desert of New Mexico; a Mexican drug dealer who reads Lao-tzu; several elderly men and women in Britain who ordered lethal drugs on the Internet; and a former corporate executive who travels around the US teaching strangers how to take their lives with gas canisters and plastic bags. In the time we spent together, these people considered the impulse to live and the impulse to die, and the way those inclinations can bend around each other. In the end, I devoted very little attention to the experiences of politicians battling in state legislatures and religious figures who oppose assisted death on theological grounds. Those stories felt too tired, too obvious. Instead, I focused on six personal stories, which make up the six chapters of this book. Two are about doctors: one a physician in California who opened a clinic specializing in assisted death, and the other an Australian named Philip Nitschke who lost his medical license for teaching people how to "exit" at "DIY Death" seminars. Nitschke's organization, Exit International, and his published suicide manual, *The Peaceful Pill Handbook*, make appearances throughout this book. The other four chapters belong to people who told me that they wanted to die because they were suffering unbearably—of, respectively, old age, chronic illness, dementia, and mental illness.

Many of the people I met had stories that were messier and more tangled than those I read in daily newspaper reports about physician-assisted dying: tidy narratives about terribly sick people in the US or Belgium who, after receiving their terminal diagnoses, made tortured but lucid choices, in direct and exclusive response to that tumor, or this lung disease, or that neurological failing. The people I met were certainly motivated to die because they were sick, but also because of mental anguish, loneliness, love, shame, long-ago traumas, or a yearning for the approval of Facebook followers. Some were driven by money, or a lack of it. The peo-

ple I met were not, in other words, pure characters. They weren't always
likable or relatable, or even emotionally legible. They were not always
brave in the face of death. And their suffering did not always yield meaningful lessons to impart to the world around them. Sometimes, their pain
was just pointless and awful.

My reporting was not straightforward. In several cases, I knew that
people had the intention to end their lives before they carried out the
act—alone at home, without a doctor's help or knowledge—and I did not
intervene. This work was ethically knotty. I was often unnerved and uncertain, both as a journalist and as a human. As any reporter knows, the
story changes as soon as she appears with her notebook and recorder, no
matter how unassuming she is or how delicately she navigates the scene.
I never wanted my presence in someone's life to nudge her toward death.
I didn't want anyone to die for the sake of a story, or for the sake of *my*
story. I tried to be careful. I was selective about whom I met with. When
possible, I spoke with family members, friends, doctors, therapists, and
caregivers. I reminded people, over and over, that they owed me nothing
and that I expected nothing. They could speak with me for as long as they
wanted to and then tell me to back off. If it was easier, they could just stop
answering my calls. Some did, and I let them go.

Over the years, I found myself discussing this book at dinner parties
and work functions and crowded bars, and then being sought out later for
private confession. It seemed like everyone had a story and was starved to
tell it. Why? Near strangers described terrible endings they had witnessed.
Unruly. Slow. Embarrassing. Others told me about deaths that had been
planned. A friend said his grandfather had hoarded cardiac medication to
kill himself with. Another described how her sister had crushed pain pills
to stir into an elderly aunt's yogurt. A colleague told me that his ninety-
something father had opted for a needless and risky surgery in the feverish
hope that he would die on the operating table. The man was too weak to
kill himself, but he hoped that he could make his doctors kill him.

What does this all mean? This hunger for absolute control—or maybe just a shred of control—at the end of life, and this revolt against the machines that sometimes sustain a spiritless version of it? It is about the desire to avoid suffering. It is about autonomy. It is also about the right to privacy and the negative right to not be interfered with. But for most of the people I met, choosing to die at a planned moment was principally about "dignity."

Dignity, of course, is a muddy sentiment—and some philosophers take issue with the very idea of it. They argue that dignity is, at best, conceptually redundant: another way of saying respect for choice or for autonomy. Others resent its use in this particular fight. Aren't all humans endowed with an intrinsic dignity, they ask? Isn't everyone, by extension, dignified when they die? Proponents of medical aid in dying have absorbed the word into their catchphrase euphemism "death with dignity" and so claimed a monopoly on it, but opponents have made their own dignity appeals. "We oppose euthanasia and assisted suicide," read the 2008 Republican Party platform in a paragraph titled "Maintaining the Sanctity and Dignity of Human Life." For others, dignity is not found in escaping physical pain, but rather in being calm and courageous and self-restrained in the face of it. Dignity, in this view, is reflected in composure—and earned through endurance.

When I interviewed sick and dying people for this book, I sometimes asked them about dignity. In the beginning, I admit, I found myself expecting a kind of transcendent wisdom from them, as if, by virtue of being especially intimate with mortality, they would understand things in a way that I couldn't. It wasn't like that. A lot of people I interviewed equated dignity precisely with sphincter control. Their lives would be dignified, they said, until they shit their pants or had to have someone else wipe their ass. It was really that straightforward. It seemed that even when people had trouble defining dignity in a precise way, they knew intrinsically when something felt undignified. For them, planning death was often about avoiding indignity, something they imagined would be humiliating, degrading, futile, constraining, selfish, ugly, physically immodest, financially ruinous, burdensome, unreasonable, or untrue.

"HOW CAN I explain this? I think it's virtually impossible for any human being, no matter how old they are, to imagine their own death," Betty said. We were seated in her dining room, in straight-backed wooden chairs, eating fruit salad. She had just told me about the trip to Mexico and the drugs and the suicide pact. "The resurrection was the best idea to get people to sign up to Christianity that ever existed." But Betty did not believe in resurrection. The best she could hope for, and the only thing she could plan for, was "a peaceful death," which she hoped she could achieve by cutting short the very last stretch of her life. She would die before she became so ill or demented that she lost herself. The deep slumber of a barbiturate overdose seemed easy enough.

It was strange, Betty thought, how humans were left to suffer in the end, while dogs got to be put out of their misery with a quick shot of medicine. Strange, too, how the putting down of dogs was seen as an act of mercy. Strange to be envious of dogs! There was a slogan that Betty liked that was shared by right-to-die enthusiasts online: "I would rather die like a dog."

Modern Medicine

The first thing Dr. Lonny Shavelson thought when he stepped into the room was, *This is a bad room to die in*. It was small and stuffy and there weren't enough chairs. He would have to rearrange things. He would start by pulling the hospital bed away from the wall, so that anyone who wanted to touch the patient as he died would have easy access to a hand or arm or soft, uncovered foot. But first, there were loved ones to greet. They all stood stiffly by the doorway, and Lonny hugged each of them: the three grown children, the grandson, the puffy-eyed daughter-in-law, and the stocky, silent friend. Then he sat his slight body down on the edge of the bed. "Bradshaw," he said gently, looking down at the old man lying under the covers. Bradshaw blinked his eyes and stared vacantly at the doctor. The room smelled sour and institutional, like evaporated urine. "You don't know who I am yet, because you're still waking up," Lonny said buoyantly. "Let me help you a little bit. Do you remember that I'm the doctor who is here to help you die?"

The old man blinked again. Someone had combed his gray hair back, away from his forehead, and he wore a brown cotton T-shirt over thin, age-spotted arms. "It's the prelude to the final attraction," Bradshaw said at last.

Lonny, who is small and slim, with a receding hairline and wire-rimmed glasses, left his Berkeley home office that morning at 9 a.m., with a canvas medicine bag in one hand and a pair of black dress shoes in the other. He always wore house slippers when he drove, for comfort, and then changed into nicer shoes when he got to the patient's home. This would be Lonny's ninetieth assisted death. Everyone said there was no doctor in California who did more deaths than Lonny. He would say that this had less to do with his particular allure as a physician and more to do with the fact that other doctors in California refused to do assisted deaths or were forbidden to do them by the hospitals and hospices where they worked. Sometimes, Lonny said, he got quiet phone calls from doctors at Catholic health systems. "I have a patient," the doctors would say. "Can you help?"

Lonny drove north, through residential Berkeley, past tidy streets lined with bungalows and blossoming cherry trees, and then along un-attractive stretches of highway dotted with drive-through restaurants and Chinese buffets. After a while, the urban sprawl gave way to water-soaked rice fields. Lonny took tiny sips from his water bottle and tried to memorize the names of the patient and his children. I quizzed him until they came easily. The patient was Bradshaw Perkins Jr. and he was dying of prostate cancer.

Three years earlier, when Bradshaw was living with his son Marc and his daughter-in-law Stephanie, he had tried to gas himself to death in the garage. Later Bradshaw would claim that he sat in the driver's seat for an hour, waiting to die, but that nothing happened. He had messed something up. Marc wasn't sure if his father had really meant to die that day. Was he for real? Was it a play for attention? "Hard to say," Marc said. "He always claimed he was never depressed and that it wasn't an issue. He was just tired of life."

In the three years since, cancer had spread through Bradshaw's body with a kind of berserk enthusiasm, from his prostate to his lungs and into his bone marrow. At the nursing home where he had once been happy enough—watching TV, eating take-out KFC, flirting with his nurses—he had grown restless, bored, and despairing of the hours before him. When Marc came to visit, he would find his father staring at the wall. Bradshaw's body began to ache. His bowels cycled between constipation and diarrhea, so that he always felt either stuffed or hollow. Eventually, after a lifetime of refusing to take so much as an aspirin, Bradshaw gave in to the medication protocols recommended by his hospice doctors. He felt less pain on drugs, but he grew loopy and started falling when he got up to pee. His arms sprouted purple bruises and his left leg felt funny all the time. Nurses had trouble picking him up when he fell, and Bradshaw worried about hurting them. He stopped leaving his bed. In May 2018, doctors told Bradshaw that he was nearing the end and that he likely had just two or three months left to live. Marc was in the room and thought he saw his father smile. "People try to help me," said Bradshaw. "But I think I am done needing help."

Bradshaw told Marc that he had lived a good life, but that after eighty-nine years, the bad was worse than the good was good. He missed running. He missed fixing up cars. He missed taking his body for granted. "I want to pass," he said.

"Whoa-kay," said Marc. And right there, in his father's little nursing home apartment, Marc took out his phone and Googled "assisted dying + California." He found a page describing the California End of Life Option Act, which passed in 2015 and which legalized medical aid in dying across the state. It seemed to both men that Bradshaw met the requirements: terminal illness, close to death, mentally competent.

Bradshaw said he had already asked his nurses, twice, about speeding up his death, and that each time the nurses had said that they couldn't talk about it because it was against their religion. When Marc called VITAS Healthcare—the national hospice chain that managed Bradshaw's care, dispensing all the nurses and drugs and equipment that Medicare pays for when someone is within six months of death—a social worker explained that while the company respected Bradshaw's choice, its doctors and staff members would play no part in it. VITAS had prohibited its physicians from prescribing drugs or consulting with patients in aid-in-dying cases, as had many other hospices in the area, along with the state's dozens of Catholic hospitals and health systems. On the phone, Marc asked the social worker whom he should call for more information, but the social worker said she wasn't allowed to help him with that either. (VITAS's chief medical officer told me later, in an email, that VITAS staff can in fact "discuss and answer any questions on eligibility requirements" and can help refer patients to prescribing physicians.)

It was the hospice chaplain, Marc said, who took him aside and told him to look up Dr. Lonny Shavelson. When Marc searched Lonny's name, he saw that the doctor ran something called Bay Area End of Life Options. The medical practice was the first of its kind in California, if not the whole country: a one-stop shop that specialized in assisted death. There were articles on the Internet that praised Lonny as a medical pioneer. Unlike other doctors, who prescribed lethal medications for patients to take on their own, Lonny or his nurse was present at every single death; it was part of their standard package, which went beyond the requirements of the law. Other articles, though, were less kind. Some criticized Lonny for running a boutique death clinic. He charged $3,000 and didn't take insurance, and he didn't offer refunds if people changed their minds. "Less than you pay for a funeral," Lonny told me when I asked about his rate.

Marc did some research and found that neither Medicare nor the Department of Veterans Affairs would pay for Bradshaw's assisted death. Under the 1997 Assisted Suicide Funding Restriction Act, Congress had, with bipartisan support, banned the use of federal funds "for the purpose of causing or assisting in the suicide, euthanasia, or mercy killing of any individual," a move supported by then president Bill Clinton, who had pledged during his first campaign to oppose death with dignity legislation across the country. Marc didn't care about the politics. He could pay.

He sent an email to the address listed on Lonny's website: "We would like to enlist your services in this regard."

Bradshaw formally requested to die on January 9, 2019, starting the clock on California's mandated fifteen-day waiting period. Afterward, Lonny's nurse sent over the paperwork. Bradshaw had to sign a state of California form titled "Request for an Aid-in-Dying Drug to End My Life in a Humane and Dignified Manner," pledging that he was "an adult of sound mind" who was making his request "without reservation, and without being coerced." Bradshaw told Marc that he wanted to sign his name perfectly—every letter in its proper place—but midway through, his handwriting gave way and looped upward into a wispy scrawl.

It seemed to Lonny that if Bradshaw let the cancer take its course, it would probably kill him in a few weeks' time. It was hard to say exactly what the death would look like, though it's possible that he would feel some pain in the end and that hospice nurses would offer him heavy painkillers, probably morphine. On the way out, he might pass through a period of what doctors call "terminal restlessness" or "terminal agitation," which can induce confusion, disorientation, insomnia, angry outbursts, paranoia, and hallucinations. Some dying people dream that they are underwater and trying hard to swim to the surface to *tell you something*, but they can't get there. Many dream of travel. Planes, trains, buses. The metaphors that fill a dying man's dreamscape can be callow and obvious. For others, delirium is more pleasant; they see angels on the ceilings and the walls. Benzodiazepines could help with the unrest and anxiety. Antipsychotics could ease the visions. Drugged or not, Bradshaw would likely fall into a coma. Maybe he would stay that way or maybe he would dip in and out of consciousness for a while. After a few days or weeks, he would die. The cause of death would technically be dehydration and kidney failure, but the death certificate would recognize his cancer as the underlying killer. Perhaps his children would be at his bedside, but perhaps they would have gone home for the night to get some sleep when Bradshaw took his final breath. Death isn't always poetic. People die while nurses are adjusting their bodies in bed, to ease pressure off their bedsores. They die when they get up to pee. One hospice nurse told me that men often let go after their wives leave the room for a bite to eat.

The nursing home was painted pale yellow and it looked like a life-size dollhouse, tucked into a street of suburban bungalows in a city called Citrus Heights. The parking lot outside was full, so Lonny pulled into a space next door, which belonged to the Christ Fellowship Church. "We'll tell them we're just going to kill someone," he said brightly as he changed his shoes. Marc was waiting outside, a middle-aged man with a broad frame and black rectangular glasses. He squinted at us, uneasy.

Inside Bradshaw's room, someone had hung framed photographs on the wall: collages of children and grandchildren, close friends and their grandchildren. There was a certificate thanking Bradshaw for his military service. On the countertop were half-eaten bags of Halloween candy and half-used bottles of hand sanitizer and a plastic cowboy hat—maybe left over from some nursing home theme night. I imagined it sitting atop a nimbler, more alert Bradshaw. "Hi, sweetie," Cheryl said, sitting at the edge of her father's bed. She was as slender as her brother was robust, in a peach-colored sweater. "Everyone is here." Cheryl had flown in from Maryland and Sean had come from Washington State. Marc and Stephanie had driven from nearby and had brought their son. They had all scheduled time off work for the death.

Lonny could see that Bradshaw was a more diminished man than he had been just a few days earlier. When California's aid-in-dying law passed, opponents imagined that plucky cancer patients would soon be marching into their oncologists' offices to demand lethal drugs, but that wasn't what Lonny was seeing. Most of his patients were almost dead by the time they ended their lives; they were weak and a little hazy. Sometimes, this was because their primary doctors had dragged their heels—delaying the process for weeks or months. About a third of people didn't make it through the state's required fifteen-day waiting period because they died naturally or lost consciousness, or because they grew too weak to lift a glass of medication to their lips. Or because, when the day arrived, they were too disoriented and confused to fully consent to their own deaths. Bradshaw was teetering on the edge.

Lonny had warned the family that confusion could set in at the end. "Let's put it this way," he said, "almost everybody, when they get really close to dying, is demented." Even so, he had to be convinced that Bradshaw knew what was going on. He didn't need to know the month of the year or the name of the president, but he had to remember what he was sick with and what he had asked for—and he still had to want it. On a few occasions, Lonny said, he had made it all the way to the bedside and then called off the death because the patient was too out of it to agree to anything at all.

"What are you dying from?" Lonny asked. Then he said it again, louder.

"I'd like to know myself," Bradshaw said.

"Dad, you have to be serious," said Marc, and the room fell silent. Cheryl rubbed the back of Bradshaw's sunken hand, like she was willing his mind to cohere.

I pressed my back into the small partition separating the two sections of the apartment and tried to breathe quietly. From where I stood, I could see into the closet, where a few T-shirts were hanging over a pile of plastic adult diaper packages. I could also see that Bradshaw's hands were bent inward and that his feet looked swollen and pale, like they were waterlogged. Behind me, his grandson looked down at his phone. Bradshaw said nothing for a while and then recalled that there was something wrong with his prostate.

"OK," Lonny said, smiling. "We have a bit of paperwork to do."

Bradshaw groaned. "Oh my God."

"As you can imagine, the state of California doesn't let you die easily." Lonny held up a document. "This little paper here is called the 'Final Attestation.' The state of California wants you to sign, to say that you are taking a medication that will make you die." Bradshaw closed his eyes.

"Dad," Marc urged. "Dad, you have to stay awake for a few minutes. . . . Daddy, you need to sign, right?"

"Dad," said Cheryl. "Sign your name."

Bradshaw opened his eyes and signed the form and Lonny said they were ready to begin. He warned everyone that he didn't know how long it would take. Some patients died in twenty minutes. Others took twelve hours. He said that he had recently been tweaking his standard drug protocol, adjusting doses and delivery schedules, and that he had managed to lower the average patient dying time to just two hours. Bradshaw would start with an initial medication mixed into apple juice. Then half an hour later he would drink a cocktail of respiratory and cardiac drugs and some fentanyl. The drugs would work to kill Bradshaw in different ways. The respiratory suppressants would likely kick in first, to stop his breathing, but if they didn't, then the high-dose cardiac medications would eventually stop his heart. Either way, it would feel the same to Bradshaw, who would fall unconscious just a few minutes after taking the final dose. New patients were always asking for "the pill," Lonny said, but there was no magic death pill. In fact, it was surprisingly hard to kill people quickly and painlessly; the drugs weren't designed for it and nobody taught you how to do it in medical school.

At the sink, Lonny opened a small lockbox that was filled with $700 worth of medication. I stood beside him and watched him unpack it. He pointed to a green glass bottle. "That's the fentanyl," he whispered. Fentanyl, a synthetic opioid, wasn't part of the usual drug protocol, but Lonny had added it to the mix to see if it would speed up his patients' deaths. He had got the idea from a *New York Times* article about an opioid addict who overdosed after sucking the fentanyl out of some prescription pain patches and letting the solution dissolve in his cheek. "Wow, why can't we do that?" he had wondered.

Lonny mixed the first powdered drug into a plastic bottle of juice and passed it to Bradshaw, who drank it quickly. Marc exhaled. "You did good," said Lonny, who noted that the time was noon.

At the bedside, everyone was teasing Bradshaw about the women he was going to kiss in heaven. "I hope he gives *all* the girls a kiss," said Sean.

"Well, that's a given," said Marc's wife, Stephanie, who couldn't stop crying.

Bradshaw's flirting had always been a source of family embarrassment. Even in his final years, he was forever hitting on his nurses and vocally appraising their figures. Marc told me that if it had been any other occasion, and if Bradshaw weren't quite so sleepy, "I mean, he would have been hitting on you like crazy." Now, on the day of his death, the old humiliations had softened into a hokey inside joke. "When you're dying," the writer Cory Taylor observed in *Dying: A Memoir*, "even your unhappiest memories can induce a sort of fondness, as if delight is not confined to the good times."

"Well, Dad," said Cheryl, her voice honeyed and uncertain, "I love you. And I've enjoyed being your daughter."

Bradshaw's eyes opened, and then they were wide open: pale blue and, for the first time all morning, unclouded. I had read that people sometimes experience a "surge of energy" just before death and I wondered if I was seeing one. "I have never been around a more delightful girl in my life," Bradshaw said to Cheryl. "You're the most glorious girl."

"Who is going to help me fix my car when it breaks down?" said Marc, who started weeping and turned his face away. "I know we didn't always get along, but I always knew that you loved me."

"I always have and I always will," said Bradshaw.

"When you get up there, if there's a way to let me know, I want you to do it."

"I'll try," said Bradshaw.

"You've got a smile on your face," said Sean.

"Oh boy."

Bradshaw had raised his three children without religion. Marc said his dad never brought them to church. Not even once. They were a family of devout nonbelievers. Still, in this final stretch, everyone was talking about afterlife reunions. Maybe Bradshaw's children did believe in heaven, at least a little. Or maybe they just didn't see another way to talk about what was happening. Sometimes even the firmest atheists revert to old, holy rites: not because they really trust in them, but because they are tired and sad and need the anesthetizing structure of ritual. Talking about a reunion in heaven one day might, at the very least, be a way of saying goodbye that wasn't so unbearably sad. "The road to death," wrote the anthropologist Nigel Barley, "is paved with platitudes."

At his patients' bedsides, Lonny also liked to think about ritual. He thought about how physician-assisted death was a brand-new kind of dying, and how any traditions that developed around it would also be new. As it was, everyone did things differently. Once, a family ordered Chinese food while the patient faded away. Another time, a Latino family ate nothing for hours and hours and instead stood quiet vigil, with fistfuls of shaking rosary beads. One Korean family set up rows of chairs in front of the hospital bed, which made the death seem like a spectacle. Because his patients' deaths were scheduled, they could also be choreographed. Loved ones could compose their final words. Old family customs could be dug up and played out. Most families, in Lonny's experience, managed to pull themselves together and be pleasant at the bedside. Only a few times had someone freaked out.

Lonny stirred the second drug mixture, which had the consistency of tomato juice. "This is the final drink," he said. "This is important stuff." Lonny explained again that, according to the California law, Bradshaw had to drink the medication himself—which meant that he alone had to lift the cup to his lips. If he spilled, there was no backup. "Ready to roll?"

"Ready to roll," said Bradshaw.

"Dad, you have to drink again," said Marc.

"I'll make it," said Bradshaw. It took him a few sips to finish everything. Afterward, he coughed and gave a thumbs-down sign because the taste was bitter.

"This medicine has a little bit of a euphoric, pleasant feeling," Lonny said. "Go with it. Enjoy it." He attached a plastic pulse oximeter to Bradshaw's index finger and then stuck three small, adhesive-backed sensors to his chest. Together, they would feed information about the old man's heartbeat and oxygen levels to a small cardiac monitor. Most doctors didn't do any of this, but Lonny liked to track exactly what was happening as his patients' bodies wound down.

"So far, so good," said Bradshaw. Then he closed his eyes and his forehead went slack. A few minutes later, he started breathing in a raspy way, and then in a gurgling way, like water forcing itself down a wet sink clogged with hair. Lonny said that everything was normal. This was just the way that dying sounded. There was nothing to be done, even though it felt like the right thing to do was to pound on Bradshaw's chest with a tight fist—as if doing so would free some sticky knot of phlegm and make him quiet again. A half hour passed, and then an hour. Bradshaw's lips turned beige. Cheryl leaned over to smooth the front of his brown T-shirt. Some of Lonny's patients got dressed up for their deaths, in formal clothes, but most people didn't; they died in their pajamas.

"It's a great thing you do," said Stephanie, turning to Lonny.

"How many states allow this?" asked Marc.

"Seven," said Lonny. "And DC."

"This is peaceful," said Cheryl.

Marc said he wished they had done it all earlier. "He hadn't wanted to be sick."

Lonny looked down at the cardiac monitor. Flatline. "Here's how this works," he said after a while. "I'm going to give you a time of death of 1:45 p.m."

In the hallway outside, Lonny sat on a bench and leaned back against the beige wall. Soft jazz was playing in the front lobby, and a woman in a purple velour jumpsuit shuffled by with a walker. "Hi, baby," she said to another resident, who was drinking quietly from a plastic Dunkin'

Donuts cup. Lonny called the funeral home and said he had a death to report and that it was a medical aid-in-dying death. "Is that legal?" the woman at the funeral home asked.

Within thirty days, Lonny told me, he would have to send an "Attending Physician Follow-Up Form" to the California Department of Public Health. He would record the date of death and the number of minutes it took for Bradshaw to die. He would check a box, affirming that there were "No Complications." And then he would answer a series of questions about Bradshaw's motivations at the end. Had Bradshaw worried about "a steady loss of autonomy"? Or "a loss of dignity"? Lonny thought the form was stupid. How could he really know what Bradshaw had been thinking? How could any doctor know, of any patient? Also, the wording of the paperwork annoyed him. One question asked about "persistent and uncontrollable pain and suffering." That didn't make sense, Lonny said, because "pain" and "suffering" were two different things.

On the way out, Lonny told Marc that they should all go for a walk. Go for lunch, he said. Go for a drive. Do whatever—but try not to be there when the funeral home workers arrived with their transport bags.

LONNY ASKED FOR my impressions of the death, like he might have asked for my opinion of a painting. "What do you think?" It was a few hours later. We were sitting in his large backyard, in the small cottage that he had renovated into an office. The walls were lined with filing cabinets and the sliding glass doors looked out on a large wooden birdcage, which was filled with pet doves. Sometimes, Lonny said, a neighborhood cat came to sit on the fence and look down menacingly at the caged birds, but the birds were always too stupid to notice and be frightened.

"The noises. They were awful," I said hurriedly. Lonny nodded and ran a hand over his forehead. I tried again. "They were a nice family. They seemed very grateful."

When Lonny first started thinking about assisted death, he read the work of the American philosopher Margaret Pabst Battin, who argued that when a sick patient wanted to die, his physician was morally obligated to help him achieve "an easy death, to whatever extent possible." In Battin's view, the physician's pledge to do no harm was about more than not hurting; it meant actively working to relieve suffering. Maybe it even meant moving preemptively to stave off future, anticipated suffering. "Which is the greater evil, death or pain?" Battin wrote. "It is the patient who must choose."

Battin's work also considered the evolution of the doctor's role at the deathbed. In medieval Christian households, she wrote, the doctor was wholly absent. The dying person's final communications were reserved for God and focused on preparation for the afterlife. Final moments were final bids for repentance and salvation. But contemporary, secular deathbeds functioned differently. In the absence of God, the last stretch of life was recast; it was no longer a means to eternity, but an end in its own right. The point was not salvation, but closure. Today, Battin wrote, final moments "can be viewed as the conclusion, the resolution, the culmination of a life now completely lived. That is the reason some people choose to end their lives directly, so that they can finish their lives as themselves, able to think, communicate, and (for some) to pray, rather than be overtaken by pain or sedated into oblivion." A modern physician could use his tools to facilitate this new kind of ending.

That evening, alone in my rented Airbnb room, I thought about Bradshaw's final hours. I was already dismissive of idealized deathbed scenes—at least, the ones often rendered in novels and films. They seemed to feature very cogent old men or very flushed young women who, surrounded by loved ones, offered some carefully selected words or a consequential gaze before drifting off, gently, gently. Solemn and meaningful. I knew that real-life deaths don't always look that way. Final moments are not always transformative. And when they aren't, they can disappoint the people left behind, making them feel as though they have failed or been failed. As if they have been robbed of something they never

quite possessed, but still deserved. Was it possible that, in some way, assisted deaths came closer to the romanticized ideal—because they were
anticipated and so could be staged? And what of the final scene in the life
of Bradshaw Perkins Jr.? At least he had died with his three children in
the room: all of them touching his body when his heart stopped beating.
At least he had known when it was time for last words and could mumble something sweet to his daughter. Maybe that was a good death. Or a
good enough death. Or the best there is.

LONNY GREW UP in the wake of one bad death and under the threat of
another. The first took place two years before his birth. The dying person was his mother's mother, who was just fifty-nine years old and had
survived pogroms in Russia before moving to the United States. The
woman was reeling from a second heart attack: bedridden, on oxygen,
unable to feed herself. At some point, she stopped speaking—willfully,
her family thought—except to sometimes cry out in Yiddish, *Rateve
mir, rateve mir!* Save me, save me. Then she had a stroke and went blind.
She swung her arms violently and searched for people in the room who
were not there. A doctor was called. He was a tall man and he stood over
the bed, looking down at the patient. Then, with barely a word, he drew
up a syringe and pushed it through the dying woman's skin. After about
ten minutes, her pulse stopped. Lonny's mother screamed and "carried
on like a lunatic" until she was taken from the room. Later, everyone
would agree that the doctor had acted in mercy. But then again, no one
had asked for it.

The other bad death: For as long as Lonny could remember, his
mother had spent much of her life housebound, with Crohn's disease and
strange fevers—and, Lonny would eventually understand, with depression. From a young age, it was impressed upon him that he should grow
up to become a physician and find a cure for all the things that ailed her.
Failing that, he should kill her, preferably with an intravenous injection

of potassium chloride. Lonny was fourteen when his mother first asked him to be her murderer. "I would have jumped out the window right then if I'd had the courage," she told him later. "But I needed help—and you were the logical one to do it."

Lonny did go to medical school, but when he graduated in 1977, he chose to enter the then developing field of emergency medicine. He liked the idea of being able to save people quickly and decisively and then, at the end of a shift, to leave them at the hospital doors and forget all about them. He trained himself to forget his patients' names. It was only later that Lonny started thinking about people who did not want to be saved.

In 1992, a suicide manual called *Final Exit: The Practicalities of Self-Deliverance and Assisted Suicide for the Dying*, by Derek Humphry, made its way onto the *New York Times* best-seller list. It contained descriptions of different suicide methods and advice on how to trick doctors into prescribing lethal drugs. It was full of names and numbers, doses and drug combinations. Lonny heard about the manual and wondered why so many Americans wanted to know, in a specific way, how to kill themselves. What could it mean? He looked for books about suicide and read what he could find. He liked *The Enigma of Suicide*, published in 1991 by the journalist George Howe Colt, who ridiculed the notion that suffering at the end of life was an opportunity for eleventh-hour spiritual ennoblement. Colt wrote, "While some may find the last stages of terminal illness spiritually rewarding, ethicists question whether it is a person's duty to stay alive because others insist that pain is good for him."

Around that time, he started reading more about a doctor in Michigan named Jack Kevorkian, who in 1990 had helped a dementia patient kill herself in the back seat of his dirty old van. Kevorkian was charged, but then acquitted, and then went on to assist in more than one hundred deaths, many of which Lonny read about in the newspaper. It seemed to him that Kevorkian, who never tried to hide what he was doing, was in the headlines every day. People were obsessed. They followed the Kevorkian suicides like they were episodes in a soap opera, and they talked about them everywhere. Lonny read the news articles, like everyone else, but he was irritated by them. He thought that journalists were way too interested in Kevorkian, the man and myth, and not focused enough on his "patients"—and the larger question of what drove them into the hands of the weird "Dr. Death."

"I realized," Lonny would later write, "that, secretly, in darkened bedrooms across the country, thousands of parents, children, husbands, wives, sisters, brothers, lovers, and friends were deciding whether or not to aid in the death of a loved one." Lonny wanted to understand those darkened bedrooms and the ways that people inside them were hurting, and plotting. He started contacting hospice doctors and nurses in San Francisco and asking for on-the-sly introductions to their patients.

In 1995 Lonny published *A Chosen Death: The Dying Confront Assisted Suicide*. In it, he told the stories of five suicides, of five people whom he followed in the last weeks of their lives. One chapter was about a profoundly disabled man who tried and then tried again to starve himself to death—until finally, at his rabid insistence, his mother agreed to drug him and hold a plastic bag around his head. In another, Lonny admitted to watching a right-to-die activist smother an elderly man who claimed to be very sick but whose symptoms Lonny did not quite trust. Over several excruciating pages, Lonny described his indecision over whether to intervene. He wondered if he should pull the woman off the old man's jerking body.

In an especially aching chapter, Lonny told the story of a thirty-two-year-old trapeze artist named Pierre Nadeau, who was gay and had AIDS and who had fallen into a cavernous depression. Through Pierre, Lonny connected with a shadow network of AIDS sufferers who, "isolated by a society that had rejected them . . . were making their own rules" and helping one another to die. Lonny heard of AIDS patients who bequeathed leftover prescription drugs to other dying AIDS patients, so they could use them for planned overdoses; gay men who, at the sight of those foretelling purple skin lesions, started exchanging recipes for suicide cocktails "as casually as housewives swap recipes for chocolate-chip cookies," in the words of the reporter Randy Shilts. In Lonny's telling, these networks were careful and self-regulating, with their own procedures and safeguards. Nevertheless, the technology sometimes failed them. Some assisted deaths were not completed, or they were agonizing, or they took hours—and sometimes panicked bystanders resorted to pillows, or knives, or guns.

It made sense to Lonny that AIDS patients were the first to organize in this way. San Francisco was full of young and beautiful men who had watched other young and beautiful men slip into long, viral declines, into sores and bleeds and wasting muscle tissues, and then into tuberculosis and pneumonia rattles. Their sufferings were immense, their deaths were slow, and their fates were fixed from the moment of infection. And yet, for many of these men, just having a lethal drug—or knowing they could get one, if and when they wanted one—appeared to make them feel better. It seemed to Lonny that a mix of the right drugs was, in and of itself, a kind of cure. It let a sick person look away from his pain and move on with life for a while.

Twenty years after *A Chosen Death* was published, California passed the End of Life Option Act, becoming the fifth state in America to legalize medical aid in dying. Governor Jerry Brown, a former Jesuit seminary student, had publicly struggled over whether the legislation was "sinful" before reportedly being persuaded by, among other things, the writings of South African archbishop and Nobel peace laureate Desmond Tutu, who announced on his eighty-fifth birthday that he wanted the option of an assisted death. In 2016, 191 Californians received lethal prescriptions under the new law. In 2017, the number went up to 577. What happened in California, advocates knew, would be decisive for the broader movement. California was the first large, diverse state to legalize aid in dying. If things went well there, the California example could inspire legislators in other powerhouse states, like New York.

In 2018, I bought a used copy of Lonny's book online. It arrived with the stamp of a public library in Ohio, from which it had presumably fallen out of circulation. I read it through, and then I called Lonny, and then I flew to California to spend a month with him. By the time we met in early 2019, Lonny had written more lethal prescriptions than anyone else in the state and almost anyone in the country. Dozens of them. He had written more, even, than the doctors in Oregon who had been writing prescriptions for decades. Still, he spent most of our first day telling me all the ways that the California law was broken. It was, he insisted, a "shitty law." The right-to-die lobbyists weren't willing to say so, Lonny said, because their objective was to pass similar laws in other states—and, in fact, they sometimes pilloried him for pointing out the things that were screwy because, he assumed, his criticisms were bad for the cause. "They want New Jersey to know that this is easy. Anybody can do it! It works fine. Pass this law! Just like the other laws. There ain't no problems. . . . There's just this crazy guy in California who thinks there are some issues." Lonny said I would see it for myself. It would be obvious. He gestured toward a small chair beside his desk. "Just sit here and listen."

TO DIE WELL, YOU need the right drugs, but there were problems with the drugs. When the Death with Dignity Act came into effect in Oregon in 1997, prescribing doctors often used pentobarbital, a fast-acting barbiturate, as their lethal agent. It came in a liquid form called Nembutal that a patient could drink, and if he drank enough, he would fall asleep. "It's very gentle," one doctor who prescribed it back then told me. People who took pentobarbital almost always fell asleep quickly, within five or ten minutes. Soon after that, the drug would suppress a part of the brain that controlled respiration, slowing and then stopping the breath. This often took less than thirty minutes, though in some instances it could take longer: once, in Oregon, 104 hours.

By 2011, however, pharmacists were struggling to get their hands on the drug, in part because production had shifted offshore and the main European manufacturer—a Danish company called Lundbeck, which sold FDA-approved pentobarbital for the treatment of epileptic seizures—began restricting sales to the United States, under pressure from criminal justice advocates who noted that it sometimes ended up in prisons and was used to execute death-row inmates. That same year, the European Union placed an export ban on the drug. Then Akorn Pharmaceuticals, Lundbeck's American partner and the only domestic producer of pentobarbital that was approved for human consumption, introduced heavy restrictions on the medicine's nontherapeutic uses and stopped selling it to pharmacies for use in assisted deaths. The price of liquid pentobarbital rose from about $500 to more than $15,000.

Many American doctors switched to secobarbital, another barbiturate, which came in a capsule form called Seconal. It was a bit more complicated; patients had to open dozens of capsules and shake out the powder inside, then stir the medicine into yogurt or applesauce or pudding. Still, it worked in a similar way. But then the price of Seconal started rising, too. Just after the California law came into effect, a Canadian company called Valeant Pharmaceuticals (now Bausch Health) bought the manufacturing rights to the drug and doubled the price. A lethal dose of Seconal that had sold for $200 or $300 a few years earlier now went for $3,000 and sometimes more. A *JAMA Oncology* article called the price hike "one of the most poignant examples of pharmaceutical company profiteering from sales of older niche drugs." Medicare wouldn't pay for it. Medicaid would, in a few states, but not in others—and only for a fraction of the lowest-income patients. Most people who wanted an assisted death had to pay privately and up front, and many couldn't. One Oregon oncologist, Dr. Devon Webster, told me that she met patients who wanted to die and who qualified under the law but who couldn't afford the medications, and in some cases couldn't even afford gas money to get to the pharmacy. "I guess I'll take out my rifle and shoot myself," one of those patients told her. When aid in dying was first legalized, some opponents worried that poor people would be bulldozed into early deaths, but now it seemed like things could work the other way. Poor patients sometimes had to live, while richer patients got to die.

Back in California, Lonny heard that supplies of Seconal were running low and that the drug was getting harder to find. "What the fuck do we do now?" he asked his colleagues. In Washington State, some doctors hypothesized that a certain sedative could end a person's life if consumed in high enough doses, and they started prescribing it, but a few patients reported burning in their mouths and throats after swallowing, so they stopped. As it was, there wasn't much research about medicines that could painlessly kill patients by oral administration. Or, really, any research. No pharmaceutical drugs were explicitly designed to kill humans. And you couldn't exactly run a double-blind clinical trial with patients who were dying and wanted to die now.

In June 2016, a handful of anxious physicians—an anesthesiologist, a cardiologist, and two internists—met in a conference room in Seattle and vowed to work things out. Once they were settled, they called a few others on speakerphone: a second anesthesiologist, a pharmacologist, a toxicologist in Iowa, and a veterinarian who regularly euthanized animals. The goal of the collective was to find a drug that ended life reliably, was entirely painless to consume, and cost less than $500. The drug's component parts should be widely available in powdered form so that they could be purchased by specialty pharmacists and compounded together. So-called compound drugs had a particular advantage: they wouldn't be subject to FDA regulation, which meant that if the doctors in Seattle came up with a drug formula they liked, they wouldn't have to put it through years of randomized control trials and state oversight. They could simply start testing it. It was sort of wild, Dr. Carol Parrot, the anesthesiologist in the room, thought, how something this important was being figured out on the fly, in a little room in Washington State. But that was the thing with the law; it legalized a new kind of dying but didn't specify exactly how the deaths should be accomplished—or who was meant to figure that out.

At the end of their meeting, the Seattle doctors decided on a combination of sedative narcotics and cardiac medications: a compound that they called DDMP, for a mix of diazepam, digoxin, morphine, and propranolol. At first, they agreed to be guarded about their invention. They didn't want people to think that things were chaotic behind the scenes, or that doctors didn't know what they were doing. Instead, Carol prescribed the formula to ten of her own patients and sat by their bedsides while they died, making notes. The patients seemed to fall asleep about as quickly as people who took Seconal, and though the time it took for them to die could vary, they all died. The drugs worked. Afterward, Carol and the other physicians agreed to start sharing the recipe, informally, with colleagues across the state and beyond. They found compound pharmacists who would agree to make the new mix and started sharing their names, too.

In Berkeley, Lonny heard about DDMP and started using it, but he was surprised by how long it took for some of his patients to die. Sometimes he had these little old lady patients—they were so weak, they looked like a gust of wind might shatter them—and he would give them crazy amounts of toxic drugs, and still they would take hours and hours to die. Even the frailest life sometimes clung on to itself. Some of the slowest-dying patients were opioid tolerant, after months and years of pain treatment. Others were overweight, or on nausea medication that delayed gastric emptying, or were so constipated that the drugs got kind of stuck inside them. In very rare instances, Lonny learned, aid-in-dying drugs could fail, no matter what drug protocol was used. Patients got nauseous and vomited and didn't fall asleep. Or they fell asleep and then woke up. In Oregon, between 1998 and 2015, 991 patients died under the Death with Dignity Act, but 24 people regurgitated the drug and 6 regained consciousness. Some of those patients tried again and died successfully. Others did not. One awoken person reportedly gave up his death plans and went on to write a collection of poetry.

Lonny knew that American doctors were in a bind. In almost every other place where physician-assisted death is legal, euthanasia is also legal. This means that patients who qualify can choose between two kinds of dying: a lethal solution, prescribed by doctors, or an injection. In Canada and Belgium, patients almost always choose the injection. They want their doctors to manage things. Also, the injections are straightforward and quick, and they always work. No stress about mixing the solution and swallowing it. No chance of vomiting or waking up. But that has never been allowed in America. In the 1990s, Oregon legislators added a "self-administration" requirement to their proposed law as a way of winning over skeptics who worried that if a Death with Dignity Act passed, rogue doctors or bad-apple family members might euthanize sick patients against their will. If patients had to drink the drugs, the thinking went, they were less likely to be abused or coerced. The act of swallowing could be taken as final proof of the patient's consent, an autonomous gesture for an autonomous choice. The same logic has been applied in every other US state with legal physician-assisted death—to the horror of some European and Canadian doctors, who think it is unreasonable to make people drink liquid drug cocktails when much better, intravenous options are on offer. In fact, in other countries, if an aid-in-dying patient opts for a lethal drink, his doctor is legally required to have a backup injection on hand, in case something goes wrong or the death takes more than a few hours. In the United States, not even backup shots are allowed.

Lonny hoped that he could, at least, improve the lethal drug formula. He had never worked in experimental pharmacology or research before, or even in palliative medicine, but he started tinkering: making small modifications to the DDMP mix and using his tiny pulse oximeter and electrocardiograph to monitor the effects on his patients. He tried giving people one of the cardiac medications before the others. Then he doubled the dose and added an antidepressant drug that he liked because of its ability to "irritate the shit out of the heart." Later, he replaced the propranolol with another drug. He kept careful track of his research but was careful not to call it "research." Proper medical research, he knew,

required institutional oversight and ethics committees and formal exper-
iment setups, and Lonny didn't want to deal with all that. He imagined
that if he had lived in another era—an era without so much institutional
red tape—he might have been a revolutionary scientist, like the Canadian
researchers who discovered insulin in the 1920s: in part, by experimenting on stray dogs that they captured in the streets. Those doctors hadn't
asked for permission either.

Some other doctors in California heard about Lonny's amateur ma-
neuvering and were upset by it. What if he got things wrong? What if
one of the cardiac drugs kicked in too soon, and the patient had a heart
attack before he fell unconscious? If that happened, the death would be
violent and terrible. One palliative care physician told me that he saw
Lonny's work as "pseudo-science": imprecise and lacking in scholarly
rigor, and fundamentally dangerous. Others were just confused by Lonny's obsessive quest to lower his patients' death times—even if it meant
complicating the protocol and making it harder for families to follow
on their own. What did a few hours matter, if the patient was unconscious anyway? Lonny insisted that speed mattered. People wanted to die
quickly. That was literally the point.

"We are the first practice that ever looked at the pharmacophysiology
of death from medically aided dying. It had *never* been done," Lonny told
me one day in his backyard office. "The data I'm going to show you now
is the first time you'll ever see anything like that, because nobody has *ever*
done it." We were seated side by side in front of his computer, looking
at an Excel spreadsheet. Lonny wore a pair of glasses on the bridge of
his nose and had a second pair tucked into the front pocket of his dress
shirt. The graphs on the Excel sheets were color-coded and showed time
from drug ingestion to death. The lowest peaks, Lonny said, generally
belonged to his ALS patients. "I tell ALS patients jokingly, 'There's only
one good thing about ALS: You'll die quickly.'"

I pointed at a taller ALS peak. "What about that one?"

"It's a good question," Lonny said. "She was an ALS patient who decided that she hated her disability and she died early." He paused. "She was still walking." Often, Lonny said, tall peaks meant that the patients had been athletes whose hearts were strong and tended to beat for longer. "This guy here was a swimmer."

The goal, Lonny said, was to make the patients' deaths quick but not too quick. "Our sweet spot is about forty-five minutes. . . . The family has done their thing. The patient is deeply unconscious. You get to see how comfortable they are. Their eyes are closed. 'That's the first time I've seen Uncle John be comfortable in the last three years.' They get to observe that a little bit. . . . Then they crawl into bed and they hold him and all that. In about forty-five minutes, I say, 'His heart has stopped,' and we're done."

But Lonny knew that even a perfect drug protocol wouldn't fix everything. As he took on more patients, he started meeting people who couldn't self-administer the drugs in the way that they were legally required to: with an "affirmative, conscious, and physical act." Some were too weak to lift a cup of medicine to their lips or had gastrointestinal systems that were too ravaged by disease. Some of the ALS patients couldn't even suck up liquid through a straw. For years, lots of doctors in Oregon and Washington had turned these patients away, with wistful references to American legal requirements, but Lonny didn't want to do that. He hated the idea that someone would lose a legal right just because he couldn't drink something or lift his hand up: that effectively, a man with prostate cancer might have more rights than a man with esophageal cancer, just because the former could swallow large quantities of liquids and the latter couldn't—or that a woman with breast cancer might have more rights than a woman with brain cancer, because the latter had a tumor that prevented her from moving her limbs. That seemed so stupid.

Lonny went back to look at the language of the California law. The state paperwork said that a patient needed to "self-administer" the lethal drugs and also to "ingest" them. (In other states, patients were required to "take" or "administer" the drugs.) But what did "ingest" really mean?

Lonny emailed a few doctors he knew, but they didn't know either—so one of them emailed the California Medical Board. A few days later, the board's executive director wrote back to say that "ingest" meant anything involving the gastrointestinal system. Lonny told his doctor friends that they should get creative.

Soon, Lonny was delivering the drugs directly into feeding tubes, when patients had them. He would load up the medication into a plastic syringe and then hand the plunger to the patient, who would press down on it to "self-administer" and "ingest" the drugs. Sometimes, if a patient was feeling weak, Lonny would hold the plunger himself and place the patient's hand on top of his. "If I feel you pushing on my hand," he would say, "we will push together." They were lovely deaths. And legal deaths. But in a way, it was all ridiculous. Later, I read online about an ALS patient in Oregon who was too weak to even manage the plastic syringe. In the end, she had to deliberately drive her electric wheelchair into a wall, allowing the impact to depress the feeding tube plunger and deliver her lethal dose. The writers of the California End of Life Option Act had been attentive to the potential for abuse and coercion, but they were less focused on more abstract questions of decency and what a person might find to be decent as he lay dying.

Later, Lonny started using rectal administration for patients with disturbed intestinal systems. He would snake a catheter up the person's rectum and inflate the little balloon on the end of it, to seal the passage—then load up the drugs and hand the patient the plunger, to press down. I asked Lonny if he thought that these deaths were dignified and he looked at me strangely, as if I'd said something deranged. "It's not undignified at all."

ONE LATE MORNING, Lonny sat at his desk, preparing for a phone call with a patient. He read through notes that his nurse, Thalia DeWolf, had written about her and shook his head. Her name was Christine,* seventy-five, mother of two, with a degenerative vascular disorder. The blood vessels

lining her intestinal walls were swollen and breaking down. She was
bleeding so much that she had become anemic and needed blood transfusions every few days. "Torturous little blood vessels," Lonny muttered.
Christine's doctor had cauterized the site, burning dozens of the vessels to
create scar tissue that would stop the blood flow, but the colon kept bleeding.

"Would it be a bad death?" I asked Lonny.

"Could be long," he said.

Christine had asked her own GP about aid in dying, but he told her to
ask her hematologist. She called the hematologist's office, but one of his
nurses told her, bashfully, that the doctor didn't really *do* assisted death.

Christine, who had a narrow face and wisps of dyed black hair, told
Lonny over the phone that her doctor had tried everything but that he
couldn't make her better. "There is nothing more he can do." She now
saw blood whenever she went to the bathroom. It wasn't gushing blood,
but it was still blood. Christine said she hated going to the hospital for
transfusions. The whole thing was awful. The drive. The finding a parking spot. The lighting inside. The noise. In between transfusions, Christine's hemoglobin would drop and it would be hard to get out of bed.
It would be hard to get interested in living. "The will to live goes with
one's energy," she said. When she was in bed, Christine thought about dying there, slowly, slouching toward it. "And I'm going to poop and pee
in my bed." Christine said she wasn't especially eager to die, but "I think
I can do it when I'm miserable enough. . . . OK. Why be miserable?" She
could probably do it on a bad day.

"Some patients have a specific line in the sand," Lonny said. "Do you?"

"I don't want to lie in bed and die and poop in my pants and have
someone drag me to the hospital," Christine said. "No. No. No. No. I
don't want to live like that."

Lonny asked Christine if she wanted to make an official request for
aid in dying, to start the fifteen-day countdown, and Christine said that
she did. "But what if I feel so good on the day that I can't do it?"

"That would be OK," Lonny said.

After the appointment, Thalia came into the backyard office to check on us. She was tall and beautiful, with sharp cheekbones and long fingers, and she always wore black—except on days when she was attending a death, because then black seemed too morbid and she would wear navy or gray instead. Lonny told her about the call with Christine.

I told Thalia about an academic paper I had come across in *JAMA Internal Medicine*, which included a survey of seriously ill patients over sixty years old at a Pennsylvania hospital. The vast majority of patients, 68.9 percent, told researchers they considered bowel and bladder incontinence to be "as bad as or worse than death." The paper had deeply depressed me. What had we done to make people so ashamed? To make them prefer nothingness to padded underwear?

Thalia nodded. "A lot of people are weird about poop and pee." People were embarrassed by their bowels. They felt reduced and betrayed by them. "It's a really common line in the sand: 'When someone has to change my diaper, I don't want to live.'" Adult patients often felt worse about having their diapers changed than their caregivers felt about changing them. When Thalia met with patients in advance of their assisted deaths, they often asked her if they would defecate while they died, or after they died. Really, they asked her that more than they asked about anything else. "Everyone wants to know that! I'm like, 'No. Not likely. But if you poop, I will clean you up so fast no one will even notice. I'll just whisk that little turd away.'"

On her way out of the office, Thalia asked Lonny who Christine's hematologist was. When Lonny said his name, Thalia snorted. "He will pry the lid off a coffin to try another treatment, I swear."

I asked Lonny to tell me about his other patients. I wanted to know what they were like. Some of them, he told me, were similar to Christine: the well-off, educated, white, in-control people whom researchers always talked about in Oregon. But not all were. Sometimes people came to Lonny who were too poor to pay his fee and he would agree to treat them for less or for free. On rare occasions, patients were black or brown.

With elderly black patients especially, the conversations were delicate. Sometimes, the patients were very religious, and their families were still holding out for a miracle. Sometimes, they called Lonny after refusing hospice care—because they thought hospice might be a trap. In part, they remembered a time when white doctors did awful, unethical experiments on black bodies, and they worried that physicians were pushing them to end treatment prematurely in order to ration their healthcare and save the system money. As a class of patients, African Americans were already less likely to enter hospice or to write living wills, or to access certain kinds of palliative care. Lonny tried to be sensitive to their fears and to assuage them.

Most people told Lonny that they wanted an assisted death because they didn't want to die slowly, but others told him different things. One man had terminal cancer but said he really wanted to die *now* for financial reasons. He was a Vietnam War vet, he said, and he couldn't stop thinking about the Agent Orange attacks against Vietnamese farmers. He wanted all his savings to go to Vietnamese victims—not to pay his way through some shitty American nursing home. Other patients had already tried to end their lives: overdosing on the morphine left by their hospice nurses and then waking up a few days later to find everyone around them flipping out.

In most cases, Lonny could tell pretty soon after meeting a person whether he qualified to die under the California law, but sometimes he met someone who stumped him. The law set broad legal parameters but left doctors to make their own calls on individual patients. Lonny sometimes felt like he was refining the rules as he went. What if, for instance, a 103-year-old wanted to die but didn't have a specific illness or condition? Could you reasonably assume that he had just six months left to live? Sure, Lonny thought, as long as he scored high enough on a "frailty index" text or demonstrated what doctors call a "failure to thrive." What about a woman, say, a cancer patient, who was predicted to live another two years—but who refused food and water and vowed that she would never eat or drink again? Could she qualify, once she was so starved and dehydrated that she was days from death? Did it matter if she was ninety years old or thirty? Lonny had thought hard about that one and decided that he wouldn't treat someone who starved herself into a terminal state. If he did, where would it end? People could qualify who weren't sick at all. A young person. A depressed person. An anorexic person.

Sometimes, patients tried to convince Lonny that he should help them die because of their mental illnesses. "We get *a lot* of calls from people with depression," he told me. "Here's their argument: 'I'm depressed. I'm going to kill myself because of my depression. Therefore, I have a terminal illness. Therefore, I qualify for medical aid in dying.'" There was a certain logic to it. "But we say no, obviously." He turned down depressed patients all the time.

"Here's an interesting thing," Lonny said, leaning toward me. "If patients are willing to stop treatment and *that* will make them terminal—so, say, turn off a pacemaker—we don't actually have them do it." All the patients had to do was say that they were planning to turn off their pacemakers and Lonny would consider them eligible. They became eligible at the moment their intention crystallized. "Is there anything in the legislation that says that? No. We're winging it here, because that's what we've been doing from day one. . . . We're making shit up as we go because nobody has had enough cases to figure it out." Lonny paused. "This is a beautiful and rare opportunity to invent a new field. . . . We don't have people with fancy degrees and university backing controlling it. I am inventing an entire new field of medicine. I'm not trying to exaggerate this." He shook his head. "Nobody else wants it."

BEFORE THE CALIFORNIA End of Life Option Act passed, Dr. Sally Sample, a hospice doctor north of San Francisco, had hoped very much that it would fail. "It just didn't feel right," she told me, in an office at Hospice East Bay, on the side of a highway in Pleasant Hill. "Not because I don't think a person has a right to choose. I think it's like abortion, but . . . I was just hoping we wouldn't have the option." When the law did pass, Sally decided that the right thing to do was get over herself and become a prescriber. She wrote a prescription and then another. But then she had to stop. "With our first few patients," she said, "it felt like an execution."

"Really?"

"Yes."

"Just because it was so antithetical to what you had been practicing?"

"How do I articulate it?" Sally frowned. She had black hair and black cat-eye glasses and was wearing one scarf on top of another. She said that she was not religious but that she saw the act of dying as fundamentally regenerative. Through the process of losing consciousness and becoming dead—naturally or with a nudge from pain medication—patients could make peace with their lives and any lingering sense of unfinishedness. So could their loved ones. It would be a shame, Sally said, to miss out on that. "I felt like this is definitely not right with the circle of life. . . . It's especially when people are at the very end of life or they're unconscious that I think some kind of spiritual work goes on. I have no idea what it is. It's between here and the next thing." She said she could feel it in her patients: a kind of existential negotiation. With the cosmos? "It's peaceful. Usually. Not always. Some people go out kicking and screaming." Sally looked up at me. "I have talked to Lonny about it. He doesn't agree with me."

Sally heard about Lonny through the hospice grapevine and started sending her patients to him so that she could act as their second, consulting doctor instead of their prescriber. She liked that Lonny had done so much research on the drugs. She also liked that he sat with people while they died, instead of just arranging for the drugs to be dropped off at their homes, like most doctors. That idea stressed her out. If a doctor wasn't at the bedside, who would make sure that the state of California's many legal requirements were being adhered to—and that family members weren't pushing ambivalent or demented patients into premature deaths?

Lonny felt like the safest option. After referring ten or so patients to him, Sally had even come around to the California law. "Having this as an option lets people relax," she said. "Not even getting the drugs, but knowing, 'I *can* get these drugs.'" In the end, she thought, Lonny was weird, and she definitely didn't get him *at all*—but she was glad he existed.

But other doctors were wary of Lonny and disturbed by what he and other prescribers were doing to their patients. Some argued straight from first principles. They said that physician-assisted death was morally wrong, without exception, and that it was incompatible with a physician's duty to heal. A doctor was meant to do no harm. Others worried about what assisted dying would do to the physicians who performed it. They imagined doctors becoming ethically broken and ontologically confused. "What are we asking of our medical profession?" asked Dr. Daniel Sulmasy in a 2017 book, *Euthanasia and Assisted Suicide*. Sulmasy argued that doctors feel a natural and correct "moral resistance" when they are asked to hasten a patient's death, but that this resistance can be ground down and subdued over time, and by repetition. "Repetition of the act becomes, of itself, a powerful means of such justification." Sulmasy warned that this moral quieting was perilous, because it could leave the physician numb to his once instinctive distress—but that it was exponentially perilous, too, because once he was numbed, a physician would be more likely to see more kinds of patients as candidates for hastened death. "This is what is meant by the psychological slippery slope. Once one crosses a moral barrier, a practice that is initially difficult becomes easier," Sulmasy wrote. He quoted a Dutch doctor who offered euthanasia to patients in the Netherlands: "The first time you do it, euthanasia is difficult, like climbing a mountain."

Another group of skeptics protested from inside the field of hospice care. Since the 1970s, the goal of hospice had been to guide people through the dying process at home, in a holistic way: using interdisciplinary teams of doctors, nurses, social workers, and chaplains who would work together to ease physical symptoms and also provide social services and spiritual guidance. In 1982, the US federal government agreed to start funding at-home hospice care for people who had six months or less to live, on the condition that they give up treatments aimed at a cure and instead shift to pain management. By the time assisted dying was legalized in California, the United States had more than 4,000 hospice agencies treating 1.5 million patients, at an annual Medicare cost of $17.8 billion. From the start, though, that hospice infrastructure was pitted against the right-to-die cause, which many practitioners saw as an affront to hospice's core mission. Some palliative care doctors rejected the very idea that Americans were dying badly and in pain. They argued that advances in science and medicine allowed them to control end-of-life symptoms like never before, and so made physician-assisted death unnecessary. The National Hospice and Palliative Care Organization (NHPCO), a national umbrella group, declared itself opposed. Its whole purpose was to help patients through dying, not to short-circuit natural death.

But during the 1990s, voices of dissent grew louder, in favor of physician assistance in dying. In 1993, the palliative care physician Dr. Timothy Quill published a book called *Death and Dignity*, in which he reprimanded his profession for its excessive and technology-bolstered self-confidence. "Those who have witnessed difficult deaths of patients on hospice programs are not reassured by the glib assertion that we always know how to make death tolerable. . . . In fact, there is no empirical evidence that all physical suffering associated with incurable illness can be effectively relieved." Quill continued: "To think that people do not suffer in the process of dying is an illusion. . . . I am deeply troubled by our profession's unwillingness to openly acknowledge its limitations."

Gary Pasternak, a hospice doctor in San Mateo, told me that he was initially wary of the California law because he thought it fed off the failures of his craft. "I felt like, well, if the patients really need to do this, then somehow palliative medicine has failed them. We haven't figured out the key to their psychic pain. We haven't managed their pain well enough. We haven't seen their distress well enough. We haven't done enough." Gary decided that he would not include assisted death in his practice. But then one day, one of his patients, a nice gentleman with metastatic bladder cancer, shot himself on the outdoor patio of his little apartment. Afterward, Gary thought, *There must have been some other way this could have been handled*.

Gary and I met at Mission Hospice & Home Care, a ten-bed inpatient hospice house in San Mateo, where patients could stay, for a fee, if they couldn't manage at home. The house was full of fresh cut flowers. Downstairs, in the communal kitchen, a volunteer was making half a tuna fish sandwich for a dying patient who had decided that she was willing to try half a sandwich after all, as long as it wasn't ham.

When the law came into effect, Gary resolved to try an assisted death and see how it felt to him. His first case was a woman in her nineties with lung cancer. Cantankerous. A retired lawyer. "Here's the plan," she told Gary when he came to see her at her house. "You've got to help me do this."

"All right," he said. "I'll try."

Just before Gary prepared the lethal medication, and after the woman's children and grandchildren said their final goodbyes, he asked his patient softly, "Do you have any words of wisdom for us?"

"What the hell are you talking about?" the woman said. "Just get on with this." She swallowed the drink and died twenty minutes later. Gary decided it was among the most peaceful deaths that he had ever seen. "How funny," he told me later, "my uncomfortableness with my own myths."

Still, Gary thought it was part of his job to push back a little, to not let patients die too easily. Sometimes people were more uncertain than they understood themselves to be. Recently, he had treated a cancer patient named Isabel* who lived in the hospice house and was absolutely sure that she wanted an assisted death. After Gary approved her, Isabel started asking him when he thought she should die. "Do you think today is the day?"

"Well," Gary would say, "is today good enough? Is today good enough to have another day?" Isabel would say that it was.

In the end, Gary said, "it was good enough every day." Isabel died a natural death. It was a good death, he thought, apart from "some mild delirium and confusion."

More recently, the hospice movement's opposition has broadened. Today many doctors acknowledge that people are dying badly and that their profession is sometimes to blame. "Centuries from now," wrote Dr. Ira Byock, a palliative care physician and ethicist, in a 2018 essay for the medical magazine *Stat*, "one of the things our era will be known for is the plague of dying badly . . . a direct result of modern medicine's original sin: believing that we can vanquish death." Over decades, doctors had given in to their own hubris. They had promised things they couldn't deliver: an end to sickness, then an end to aging badly, then an end to aging. They had treated and treated and overtreated, until their mission to extend life had transformed into a system for prolonging death. And still, many insisted, helping patients to die was not the right way to atone for this historic transgression. Instead, doctors should work to improve healthcare. "Casting physician-hastened death as a freedom is disingenuous at best," Byock wrote. "If doctors don't communicate with you about your condition and listen to your priorities, if they are unskilled in alleviating your pain, if medical bills are bankrupting your family, asking to die may be entirely rational. As the lyric goes, 'Freedom's just another word for nothing left to lose.'"

Lonny was exasperated by his colleagues in hospice. He didn't think they made any sense. After all, they routinely did things that seemed to fall just short of euthanasia: what some ethicists call "passive euthanasia." They helped patients turn down lifesaving or life-prolonging care when they were tired of treatment. They advised families who wanted to switch off life support for comatose relatives. In other words, they cleared the way for death and sometimes helped to speed it up. "Here's my common comparison," Lonny said. "If you tell me, as an oncologist, that you have breast cancer and you're tired of chemotherapy and you're deciding to stop, I have a half-hour conversation with you and we stop chemotherapy. That's how it works. That's a life decision. You are deciding to die. But if you tell me you want medical aid in dying, I'm like, 'Well, you need three more appointments and . . .'"

Sometimes doctors went even further than those acts of omission: administering such high doses of morphine that their dying patients fell unconscious and never woke up again. Back in 1997, the US Supreme Court ruled that there was no constitutional right to physician-assisted death—but at the same time, it affirmed that dying people had the right to as much pain-relieving medication as they needed, even "to the point of causing unconsciousness and hastening death." From then on, "palliative sedation," which had always occurred behind the scenes, became a mainstream medical intervention. It was formally endorsed by the NHPCO, which permitted the "lowering of patient consciousness using medications for the express purpose of limiting patient awareness of suffering that is intractable and intolerable." Palliative sedation was reserved for imminently dying patients. Doctors were meant to administer the drugs gradually, using the smallest possible dose.

Today it's hard to say how often palliative sedation is used. Nobody is collecting national data, and rates vary widely from city to city, hospital to hospital. Even NHPCO estimates are comically imprecise; the organization says that the "prevalence of the use of palliative sedation in terminally ill patients has been reported between 1% and 52%." There are also no national protocols that advise doctors on exactly what drugs to use and how quickly to use them—and no consumer guides that tell patients which doctors, at what hospitals, offer what palliative interventions. A patient has no way to know, until she gets there. Some doctors use palliative sedation only to relieve physical symptoms, while others use it to settle restlessness and delirium and existential distress. Some doctors ask patients if they want to be sedated; others just sedate. "I don't think of palliative sedation as a procedure that you have to get informed consent for," Dr. Pasternak, the San Mateo hospice doctor, told me. "It really is, in the context of a patient's symptoms, just good palliative care." Most controversially, while some doctors will sedate only in a proportional way—titrating drugs slowly and observing their effects—others, in dire situations, are willing to administer a large amount of medication at once, with the express intention of drugging a patient unconscious.

For the dying person in the hospital bed, the distinction between "palliative sedation to unconsciousness" and straight-up euthanasia can seem awfully thin. Either way, the patient ends up dead: maybe right away, or maybe after a few days of deep sleep—during which the patient is dead to the world anyway. But bioethicists have long insisted that there is a meaningful difference and that it can be explained by the principle of "double effect." The idea dates back to the Italian philosopher Thomas Aquinas and his thirteenth-century religious text *Summa Theologiae*, which argued that killing could be justified if it was done in self-defense and was not *intended* to kill the attacker. Later, the doctrine of double effect was taught in war colleges to excuse the accidental killings of civilians in military combat. Later still, it was deployed in medical schools by instructors who used it to justify the life-shortening effect of palliative sedation on consenting patients. What mattered, according to the double effect theory, was the intent of the physician. Palliative sedation was acceptable if physicians intended only to alleviate pain and not to bring about unconsciousness and death—even if those physicians could anticipate, all along, that their patients would likely fall unconscious and die. If those conditions were met, then what a doctor did was ethically permissible. And definitely not euthanasia.

"What a bunch of shit," Lonny said when I asked him about the double effect doctrine. He thought the whole thing was a sellout and that it gave doctors a cover, both to mollify their own moral queasiness and to do what they personally thought was right. "Doctor knows best." He thought that most doctors were so busy with diagnostic algorithms and paperwork that they never even stopped to think about it: the fineness of that dividing line. Why did it make sense that a patient had to wait until he was almost dead and suffering terribly—and sometimes unable to express his own desires—before he could get relief from his doctor? And once a doctor was committed to providing relief, why did it make sense to go through an elaborate charade of titrating morphine until the patient fell asleep? Why couldn't the patient just ask for what he wanted and get it? It seemed to Lonny that the system was designed to keep patients and doctors from being honest with each other, lest either side say too much and expose the double effect charade too clearly.

Soon, though, Lonny grew tired of my questions. "I'm not in any way trying to shoot you down," he said kindly. "We don't need to talk about far-off philosophies. Let's talk about reality. Not something about the double effect or whatever. That's all irrelevant shit. We're out here seeing patients." What I needed to understand was that there were rules about who could be helped and who couldn't and sometimes they made no sense at all. Sometimes a doctor's hands were tied.

ROBERT* WAS EIGHTY-ONE and he was sitting on the brown couch beside his husband, Oliver,* who was a few decades younger. Robert looked like a standard-order old man: soft and loose and balding. Oliver looked cool, with a styled mustache. Behind them was a painting of a lion, its legs stout and sinewy. Robert and Oliver were very still.

"One of the parts of the law is that you have to have less than six months to live, in the opinion of two doctors," Lonny said, speaking loudly because Robert had trouble hearing. "My job with you folks has been to go pretty thoroughly through your medical records. . . . It can be complicated with an older person with many diseases." He looked up from his papers. "Robert, can you tell me about your understanding of your cancer?"

"I don't know much about it," Robert said tautly. "I don't think I know what kind of cancer it was."

"It was non-Hodgkin's lymphoma," Oliver said.

Lonny nodded. "It is fair for me to say, Robert, that your memory issues are making it hard for you to remember the cancer?"

"That's right," said Robert.

Lonny told Robert that his cancer was in remission. "I don't think the cancer is going to harm you anymore."

"But the doctor said the cancer could come back," Oliver said.

"Yes, but you're about twelve years out. That makes it less likely." Lonny turned back to Robert. "It doesn't look like the cancer is going to kill you and certainly not in six months. . . . Do you tend to feel short of breath when you move around?"

"Yes, somewhat," said Robert. "I avoid moving around so it's not very prominent in my life." He had stopped driving, he said. He had stopped going to the golf club to see his friends, Oliver said.

Lonny nodded. Robert had been diagnosed with heart disease in 2009, but his cardiologist had reported that he was "stable from a cardiac standpoint" and that his heart was pumping strongly. "You have heart disease," Lonny said, "but it's not going to kill you either."

"OK," said Robert.

"You have some memory changes. I understand that this is the most frustrating thing you're experiencing in the moment. Is that a fair guess?"

"Yes," Robert said. "Everything is going downhill."

"I think that's exactly the right summary," Lonny said. "Everything is going downhill. What makes you get to the point where you're ready to die?"

"I really don't want to live anymore," said Robert. "I'm not finding it an interesting thing. Umm . . . you know. Everything is closing in and there is not much left to be looking forward to." He paused. "I don't want to make people unhappy in any way. But I don't want to make me unhappy. I spend more and more time in bed. Trying to be sleepy. Trying to be asleep. What's going to happen if I get up?"

"Hmm."

"I really don't want to go and jump off a bridge. I would much rather take a pill and just go out of it like that."

"I understand that," said Lonny. "Would you use the word 'depression' for what you're feeling or just being sad?"

"I think both," said Robert.

"I would agree with that," said Lonny. He coughed. "So let me see if I can sum it up, if I may. Robert, the way I look at all of your illnesses, in terms of physical illnesses, is none of them are likely to cause your death in the next six months or so. Which is not to say that you will necessarily live for the next six months. I don't know if you'll have a sudden heart attack or a stroke, but there is nothing that says to me that it's likely. So I'm going to tell you what may be bad news for you, based on your desire that you just want a pill and don't want to jump off a bridge. I certainly agree with you on the not-jumping-off-a-bridge part. Uh, let me just ask a quick question: Do you have any weapons in the house? Any guns? No? Well, that's good. Thank you for not having them. They're dangerous things. So now that we're done with that . . . Unfortunately, we cannot help you at this point in time to die legally."

Robert and Oliver were quiet. Lonny told them that things could change. Something could come up out of the blue that would make Robert eligible. "It may well be that you develop a pneumonia in three months and, boom, you're eligible. So I'm not abandoning you." Lonny said he thought that Robert should see a geriatric psychiatrist who could talk to him about his sadness. Also a physical therapist, who could help with his walking.

Oliver interrupted. They had seen a physical therapist, he said. In fact, they had seen several, but Robert always refused to do the exercises.

"It's going to be frustrating," Lonny said with a half smile, "because nobody is going to make you walk normally again and you might not like that. . . . You're going to be an older, frail man. And sometimes you have to come to terms with that."

"I don't really want to come to terms with it," said Robert. "I'd like to stop it."

"Well, at this moment, as the doctor who does aid in dying, I cannot help you stop your life."

"OK," said Robert.

"Any other questions, or are we OK?"

"If you were going to prescribe a pill," said Robert slowly, "what would it be called?"

Lonny sighed. "It's actually not a pill."

2

Age

In the late morning, on the day she planned to die, in April 2016, Avril Henry went to get the poison from the downstairs bathroom. She walked past the mustard-yellow curtains and the frosted-glass doors of the parlor, past the padded rocking chair where she sometimes sat for hours with her feet tilted above her head—to ease the swelling in her ankles, she said. When she arrived inside, she steadied herself against the countertop before reaching up to the top shelf and feeling around for the glass bottles that she had hidden there, behind the toilet cleaner and the baby powder. Two of the bottles were small, like jars of cough syrup, and had Spanish writing on the labels. They contained the drugs. A third bottle held orange liqueur. Avril's suicide manual warned that pentobarbital had a bitter aftertaste and recommended chasing it with a bit of spirit.

"I got it imported illegally," Avril had said of the drug supply. "It's quite easy to do, but very risky." She was at her home in Brampford Speke, a small village in southwest England with three hundred residents, a pub called the Lazy Toad, a Church of England parish church, and a town council on which Avril had served several terms, earning a reputation as brilliant and steadfast, if sometimes needlessly querulous.

In her eighties, Avril had a loose, unformed aesthetic: all soft beige
sweaters, soft beige skin, plastic clogs, walking aids. Often, dangly silver
earrings. Sometimes, a dash of lipstick. By the time she planned to die,
her white hair was so long that it nearly reached her waist. Things got
stuck in it: some fluff, a twig from the garden. In the mornings, it took
no small effort for Avril to pull the hair back from her face and impose
a kind of order on it with hair elastics and bobby pins. By late morning,
wisps of it would have escaped their restraints and fallen down around
her forehead.

Avril climbed upstairs slowly, as she always did: bent over and clinging to the banister—nearly crawling, so that if she fell, she wouldn't fall
far. Her walker was waiting at the top of the staircase, but she didn't need
it. She was only going as far as the bathroom. It had always been Avril's
intention to die in her bathtub, reclining and fully clothed. For weeks, she
had worried that, in the throes of dying, her bowels would give way and
she would make a mess of herself, and then that the house would smell
for weeks. By dying in the bathtub, she hoped to contain the mess. Just
in case, she left a bottle of Dettol cleaning fluid under the towel rack, for
whoever came to mop up after her. She explained all this in the suicide
note. *I am about to take my own life*, the letter read. *I am alone. The decision
is wholly mine. . . . This has been laboriously planned.*

When everything was ready, Avril called her Internet provider to explain that even though she planned to kill herself at 7 p.m., she wished
for her account to remain active until the executors of her estate had time
to tie up loose ends around the house. Her longtime lawyer, William Mi-
chelmore, would later agree that this was a reckless thing to do, all things
considered. But by then, Avril had already told her friends, her handyman, her caregiver, her gardener and his wife, and her acquaintances
from the local swimming pool. She had read in some online forums that it
was best to tell people about your death plans in advance. That way, they
would be less traumatized by your suicide. Also, they would understand
that you hadn't acted rashly, on a very bad day; rather, you had really

meant to die and wanted to be dead. When Avril told her lawyer, he wasn't entirely surprised, knowing Avril's personality as well as he did. "Her dignity was fully compromised by the disease, which attacked her nervous system," he told me later, as if dignity was a thing that could be broken by a body.

Most people, Avril said, had taken the news well, though a few had not. One friend, a former colleague at the university, had even argued with her. "Have you considered the effect of this on your family?" he asked.

"Of course I have bloody well considered the effect," Avril said. Then she told him about all her aches and pains and untreatable conditions—and about her flagrantly incontinent bowels. "He was appalled!" she said later, delighted. "And I'm glad he was."

Her handyman, Geoff—who had observed in recent years that Avril was spending less time in the garden than she used to—found the whole conversation a bit "surreal" but told Avril over a cup of tea that he did not, on principle, object to her decision. "I have no moral qualms about this at all," he said. Still, he asked whether "the pain was *that* bad?" Whether this wasn't all a bit drastic? Avril brushed him aside. She said her suicide confessions were serious and final; they were not pretexts for sympathy and they were not invitations for anyone to try to stop her.

Mona* handled things better. They were in the women's shower room, beside the community center swimming pool, and Avril said it abruptly: that she would soon be killing herself. Mona, an affable German woman, burst into tears. Eventually, though, she came around. Avril explained that she was tired of life and ready to go. In her old age, the pain eclipsed the pleasure. It was really that simple. She was old. She was worn down. She was played out.

In March, Avril and Mona had met for lunch to discuss the suicide matter in more detail. "You're not going to argue with me and say, 'Please change your mind!' Are you?" Avril demanded. She and Mona were sitting in the Crediton community center café, as they did twice a week, eating meat pies out of brown cardboard boxes.

Mona shook her head. "I think I would do the same, if I were in pain all the time," she said. "I would do this, too. I'd do it my own way."

"That's a girl!" Avril said. Then she cocked her head to the side. "You say you'd do it your *own way*. Do you know that most suicides fail?" Mona shrugged. "No. You didn't, because nobody ever does and the reason they don't is that the people who are mindless and quadriplegic and helpless as a result of a failed suicide don't publicize the fact."

"But I can take an overdose of pills," Mona protested.

"No, you can't."

"Of course I can."

"What pills would you take?"

Mona hesitated. "Acetaminophen?"

"That won't do," Avril said. "That will just destroy your liver.

"People think it's easy to hang yourself," she went on. "It can take over three minutes to die. And if you just happen to partially break your neck, you will end up a paraplegic. Killing yourself, especially if you are disabled, is very difficult. Very, very difficult. Indeed, I made a list of all the ways I could kill myself at home." Every method, Avril told Mona, had its particular shortcomings. If she jumped from the roof, she might survive the fall. If she unscrewed the panel covering her house's electricity source and touched the wires, she could end up being roasted alive. For a while, Avril had thought seriously about eating some of the lethal fungi growing in her garden. On the upside, there was no known antidote. On the downside, death by mushroom could be slow, messy, painful. The Nembutal would work better. Avril told Mona that, online, she had read about a concept called the Completed Life. "That's when you feel that your life is shaped and finished. And the direction thereafter is down. I did have a complete life. It was a great life."

"I can understand that."

"I don't want to be negative."

"The pain . . ."

"I dread waking up every morning," said Avril. "That's the worst."

Mona put her fork down and said that she wanted to be there when Avril took the medicine. She could at least hold her friend's hand. "I would."

Avril smiled and touched Mona's arm. "I don't want to see you in prison."

"It's just so sad."

"Mona, it's not sad."

"I just want you to stay alive!"

"Very selfish!" Avril clucked. And then it was time to go. "I want to thank you for your friendship. You've been a great support."

Mona looked away and started to cry. "Don't . . ."

MY COLLEAGUES AND I had found Avril while researching our documentary film and arranged, in February 2016, to take the train west from London to meet her. She sent us long, perplexing directions to her house and told us to bring slippers. "I do ask visitors to remove their shoes for the sake of my poor carpet. I hope you don't mind." When she answered the door, in a gray turtleneck sweater with a gray cardigan sweater on top, she offered, "Coffee? Tea? Double brandy?" In her own mind, Avril was dying of everything and of nothing in particular. Death by what we euphemistically call "old age"; what William Osler, in his classic *The Principles and Practice of Medicine*, referred to as those "cold gradations of decay."

A few weeks earlier, Avril had written an essay detailing her many symptoms, and she offered to read it aloud, as a kind of state-of-the-body address. She warned everyone that the treatise would be "tedious" and "disgusting." Then she pulled her plastic-framed glasses down the arch of her nose and started reading.

"I've lived for eighty-two years. I'm now dysfunctional in spine, feet, hips, peripheral nervous system, bowel, bladder, elbows, and hands. All combine in pain and failure to work," she read. "The future is bleak."

Avril had rotator cuff injuries, arthritis, and a tender back. Her feet burned from peripheral neuropathy. One doctor had said he could operate on them but that it would be a difficult surgery and that Avril wouldn't be able to walk for weeks. Well, what was the point of that? "Not practical," Avril said. It was getting harder to stand straight. It was getting harder to see and to hear people. Strangely, she could hear vowels just fine but was losing her consonants. "To me, 'The cat sat on the mat' sounds like *uhaaouha*," she said.

Her personality had changed, too. She had become less likely to laugh. More rigid. Her moods lost their elasticity. And she fretted too much. Avril nagged Geoff and hovered over him while he worked, assigning him increasingly ludicrous tasks: to straighten out a small kink in the plastic hose of the vacuum cleaner, to plaster over barely perceptible cracks at the back of the fireplace. She nagged the gardener, too. "I have become querulous, introverted, angry, fearful," Avril read. "I was none of these things." She had been an artist. An intellectual. Happy.

Nights were the worst. Because it hurt everywhere, it was hard to find a position that was comfortable enough to let her sleep. She tried lying flat on her back, with her orange quilt tucked in around her rose-colored pajamas. She tried supporting her neck with a foam pillow. Because her breathing was labored, Avril slept with an oxygen mask on, its blue straps pulled tight around her forehead and cheeks. In that way, she would lie for hours, marinating in her pain. It would occur to her that she would never find relief. There would only be an excess of hours, a punishing profligacy of time.

Sometimes, Avril said, she was woken three or four times in a single night by her "paradoxical bowels" and her "fatal incontinence." Because she was afraid of walking, unsteady, in the dark, Avril would relieve herself in a white chamber pot tucked under the bed. But then, in the mornings, she wouldn't have the strength to carry the heavy pot into the bathroom to empty it. Instead, she would have to pull it across the room and use a long-handled soup ladle to spoon the urine into the toilet. Twice a week, on Tuesdays and Saturdays, Avril's caregiver, who was very kind to her, would come to wash the cotton diapers that she wore in the daytime. Still, in between visits, heaps of urine-soaked cloth would pile up in the bedroom. The smell was rancid. Her body was a perishable fruit that had gone sour. Or maybe a faulty machine, beset by broken parts. Avril was disgusted by her anatomy and scandalized by its leaky excesses. But she was more matter-of-fact than self-pitying. "My body served me obediently for eighty years but is now, quite suddenly, in every sense, unserviceable and well past its sell-by date."

"I'm sorry that was so unpleasant," Avril said when she finished reading the essay. "But that's how it is." She added, with a smirk, that she was thinking of sending a copy to her Member of Parliament. "Especially the nasty bits." She was still angry with the government for rejecting a bill, in 2015, which would have legalized a narrow form of assisted dying in the United Kingdom, something that, according to national polls, the overwhelming majority of British people supported. Avril had wanted very much for the law to pass, though she understood that she wouldn't qualify to die under its strict criteria—because, after all, she wasn't imminently dying of any one thing. She was, simply, old and getting older. "People with a terminal illness are the lucky ones," Avril said. "I have longed for a diagnosis of cancer."

In his bestselling 1994 book, *How We Die*, Dr. Sherwin Nuland observed that, by the logic of hospital administrators and Department of Health and Human Services guidelines, "it is illegal to die of old age." Instead, "everybody is required to die of a named entity": cancer or heart attack, stroke or traumatic injury. Plain old age—the natural wearing down of systems, the exhaustion of finite cellular life spans, the loss of internal equilibrium—did not count as a cause of death and was never a checkbox option on official paperwork. "I have no real quarrel with those who insist upon invoking the laboratory-bred specificity of microscopic pathology in order to satisfy the compulsive demands of their biomedical worldview," wrote Nuland. "I simply think they miss the point." It was age that slayed, in the end. In Nuland's view, medicine's focus on specific pathology amounted to a "legalized evasion of the greater law of nature." It was born of a twentieth-century notion, passed down to subsequent generations of physicians, that a doctor "must never allow his patients to lose hope, even when they are obviously dying." If old age does not kill, there are always more treatments to try.

More recently, the physician and writer Dr. Atul Gawande has written that "old age is not a diagnosis. There is always some final proximate cause that gets written down on the death certificate—respiratory failure, cardiac arrest. But in truth no single disease leads to the end; the culprit is just the accumulated crumbling of one's bodily systems while medicine carries out its maintenance measures and patch jobs." At the hospital where Dr. Gawande worked, physicians had even learned to avoid the erstwhile vocabularies of aging. Words like "geriatrics" and "elderly" and "senior" fell out of favor; staff spoke instead of "older adult health." In conversations between healthcare providers and their patients, the fact of death grew divorced from the aging that preceded it.

Some historians have tied this phenomenon to a larger effort, beginning in the early twentieth century, to conceptually transform old age from a natural phase of life into a stage of disease and, by extension, something to be defeated, rather than embodied or endured. In 1909, the word "geriatrics" entered the medical lexicon: a blending of the Greek *geros*, for "old man," and *iatros*, meaning "healer," which together branded a new medical specialty that was focused on the often disregarded symptoms of senility—a sort of end-of-life counterpart to pediatrics. The unusual word appeared alongside renewed hopes of a miracle cure for aging. Around the turn of the century, wayward surgeons hawked novel procedures—among them, testicular fluid injections and testicle transplants—which they claimed could reverse age-induced decline and restore youthful vigor. Nevertheless, by the 1980s and '90s it was clear that immortality was not in fact around the corner and the assurances of the medical profession grew somewhat more modest. Most researchers no longer spoke of curing old age, but, instead, of "compressing" it: of shortening the natural period of ache and pain and disability and dementia that precedes active dying. The idea was that instead of experiencing long stretches of senescence, we could mobilize the forces of science and medicine to let us live our best lives until—snap. Our abrupt end. There was, Nuland wrote, "a nice Victorian reticence in denying the probability of a miserable prelude to mortality."

Today, even this compression of morbidity seems illusory. In truth, increases in life expectancy have been accompanied by more years of age-induced disability. Aging has slowed down, rather than sped up. Still, and in spite of evidence to the contrary, the heady promise of a curtailed old age endures in the popular imagination. "Compression of morbidity is a quintessentially American idea," the physician and bioethicist Ezekiel Emanuel wrote, in a viral 2014 *Atlantic* essay called "Why I Hope to Die at 75." "It promises a kind of fountain of youth until the ever-receding time of death. It is this dream—or fantasy—that drives the American immortal and has fueled interest and investment in regenerative medicine and replacement organs." The fight against oldness has become social ritual, enforced by private fear and social momentum and a for-profit healthcare industry. Today, around a fifth of elderly Americans undergo surgical procedures in hospitals in the last month of their lives, often supported by loved ones who would do anything to help and who have come to see any option short of *do everything* as a kind of terrible abandonment.

BEFORE AVRIL FELT like she was dying, she had felt sure of herself. Arrogant and invincible. She was an only child, born in 1935, in Lincolnshire, to a moody and turbulent woman named Eileen and her older husband, Robert, a military man whom Avril adored. Avril was a studious, serious girl who learned not to ask why her mother sometimes left the house for days or weeks on end. At first, her father told her that Eileen was visiting with the aunties up in Lincoln. After a while, though, he gave up the ruse. Eileen was "disturbed," he said, and sometimes she had to live at a mental asylum for a while. When Avril was eight years old, she decided that she would never get married. She thought she was too selfish to look after anyone else. Also, she preferred the company of adults. She had always had a precocious sense of spinsterhood.

When Avril was fifteen, she found God. He was delivered to her in the form of a Jesuit priest who gave Avril a Bible and told her to read it through. Avril studied the text and was enthralled by the force of it, and she told her family that she wanted a formal Catholic conversion. Eileen and Robert did not approve. "They threw all kinds of fits," Avril said. Neither of them was particularly religious, but they certainly weren't Catholic. Catholicism was for dirty Irish people and the poor. Avril went ahead, behind their backs, and at sixteen was received at a church in Wimbledon.

When her parents found out, they flew into the most terrible rage, but Avril did not argue with them. Instead, she ran away in the middle of the night and began a new life, adrift. "I didn't go home for four years," she said. She found a job at an all-boys prep school, teaching every subject but math. Then she studied art and worked as an illustrator—and moved in with a semifamous sculptor whose name she later claimed to forget. Through her art studies, Avril acquired a new sensitivity to color, so that she started to feel, physically, her reactions to hue and tone and shade. A beautiful color could make her tremble. She also noticed pigments she hadn't seen before: different casts of cream on a wall, say, where she had once seen only white. Walking through a garden, Avril sometimes stopped just to gape at the magnolias. When she turned twenty, she stopped believing in God and told her parents that she was sorry for running away. They reconciled. Later, she would declare herself a firm atheist and celebrate the winter solstice with a makeshift pagan festival at the edge of her garden.

When Avril grew restless, she went back to school, first for an arts diploma, then for a bachelor's degree at Oxford and then for a doctorate. She didn't mind being older than the other students because it meant that she was less distracted by men and drama. The only thing she would come to regret—it was one of the biggest regrets of her life, she said— was that she didn't explore the city of Oxford very much, in all the years she lived there. All she did was work. "It's a lack of adventurousness," she said. "I'm dogged and persistent and I try to be systematic. But adventurous, I don't have." She always lived well, but never ecstatically.

In 1985 Avril's father died. She told herself that nothing could ever be worse, since he was the person she loved most. "This is the worst day. It can never recur. It can only happen once." There was some comfort in that. Avril got Robert's body cremated. A few days after she picked up the ashes, she drove up a tall hill and stood at the peak of it—and then held out the open box, so that her father could be scattered to the wind. She let herself consider the romance of the gesture. "But the wind blew back and I was covered!" Avril recalled. "He would have laughed!"

Avril worked as a lecturer at various Oxford and Cambridge colleges and then as a professor at the University of Exeter, where she specialized in English medieval studies and Christian iconography. She did translations of Middle English prose and wrote articles about their patterns and sequences, which she presented at international conferences in Greece and France and Germany. Once, she published an examination of the irregular meter and rhyming scheme in the fifth stanza of a Chaucer poem. On paper, Avril's thinking was exact and thorough, if not especially audacious. She was interested in aesthetics and form and what they revealed about the meaning of things. She also had strict ideas about what scholarly writing should look like; Avril thought that academic prose should be stripped of flourish—bare and unhandsome—and she did not hesitate to tell her colleagues so, whenever she found their papers to contain "excessive verbiage."

Outside of work, Avril was more yielding. She befriended an American professor named Karen Edwards, who taught Renaissance literature and thought that Avril was the most interesting person she had ever known. Sometimes, the two women went for garden walks and Karen would get the chills, just watching Avril study the flowers with such absorption and joy. "Her reaction to color was so powerful," Karen told me. "Avril loved being alive." During the warmer months, Avril rose early three times a week to exercise a friend's horses on the nearby moorlands. Then, in the evenings, she hosted picnics in her garden, with baskets of the nicest breads and cheeses in Exeter. All year long, she read voraciously, learning many things about many things. And so the years passed.

If her father had still been alive, Avril said, she would not be killing herself. But he was long dead. So were her mother, her aunts and uncles, and her two cats. There were still a few cousins around, and their families. "I love them all, but that doesn't in any way affect my decision," she said. "They are not that relevant in my life." They were not dependent on her, nor she on them. Avril thought it would be harder to say goodbye to the house, though it was embarrassing to think about it like that. "The house and garden are more important to me than any person," she said apologetically.

By 2015, Avril's world had grown small. Her greatest pleasure, she said, came from a daily swim at the local community center. Her doctors liked the swimming because it kept her joints loose. Avril liked it because floating in the pool was the closest she ever got to total painlessness. She started with backstroke and then switched to breaststroke. Years ago, Avril could do fifty lengths an hour, but that had fallen to forty lengths (a kilometer) and then to thirty. Sometimes less. After each stroke, a gasp. Avril started losing track of the lengths, and her own inattention riled her.

The whole thing took hours and occupied much of her day. There was the drive, alongside rolling English fields sprinkled with pretty cottages. Then the half hour it often took to lift her body out of the car, retrieve her walker from the back seat, lift her backpack, and shuffle to the front door. "All right, the worst is over," she might mumble to herself when she arrived in the lobby. Getting into her bathing suit, in the changing room, took another thirty minutes. More if she saw one of her friends and stopped to talk. Avril needed help fastening the clasp at the back of her suit, though she could manage the goggles and plastic bathing cap and customized earplugs on her own. Once, Avril asked a woman named Jenny to help her with the clasp and the two women started talking. Jenny was taking a class on Shakespeare, and over several weeks, Avril helped her to interpret some of the playwright's earlier, more difficult texts, like *Love's Labour's Lost*. But soon, Avril knew, she would lose that friendship, too, because she would lose the ability to drive to the pool. And then what? Anyway, it wouldn't matter in the end. "Does swimming make me feel good and want to live longer?" Avril asked herself. The answer came quickly: "No. I wish it did."

Philip Roth called old age "a massacre." Jean Améry, the journalist and Holocaust survivor, said it was worse even than Auschwitz. Others found it boring. That was a peculiar thing: the way a young woman's pain sometimes made her interesting, but an old woman's pain just made her tiring. The former suffers; the latter languishes and complains. The economy of sympathy never favored the elderly. Sometimes, when Avril thought about the state of her body, she was reminded of the kindly Jesuit priest who converted her to Catholicism. He had taught Avril that "hell is the pain of loss": not a place, but a condition.

Still, the idea that she should die before growing older had only come to her at the peak of a crisis, a few years earlier. Avril had been shopping at a pharmacy in Exeter when she slipped on the escalator and fell backward. The machine tossed her from side to side. Her left leg was carried upward as her body fell farther down, so that she was being pulled apart, like a wishbone. Lying with her head on the metal stairs, Avril heard a noise that was her own screaming and found it to be an ugly, harrowing sound. A staff member rushed over and pressed the emergency stop button. Someone else called an ambulance. As Avril waited, a line from a T. S. Eliot poem came to mind: "That is not what I meant at all; That is not it, at all."

When the ambulance arrived, paramedics rushed to Avril's side. "Can you hear me?" they asked.

"Yes."

"Do you hurt?"

"Not more than usual."

ON DECEMBER 10, 2009, Dr. Michael Irwin, a British physician who had worked for more than three decades at the United Nations, founded the Society for Old Age Rational Suicide (SOARS). On the group's website, Irwin, who has wispy white hair and a buttery, upper-class voice, explained that he had once been a member of the Voluntary Euthanasia Society (later renamed Dignity in Dying) but had come to feel stymied by its absolute focus on terminally ill people. "I may still not suffer from one serious specific illness—but, perhaps, from numerous, increasingly annoying health problems," he wrote. "When the burdens of living exceed the joys of being alive, I will then be close to the tipping point in wanting to die. . . . Surely this final decision should be mine, not made by anyone else." Irwin imagined a world in which people in their eighties or nineties who believed that "their lives have been fully lived" could be taken at their absolute word—and offered a physician's help to die.

The name of the group, Irwin told me later, was designed to shock. By then, the word "suicide" was effectively verboten in mainstream right-to-die activist circles—sick patients felt affronted by it, and political advocates wanted to detach their movement from it—but Irwin said he wanted to "reclaim" suicide as a "rational and positive act when a mentally competent, very elderly individual has carefully considered the main pros and cons for wanting to stay alive." Also, he said, SOARS was an easy-to-remember acronym, since many ill, elderly individuals suffer from bedsores. Practically speaking, the group would hold meetings and lobby government officials. Irwin would attend right-to-die conferences and appear on contentious television news panels. Soon, SOARS had six hundred paying members: mostly, Irwin said, older people with serious health problems who "don't have a real purpose for staying alive."

In his writing, Irwin made an effort to link his cause to a broader arc of history, reaching back to ancient Rome and Greece, to suggest evidence of "rational suicide" through the ages. The Epicureans, he wrote, felt that suicide was justified when life became unbearable. The Stoics approved of it, too. There was that brilliant Seneca quote: "I shall not abandon old age, if old age preserves me intact for myself, and intact as regards the better part of myself; but if old age begins to shatter my mind and to pull its various faculties to pieces . . . I shall rush out of a house that is crumbling and tottering." In Irwin's chronology, it was vapid Christian theologians who pulled common sense away from this reasonable position, with their insistence that suicide was self-murder, and so a kind of murder, and so a sin. Still, there were always brave thinkers who believed otherwise. Thomas More, in his 1516 book *Utopia*, wrote that in a true utopic world, a man who was suffering from an "incurable but also distressing and agonizing" disease, who had become "a burden to himself, and a trouble to others," would "free himself from this bitter life." When he did, it would be more than an act of prudence; it would be "a pious and holy action."

In the years after SOARS's launch, Irwin held small meetings across South England and wrote letters to local newspapers. He imagined that he would, for a while at least, be relegated to the narrow fringes of acceptable advocacy. But soon, Irwin started hearing echoes of the SOARS doctrine from outside the group. In 2010, the British novelist Martin Amis told the *Sunday Times* that Britain should establish suicide booths for the elderly. "There'll be a population of demented very old people, like an invasion of terrible immigrants, stinking out the restaurants and cafes and shops. . . . There should be a booth on every corner where you could get a martini and a medal." Later, after a public clamor, Amis said that he had meant to be "satirical." Still, he did not back off. "What we need to recognize is that certain lives fall into the negative, where pain hugely dwarfs those remaining pleasures that you may be left with," he said. "Geriatric science has been allowed to take over and, really, decency roars for some sort of correction." Medical science, in Amis's view, had obstructed a simpler arithmetic: pleasure versus pain.

But the loudest echo came five years later and across the ocean, at the March 2015 American Association for Geriatric Psychiatry's annual meeting. In a conference center in New Orleans, the association held a practical session—the first of its kind in the country—titled "Rational Suicide in the Elderly: Mental Illness or Choice?" At the session, psychiatrists and researchers discussed case studies "in which patients without apparent significant mental illnesses expressed a wish to kill themselves." One case study described a cheerful eighty-three-year-old woman who had undergone many operations over the previous decade and did not want another. "That's enough, I think," she said. The woman went on to acquire lethal barbiturates.

The main speaker, Dr. Robert McCue, a professor of psychiatry at New York University School of Medicine, acknowledged that in the vast majority of cases, around 90 percent, people who died by suicide had a clinically diagnosed psychiatric disorder. But some didn't. "This puts a burden on us and makes us wonder how we're going to treat someone who may not have an illness. How do you approach someone like that?" McCue said he hoped to open up discussion and perhaps encourage the formulation of new clinical guidelines. "The possibility of rational suicide is not discussed much in the psychiatric profession. Our patients may have information about it and may have opinions, but we have no training about this at all." Doctors were left on their own, to muddle through.

After the presentation, attendees in the audience had argued among themselves. One doctor observed that some of his patients were refusing medical treatment "because they want to be done." Another argued that the idea of elderly rational suicide "complicates things too much for doctors." Dr. Elissa Kolva, a young clinical psychologist who works with cancer patients, wondered if a wish to die, when someone was old and sick and compromised, could in fact be "a resilient thing" and "a sign of psychological well-being." Kolva sometimes met cancer patients who believed that something was deeply wrong with them, simply because they thought about death sometimes or imagined what it would feel like to stop their medical treatments and die. Often, she could make them feel better just by reassuring them that most people with cancer have similar thoughts. How could they not? Kolva once worked with a patient who, while getting a treatment infusion, remarked to his nurses that he might one day choose to swallow all his pills and be done with it. "He ended up spending eight hours under observation," she told me. "They took his shoelaces and his belt. . . . He's like, 'I don't want anyone to lock me up if I talk about the things I'm feeling.'"

Strictly speaking, there was no such thing as rational suicide. When suicide was mentioned in the *Diagnostic and Statistical Manual of Mental Disorders*, the profession's most authoritative guide, it was described as a symptom of mental illness. At the conference, some doctors wondered whether the first step toward a treatment solution was a change in vocabulary; professional guidelines, they said, could be updated to distinguish *suicide* suicide, or suicidal ideation, from a kind of suicidal thinking that was deliberate and reasonable and consistent with a person's long-held values. In the meantime, researchers and geriatricians could use existing diagnostic tools to help them better identify and understand rational suicidal thinking. There was the "Schedule of Attitudes Towards Hastened Death," which patients self-reported, and the "Desire for Death Rating Scale," which clinicians rated. There was the PHQ-9, which looked at severity of depression, and the "Demoralization Scale." There was the "Beck Hopelessness Scale," developed in the 1970s to measure negative attitudes about the future, and the more age-specific "Geriatric Hopelessness Scale." Psychiatrists could also draw from the "Functional Assessment of Chronic Illness Therapy-Spiritual Well-Being Scale" and its "Meaning and Peace" subscales. Through a blend of these measures, some more reliable than others, doctors and researchers could theoretically decipher "rational" suicidal thinking from the irrational kind. Of course, it was possible that all this effort would be in vain: that no amount of testing could quantify the unquantifiable—humanity, dignity, a person's understanding of the meaning of life—or even make it legible to psychiatrists who were anxious to see and appraise it. Also, none of the tests would answer the obvious next question: Then what?

After the conference, Dr. McCue and Dr. Meera Balasubramaniam, the director of geriatric psychiatry at New York University, published a volume titled *Rational Suicide in the Elderly*. "Is there such a thing as rational suicide?" they asked. "How would we know if this is the case? What would we do if it is?" The authors observed that the reasons elderly people gave for wanting to die were often identical to those listed by terminally ill patients seeking physician-assisted death, in the states where it is legal: loss of autonomy, inability to do activities that bring joy, fear of dependency, fear of being a burden on loved ones. Nevertheless, in states like Oregon, a desire to die was accepted as rational only if a patient had a terminal illness, with a prognosis of six months or less. The same wish, in an elderly patient with an unknown life span—even someone with roughly equivalent physical suffering—was assumed to be irrational. In other words, only when a patient was within six months of natural death was his psychiatrist allowed to step back and consider the specific context of the suicidal wish: to evaluate it on its own merits, rather than explaining it away as mental illness or marshaling the powers of the state to frustrate it.

In a 2018 paper in the *Journal of Clinical Psychiatry*, a small team of psychiatrists and researchers proposed a way forward. When a person had "a life-limiting physical illness" and no mental disorder and wanted to die for a sustained period of time, the authors argued, it might be appropriate for a psychiatrist to *not* attempt to prevent his death at all costs, and even to "collaborate with [the patient] around decisions to hasten death." Psychiatrists would not actively assist in suicides, but they wouldn't intervene to stop them either. They might even help patients find closure and calm, in anticipation of their planned deaths. This process could be termed "physician-unimpeded death" or "physician acknowledged death." The authors warned that further discussion of the subject was of immediate and practical importance; already, some patients were accessing lethal drugs from foreign countries.

But some doctors were anxious about these new rational suicide seekers and less assured of psychiatry's ability to help them. Even the geriatric psychiatrist Dr. Linda Ganzini, a coauthor of the 2018 paper, told me that she rejects the physician-unimpeded death model when patients don't have a serious health problem and instead want to die because they are old and have a collection of lesser, chronic ailments. To begin, Ganzini said, some of these patients might claim to be rational but in fact have an underlying depression that could be treated and eased. The opportunity for treatment would be lost if psychiatrists—perhaps influenced by their own political support for assisted death—took patients at face value. "The problem is that depression is hard to diagnose at the end of life. There is a lot of gray area," she said. "What constitutes clinically significant depression versus feeling sad and blue and just having normal grief at the end of life?" As it was, there were big, epistemological gaps in geriatric psychiatry. Doctors didn't really know how much depression and how much hopelessness was normal to see in an elderly patient, who, after all, was running out of days.

Ganzini also thinks about ageism. "To have different norms is ageist," she said. It could create a system where younger patients with dangerous thoughts are assumed to be sick and provided with urgent care, whereas older people are assumed to be rational and so denied life-saving intervention, just because they are old. Younger people would get suicide prevention and older people wouldn't. The risk felt real. As it is, geriatricians worry a lot about young doctors projecting their personal beliefs about age onto elderly patients: their fears of aging and their assumptions about what would make life unbearable—and maybe even their unacknowledged disgust with older bodies. "There is a lot of effort spent teaching primary care providers *not* just to say, 'Well, if I was ninety, I would be sad, blue, and depressed, too,'" Ganzini said. "It's not normative! If you're a thirty-five-year-old physician, you might think so. But geriatricians would say, 'That's a dangerous viewpoint. You are not going to discover and treat a lot of people with depression.'" Already, global suicide rates for elderly people are higher than for any other demographic group.

Other skeptics of the physician-unimpeded death model are more troubled by forces outside of the psychiatrist's office. The United States, they argue, has proved itself woefully unprepared, socially and economically, to deal with prolonged old age. Pharmaceutical drugs are impossibly expensive. Medical bills are bankrupting patients. Nearly 10 percent of Americans aged sixty-five and over are already living in poverty. Medicare does not cover assisted-living facilities or most at-home caregiving—driving some people into adult foster care or state-subsidized nursing homes, which almost everyone seems to fear above all else. The hard, yellow lighting. The cadres of underpaid and overworked nursing aides. The institutional food. If an older person wanted to die so that she could avoid living in one of those wretched, lonely places, would that be rational suicide? Maybe it would. Or maybe rational suicide was just a symptom of social and financial neglect, dressed up as moral choice.

Carried further, was it possible that as Medicare budgets dried up—as the population aged and the oft-cited "gray tsunami" landed on American soil—Americans might start to consider rational suicide for the elderly as an act of social responsibility, carried out by older people who understand themselves to be drains on the system and inhibitors of opportunity for the young? Already, about a quarter of Medicare spending each year is directed to patients in their very last year of life. Given all this, might we create, at least implicitly, and maybe unwittingly, what the philosopher Paul Menzel called a "duty to die cheaply"? Each elderly person, by virtue of living, would be forced to answer—for herself, if not for the rest of us—"Why are you still living?"

In early 2019, Dr. Michael Irwin started a new organization called Ninety Plus: a discussion group built around the premise that anyone ninety years old or older should automatically be granted the right to physician-assisted death. Irwin, who was eighty-eight at the time, told me that his selection of ninety as a cutoff age was somewhat arbitrary. "I don't have a good answer, I'm afraid. It seemed a kind of good target." By that age, he said, you were almost sure to be suffering. For his part, Irwin was faring relatively well. He had some lower back pain and numbness in his feet, which made it difficult to walk, and he took pills for high blood pressure, but otherwise he was OK. The hardest thing to deal with, he said, was the loss of energy. Irwin noticed that he felt pleased when long-anticipated social engagements, even ones he had looked forward to, were canceled. It meant that he could stay at home and rest and not "have to talk to relative strangers about silly things, like their grandchildren or Brexit." But then, it was useful to interrogate that feeling. Because what was the point of living if it was all so exhausting? "Why should I be forced to suffer?" he asked me. "Why should I have to drag on?"

CURRENTLY, THREE COUNTRIES in Europe have assisted-dying laws that take a patient's age into account when determining eligibility. Belgium, the Netherlands, and Luxembourg all allow elderly patients to qualify for assisted death if they suffer from "polypathology" or a "constellation of symptoms" that in the aggregate make life unbearable: symptoms like hearing loss, declining vision, and incontinence. Dr. Wim Distelmans, the head of Belgium's national euthanasia evaluation board, told me that elderly polypathology patients make up about 10 percent of euthanasias in the country. "I have no trouble with polypathology," he said when I visited him at his office in Brussels. "If you are eighty years old, you can't see anymore, you don't hear anything, you can't follow the television, you can't read a book, you need some help to eat, most of the time you are bedridden. . . . In my opinion, you can suffer unbearably."

In the Netherlands, where euthanasia was legalized in 2002, some legislators have argued that the law should go even further, so that all people above a certain threshold age can receive a physician-assisted death, even if they aren't suffering at all. In 2016, the country's health minister, Edith Schippers, proposed a measure that would have allowed elderly people with "a well-considered opinion that their life is complete" to qualify. This, she said in a statement to parliament, would help "older people who do not have the possibility to continue life in a meaningful way, who are struggling with the loss of independence and reduced mobility, and who have a sense of loneliness, partly because of the loss of loved ones, and who are burdened by general fatigue, deterioration, and loss of personal dignity."

Members of several parties applauded the minister's proposal, leaving the virulently racist and anti-immigrant populist politician Geert Wilders to emerge as an unlikely defender of communal responsibility and social grace. "We cannot allow people who are needy or lonely to be talked into dying," Wilders told the Dutch newspaper *Volkskrant*. "Combating loneliness, and investing in dignity and focusing on our elderly, is always the best option."

The minister's effort eventually stalled, but in September 2019, a parliamentarian named Pia Dijkstra announced that she would push forward an assisted-dying bill designed for elderly people with "completed lives." When I asked Dijkstra about her motivations, she answered me with typically Dutch blasé: "We think that people have the right to decide, themselves, when their life is complete. They should not have to take actions that are nasty, like putting a plastic bag over your head so you suffocate."

The logic of the completed life is a consoling one. It tells us that we will live long enough to feel existentially satiated, and that when we have reached that saturation point, we will be able to recognize it for what it is and to let go of living. But I suspect that natural end points are easier to spot in retrospect. In 2016, a number of Dutch academics published a study in the *BMJ Open*, a peer-reviewed medical journal, titled "Caught Between Intending and Doing: Older People Ideating on a Self-Chosen Death." The researchers evaluated twenty-five Dutch citizens with a mean age of eighty-two who "were ideating on a self-chosen death because they considered their lives to be no longer worth living." Each study participant "(1) considered their lives to be 'completed'; (2) suffered from the prospect of living on; (3) currently wished to die; (4) were seventy years of age or older; (5) were not terminally ill; (6) considered themselves to be mentally competent; (7) considered their death wish reasonable." On questioning, all of the participants admitted to "being torn" about their choice. In interviews, they used words like "dilemma" and "struggle" and "doubt." One woman was seriously considering hip-replacement surgery at the same time that she was making active plans to end her life. Another said she thought that she should die, in part, because of depleting global energy reserves and shrinking healthcare budgets. "In former times," she observed, "if Grandma was no longer useful to the clan, they said, 'Well, Grandma: Enough is enough.'" Ultimately, many of the study participants viewed suicide as the "reasonable" and "rational" choice, in contrast with their sometimes more emotional compulsion to live.

Still, I met people who longed for the kind of completed-life provision that the Dutch were dreaming up. One day when I was living in London, I took the subway south, toward the river Thames, to meet a seventy-five-year-old man named Tony who thought that he was nearing his own point of life completion. Tony often went for walks along the river and around the enormous National Theatre, which Prince Charles once coolly compared to a nuclear power station, on account of all the concrete. He would look at posters for upcoming productions and make tasteful selections. As a general rule, Tony went to the theater twice each month, which meant that he knew what was showing at any given time. Except, all of a sudden, the plays had stopped being interesting. Even his beloved Shakespeare. A new thought surfaced: *I have seen enough Hamlets. I have seen enough Lears.*

Tony lived alone, in a small apartment with green painted walls, a green couch, a green armchair, and a smattering of green plants. The day we met, he was dressed head to toe in maroon, a short man with curly gray hair and chubby earlobes. "I'm doddery. Going slightly deaf. But nothing untoward," he said as we shook hands. Tony had texts about Freud, Jung, and the practices of Gestalt therapy on his bookshelves. He was born to a Jewish family in Manchester and had since become "a lapsed Christian, Buddhist, Quaker. . . . I've come out on the other end as an existentialist."

It wasn't that he minded being old, he said. He was content in the role of old man, sitting in his green chair, listening to BBC Radio for hours on end. He could even tolerate the odd "gray hair moment" of blankness or confusion. Still, before long, in five years perhaps, he would be ready to go. In large part, it would be an act of avoidance. Tony wished to bypass the "leaking, smelling, bored-out-of-your-mind, severe *decrepitude*. I love that word! *Decrepitude*. Bits falling off . . ." He also did not want to end up in a nursing home, where nurses might speak to him in cooing voices, their faces frozen into sticky, grotesque smiles as they urged him to join in with the others. To play a board game. To clap along to the music. "'Oh, come on, Mr. Tony! Join in! Clap hands!'" A nursing home, he said, would be hell for an introvert like him. At the least, it would be boring, and Tony feared boredom most of all. He told me that he kept a daily journal and that, recently, he had been horrified to find himself writing the same things over and over. "When I get bored of *me*," he said, "I will kill myself."

Near the end of our conversation, Tony asked if I wanted to see his bedroom. In it, beside his bed, he had a gas canister full of pure helium and a mask made out of a thick plastic bag. He kept them in plain sight so that he could look at them, from time to time, and feel assured. "How will I know when I've had enough? Will I force myself to turn on my helium cylinder and pull the bag over my head?" He paused. "I'm interested in the philosophical concept of ceasing to be." Once before, in his twenties, Tony had thought about suicide. It had to do with a woman. He took pills but woke up vomiting a few hours later. This, he said, would be different. And it would be radical. Tony looked up at me. My face, I think, must have given something away, because he quickly looked down again. Then he told me that I was too young to be thinking about death.

IN 2015, AVRIL SAID, she had asked her doctor to help her. She was frank. Too brazen, really. "Life is not worth living anymore—but I'm not depressed," she said. So would the doctor be so kind as to give her "a nice handful of barbiturates"?

"No," said the doctor.

Avril said she asked several others, including a surgeon whom she had seen before. "They all came back and said, 'I would really love to help, but I cannot.'"

One evening, one of those doctors knocked on her front door. When she let him inside, he said that he had been thinking about things and that he wanted to explain himself. Then he started to cry. Avril said she showed him to the living room, where he sat down on the couch. She sat in the armchair, with her feet tilted up over her head. Over the course of two hours, the doctor told Avril that he had looked for ways to help her. He had even consulted a medical lawyer, at his own expense, to see if there was something he could do, but the lawyer had said that there was not. The doctor told Avril that he admired her and that it had been a pleasure to treat her. He also told her a story about one of his friends, who had tried to gas himself to death by putting his head inside an oven but had instead accidentally blown up his house. The doctor cried again.

"I fear," he said, as he rose to leave, "that this may result in you trying to kill yourself."

"Yes," Avril said. It would. Later, she told her doctors to stop contacting her. She had limited time left, she said, and they were wasting it.

Avril found the right-to-die group Exit International online. Seated in front of her office computer, in her enormous reading glasses, with a magnifying glass held up to the screen, she read through Exit's website. "Dying is not a medical process," it said. "As such, you don't necessarily need the white coat by the bed. Exit's aim is to ensure that all rational adults have access to the best available information so that they may make informed decisions over when and how they die." The website looked professional enough, with pink and purple graphics and links to news articles. Its founder was a real medical doctor from Australia named Philip Nitschke. Avril read that the average age of Exit members was seventy-five years old. She also read that for $185, she could buy an annual Exit membership and a digital copy of Dr. Nitschke's *Peaceful Pill Handbook*, which promised instruction on all the reliable and peaceful ways to end a life. Avril paid the fee and sent in an application form and was accepted. She opened the handbook right away. "In recent years, a new trend has begun to emerge," it read. "We meet elderly people who are fit and healthy (for their age) but for whom life has become increasingly burdensome."

The book was strange in its textbook formality. It rated lethal methods on the basis of reliability, peacefulness, safety to others, shelf life, and postmortem detectability. It had sections on gas canisters and cyanide and car exhaust fumes. Avril read it all, in the small office next to her living room. Beside her were stacks of paper covered with Post-it notes and a file box labeled VITAL INFORMATION FOR THE BUYER, which Avril had asked her lawyer to pass on to whoever bought the house after she died. By the end of her reading, there was only one suicide method that interested her: the one described as the best of all—Nembutal. The barbiturate apparently acted quickly, but not too quickly. Also, it created a natural-looking death. "It is the most peaceful of deaths to witness," the handbook said. "With Nembutal, you always die in your sleep." The only tricky thing was that the liquid needed to be consumed quickly: ideally, in two or three big swallows, before the coma set in. Avril wondered if she could manage that. She also worried that a bottle of poison might be difficult to open with shaking, arthritic hands.

The handbook explained that there were several ways to get the drug. Avril could buy it from a veterinary supply store in Mexico, in a liquid form that was used for anesthetizing animals before surgery. The Mexican stores sold Nembutal in standard-size doses and Exit advised members that they would need two bottles to die. Another option was China, where a powdered form of the drug could be purchased from black market chemical distributors and then mixed with water. The handbook provided email addresses for dealers in both countries. Avril decided on Mexico. She had a low opinion of Chinese consumer products—she'd bought stainless steel pots from China before and been disappointed by the quality—and she wasn't prepared to take a chance on something so important. Avril asked herself if she minded breaking the law. She decided that she didn't, because the law was "silly." As the handbook advised, Avril set up a new email address, using an encrypted service called Riseup, to use for all correspondence related to her death plans.

The Mexican dealer's name was Alejandro, and Avril wired him £460 ($575). It would have felt subversive, maybe, if it hadn't felt so ordinary. Alejandro wrote polite emails and gave clear instructions for the wire transfer. After he shipped the supply, he sent a tracking number for the package. "I am beginning to feel better," Avril wrote in an email. But when the package arrived in Brampford Speke, Avril realized that she had been sent only one dose of Nembutal, instead of the two she needed. She put the bottle in the bathroom cupboard and ordered a second supply from another dealer, for £600 ($750). When the two new bottles arrived, she put them in the white cabinet over the sink and felt an astonishing relief.

That year, I started meeting other people, in other places, who had bought Nembutal off the Internet. Some were elderly and wanted the drug for good measure, just in case. Others were very sick and had firm plans to take it. There was Jay Franklin, an Australian man in his late thirties with a congenital bowel condition, who begged for Nembutal in a YouTube video and was sent the drug by strangers. There was Bill, an elderly British man with Parkinson's, who bought powdered Nembutal from China and then hid the drug in his closet, so that his son wouldn't find it. I spoke on Skype with a twenty-seven-year-old Hungarian named Balint who told me that he was in good health and that he was generally happy with his life and his girlfriend, but that he wanted Nembutal because he was "very concerned about the direction the world is developing in." Hungary's government was not a progressive one, he said. Restrictions on civil liberties were tightening. Who knew what was next? On top of that, there were the larger issues of global overpopulation, resource depletion, climate change, war. "I just fear that I might have to *do something*. I want to ensure that if something happens to me . . . I have a way out."

"Does your girlfriend know?" I asked.

"No," he said. "But she would freak out."

Avril started refining her plans. She worried that, because of the palsy in her left hand, she would spill the Nembutal at the last moment, so she bought a plastic tray to rest on the edge of the bathtub: the kind that another sort of woman might use to hold her champagne flute while taking a bubble bath. She also found a friend who agreed to "discover" her body, at a planned time, so it would not lie there in the empty house for too long. "Gosh, I tell you," Avril said, "it's a strange thing, but it's true: The pain is less." Just having the drugs and the plans made her feel a little better. On the Exit International web forums, she had read that people sometimes felt that way.

Avril did not have much anxiety about her imminent nonexistence, but she did worry about the house and the garden and what would become of them. One day in late March, she went outside to survey the property. She walked slowly, down a winding path that cut through clusters of bluebells and apple trees. Her hair was unpinned, long and white and wild down her back. "Oh dear, don't look at the fig tree," she begged. "It's a bad year for figs and I don't know why." Her gravestone was at the back, in the garden shed. Avril had sourced the smooth, pinkish rock from the north coast of Devon and had hired a local artist to do the calligraphy: *Avril Kay Henry*. Wasn't it marvelous? Admittedly, it wasn't normal to be buried in one's backyard, but Avril had done some research and found that it could be done with approval from local environmental authorities, who needed to inspect the property and make sure that it wasn't too close to a water source. Avril's property was not too close to a water source and so she was approved. She was to be buried deep enough down that the badgers couldn't get at her corpse. "I don't mind the badgers eating me," Avril said gravely, "but the neighbors won't want to see the bits scattered around!" She had already prepaid for her funeral and left strict instructions for the attendees. There was to be a reading from Ursula K. Le Guin. No one was to wear black. They were to have a drink together afterward.

"Come April, we shall be full into spring," Avril said. "And I suspect you're wondering, as the garden is beautiful and I do love it, why I don't want to hang around for another year. Um, it's hard to explain. . . . At the moment, I can just about enjoy it, but it does hurt." She looked around. "If I stay here much longer, the garden will deteriorate just as I do."

"Do you think you'll see the garden in bloom again?"

Avril looked up for a moment and then raised her eyebrows. "You're tear-jerking, aren't you?"

AT 8:49 P.M. ON Friday, April 15, 2016, two months after we first exchanged emails, Avril heard the phone ring. The noise startled her because the phone never rang at night. Avril was sitting in her office, in front of the computer. The voice on the other end of the line was male and unfamiliar and it was hard to understand—especially the consonants. Avril told the strange voice that she was hard of hearing and asked him to slow down. "One word at a time," she begged, "with pauses in between syllables." The man told Avril that he was a police officer and that it had been brought to his attention that she was planning to end her life. Avril told him that he was correct. The officer asked if he could send some colleagues to her house to speak to her. Avril said no. He couldn't. It was dark and she never opened the front door after dark.

At 9:15 p.m., two police officers, dispatched from the nearby Heavitree Road police station, broke through the glass plate on Avril's front door and stepped into her hallway. Later, they would say that they rang the doorbell first and Avril would say that they didn't. "Oh God!" she cried aloud when she heard the glass shatter. When the officers found Avril, cowering, they told her that a member of the public had reported her as a suicide risk and that they were there to perform a "wellness check." Then the officers said something about being sent by Interpol, the International Criminal Police Organization, and asked Avril to hand over the drugs.

Avril composed herself. She began to taunt the blundering men, who didn't seem to know quite what they were looking for. Was it a powder or a liquid, or was it pills? Avril said that there were many objects and substances in her home that she could theoretically use to kill herself. There was an electric carving knife in the kitchen, for instance, and she knew the placement of critical arteries in her body. Also, she had figured out how to electrocute herself. Inside Avril's study, one of the officers found her suicide note in a folder, along with an essay describing her decision to die. According to Avril, he told her that suicide was illegal—and Avril, in turn, told him that he was mistaken: that suicide was perfectly legal and had been for decades. The officer asked Avril why she wanted to kill herself and she told him to mind his own business. She also asked if she could call her caregiver, Heather,* for support and was told that she could. When Heather arrived, Avril told her to go into the downstairs bathroom and to look inside the white cabinet. There, she would find a cardboard box holding the medicine from Mexico. Heather went to the bathroom and found the box and handed it to the officers.

Around midnight, the police called in a consulting doctor, who arrived at 12:07 a.m. The officers told the doctor that Interpol "had intercepted some information regarding chemicals coming from Mexico" and traced the package back to Avril's house. Avril was tired by then, but she sat with the physician and told him about her health problems: the back pain, the poor mobility, the deafness, the incontinence. She denied that she had ever been depressed or mentally ill. Well, once she had been depressed, but that was after her father died, so maybe that was just grief? Avril explained that she had been planning her suicide for eighteen months. She explained about the Nembutal and how expensive it had been. She said that all her affairs were in order and that her dead body was meant to be discovered, by a friend, on Monday morning. Heather listened to Avril talk and thought she sounded like a professor must sound, lecturing in front of crowds of people. Another person might have broken down, but Avril was so steady.

Later, a social worker and a psychiatrist were summoned to perform a mental health assessment. Avril took them to her bedroom and showed them the padded cloth diapers that she had to wear every day. She showed them the chamber pot under her bed and explained that she sometimes filled it up in a single night. Avril thought the social worker looked embarrassed. She also let the doctors see the goodbye letters that her friends had written her. One of Avril's Christian friends had signed her card with a *Bon Voyage!*—as if Avril were planning for some exotic trip. Avril said later that the psychiatrist seemed curious about her lapsed Catholicism. She wanted to know why Avril had left the church. "What effect does it have? Are you afraid of dying?" In notes that the doctor typed up that evening, he referred to Avril as a "very intelligent retired professor with a large number of health problems" and described her situation as "very difficult."

The two doctors and the social worker told Avril that they needed to confer privately for a moment and asked her if she could sit in the study. They stayed away for half an hour. "You have had difficulty making a decision," Avril observed when they returned.

The verdict was a good one. The three experts said they believed Avril to be of sound mind. They could not, as it were, detain her under the Mental Health Act—as "unwise" as they found her behavior to be. "Could find no evidence of depression," the doctor wrote in his report. He asked Avril if she had plans to kill herself in the next twenty-four hours.

"No."

What about after that?

"If I can, I shall kill myself."

"Crew feel she has capacity full so can't be moved to place of safety," the doctor wrote. "Crew don't feel happy leaving this lady on her own . . . will likely commit suicide.

"Long chat, agreed we cannot give back her medication (do no harm)."

As the doctor packed up his bag, he told Avril that her family physician would be in touch soon, to arrange for a more formal mental health assessment. Avril thanked him for listening to her. Then, finally, at 4:28 a.m., the doctor and psychiatrist and social worker and police officers left through the broken front door. Half an hour later, Heather left, too. And then Avril exhaled. What they did not know about—and what the police officers had not found—was her second supply of Nembutal, the one she had ordered after realizing that her first shipment did not contain enough. There were still two bottles of the drug, tucked away at the back of the white cupboard. "We won," Avril whispered to herself. Then she grew annoyed that the intruders had left the lights on in her study and the toilet seat up in the bathroom.

Later, I heard about other raids. In London, I spoke to a professional caregiver whose patient—an eighty-something woman named Barbara* with chronic fatigue syndrome—also had her front door broken down by police. As they did with Avril, officers asked Barbara if she was in possession of a life-ending substance from Mexico. They said they had been tipped off by a detective who had a "list of names." They said that Barbara was not in trouble but that they wanted her drugs.

Barbara couldn't say very much to the officers because she was very weak and needed a voice amplifier to make herself heard. She said that, yes, she had long ago ordered some Nembutal but that she had since thrown it out. The officers grew impatient and left. Afterward, the caregiver, who knew all about Barbara's illicit purchase, logged onto Exit International's website and left a note, warning other buyers about the mysterious detective and his list of names. Within weeks, Exit got reports from members about similar police checkups in Oxfordshire and Brighton. And then the visits moved abroad.

In May 2016, a woman named Janice, in Vancouver, Canada, emailed Exit's founder to say that she needed to talk about "the visit (unscheduled) of two Vancouver police detectives." Janice told Dr. Nitschke that the detectives had been wearing plain clothes and that they had told her not to panic. As she recounted it, the men told her that they were part of an "international investigation based in the States" that was looking into "online assisted suicide"—and that they knew she had ordered drugs from Mexico. Janice asked the officers if they had a search warrant and they said that they didn't. Janice told them that they could not come inside. Afterward, I called the Vancouver Police Department and the Royal Canadian Mounted Police to ask about what happened, but a VPD spokesperson told me that the department had no record of any such visit and the RCMP declined to be interviewed.

A few weeks later, a woman named Sarah logged onto Exit's website from her home in North Carolina. Police had visited her too, she wrote, and they had taken her Nembutal. Sarah was only in her sixties and she wasn't sick with anything, but she had been around very old people before, and the experience had disturbed her. It had disturbed her so much that she swore never to become very old. Sarah had ordered

Nembutal as a gift to herself, on her sixty-fifth birthday. "I just became acutely aware of what aging is. And I hate to say it . . . I just don't have the courage!"

The officers rang her doorbell around 10:30 a.m., Sarah said. At first, she ignored the noise, because she was still in bed and wasn't expecting anyone. But after the rings came loud knocking and then banging. When Sarah opened the door, she saw three young police officers staring back at her. At first, she thought she might be in trouble again for failing to mow her lawn and for allowing her garden to become unsightly. "Are you here because of my yard?" she asked. "I don't mow enough. My weeds get high and stuff." Sarah told the officers they could come inside but asked them to wait for just a minute, in her kitchen, so that she could run to the bathroom and use some mouthwash.

When she came back to the kitchen, the officers asked Sarah if she had ordered a package from Mexico. Then they said something about Homeland Security. Sarah tried to distract them with small talk—whatever came to mind, this and that. She thought they seemed nice, more embarrassed and jittery than anything else. But they kept looking at her. "You're not going to leave until I give it to you, are you?" Sarah asked. The officers were quiet. Sarah asked them if they had watched the news lately. Maybe they had seen all the shit going on in the world? Maybe they could think about whether their time wouldn't be better spent tracking down serious and important criminals? Then she opened her fridge and took out a small shopping bag and dropped it on the counter. "Byeeeee, Nembutal!"

Before the officers left, Sarah asked them how old they were. They all looked to be in their thirties or forties. Sarah told them that when they were old and frail, they should look back on that day and their decision to take the drugs from her. They should think hard about whether it had been the right thing to do. One of the male officers told Sarah that when he was old, he planned to chill on the beach, drinking beer. "Good for you," Sarah said.

Years later, in 2019, Major Keith Eury of the Concord, North Carolina, police department told me that his colleagues had indeed gone to check on Sarah at home that day. He said they did the visit on behalf of *either* Homeland Security or the Drug Enforcement Agency—but that he didn't know which federal agency had made the request, and the sergeant who was in charge at the time couldn't remember. Eury also couldn't find any paperwork documenting the event. What he did recall was that federal agents asked the Durham police officers to seize and destroy any drugs found in Sarah's home, but not to arrest Sarah. The point was not to punish her, he said. "They" were aiming, instead, to "go after someone bigger."

For its part, Exit International had no answer for the raids. Some members wondered if one of the group's recommended Mexican drug dealers had been busted by police or bought off by police or was just careless with security. In June 2016, an Exit member in Australia who had ordered a hard copy of *The Peaceful Pill Handbook* received a letter from the Australian Border Force, noting that agents had seized the book under subsection 203B(2) of Australia's Customs Act 1901. "ONE (1) BOOK DETAILING SUICIDE," border agents had written, in summary of the captured bounty. Then, that fall, the raids arrived in New Zealand, and the plot grew more fantastic. In October 2016, a handful of Exit International members, most of them elderly women, attended a group seminar and potluck lunch in Hutt Valley. Driving home afterward, a number of them hit a police roadblock that was stopping traffic through a central thoroughfare. Officers were checking IDs and conducting Breathalyzer tests: a random measure, it seemed, to catch drunk drivers. But not long after, around fifteen of those Exit members had police officers show up at their homes. A seventy-six-year-old named Wilhelmina Irving told journalists that a cop had fished for details about the seminar: "He told me he knew exactly what had been said, who was there, everything else and what did I have to say?"

New Zealand journalists would eventually report, and a judge would later confirm, that the roadblock had been a ruse, designed to ID people who attended the Exit gathering. Police had titled their effort "Operation Painter" and in the course of it had bugged the home of a sixty-seven-year-old Exit International coordinator and retired primary school teacher named Suzy Austen. In October 2016, Suzy—an avid gardener who volunteered for an Alzheimer's charity and a rape crisis program and Habitat for Humanity—was arrested after being spotted in her car, divvying up a supply of pentobarbital. After a two-week criminal hearing, she was acquitted on charges of "aiding a suicide" but found guilty of two importation offenses. "I believe I was made a scapegoat," she said; after all, there were many other people in New Zealand who were ordering the very same drugs. And then, just as soon as it all began, reports about police visits and suspiciously timed "wellness checks" dried up, for a while.

Years later, a spokesperson from the UK Metropolitan Police Service confirmed that, at the time of the 2016 visits, one of the department's "Special Inquiries Teams" was investigating Exit and its founder, Dr. Philip Nitschke—following a tip-off from a concerned citizen. In the end, the spokesperson told me, "numerous lines of inquiry" were opened, but "no action was taken."

A FEW HOURS AFTER the police left Avril's home, she slowly opened the front door and took a step outside. Her eyes looked swollen as she surveyed the bluish pane of glass that lay shattered on the doorstep and the wooden board that police had nailed over the hole. She hadn't slept. "I'm in a very odd state today," she said. "I almost burned the house down when I was making breakfast this morning. . . . It's as if my mind is going. I'm really scared. It shattered me." She was still shaking. Avril wondered if the police officers had installed listening devices in her house, to spy on her. She thought they probably had. After all, they had nothing better to do than "breaking down the door of little old ladies!"

There were things to do. Over the next few days, Avril called her lawyer and told him to file a complaint with local police authorities. She wanted the officers to apologize and promise to never bother her again. More important, she wanted them to replace her front door—and not just with any front door, but with the exact same kind of front door that she had picked out, with the exact same high-quality glass. Avril had already called several local suppliers and determined that the cost would be around £185 plus tax, totaling £222 to do the job. Avril also gave her lawyer her address book, with the names and phone numbers of all her contacts written inside. It was color-coordinated, with the different colors representing the order in which her family and friends should be notified of her death. Avril arranged for her car to be given away to the car mechanic who had long serviced it. And she wrote a letter to the future buyers of her home, urging them to hire Geoff, her handyman, because he was very reliable and knew how things were meant to be. Then she laid out a copy of her prepared suicide note. *I am alone. The decision is wholly mine*, the letter read. *I very much hope that, since the evidence here shows clearly that no murder has been committed, there will be no Post Mortem.*

Later, maybe, some people would see Avril's final note as a sign of her emotional poverty. Maybe I did. How could a final letter be so cold and so unexamined—so logistical? Of all the things to say, why talk about the bathtub and her fear of leaving it dirty? Why talk about the cleaning fluid? *PS If I have fouled the bath in death, please please be kind to wash it down*, Avril wrote. *Dettol is provided.* But suicide notes can be like that. In the 1990s, scholars who studied them observed that most are flat and economical. Maybe, in the end, it could not have been otherwise. By then, it was all so obvious to Avril. There was nothing more to say.

She planned to die in the late afternoon, on April 20, after lunch. There wasn't much to eat in the house. Avril had not gone grocery shopping that week, in anticipation of her death, so all she had left were a few frozen dinners. She was even out of biscuits. Still, she thought she would eat something before making the slow journey up to the second-floor bathtub.

But that morning, Avril's doctor's office rang to say that the police had been in touch. Was it true that she was planning to end her life that evening? A subsequent report by the local coroner, who was charged with investigating Avril's suicide, would later conclude that when Avril called her Internet provider and told the employee on the line that she would soon be dead, the employee had called the police, who in turn had called Avril's doctor, who in turn had asked his receptionist to call Avril—perhaps with a touch of exasperation because, well, everyone knew what Avril was planning, but what could be done?

Avril told the receptionist to "call the dogs off" and leave her alone. Then she hung up the phone and went to her computer.

"I better forget about lunch and get into the bath instead," she wrote in an email titled "Good traveling."

Avril opened the two bottles of Nembutal with tiny barber's scissors from her bathroom. They were difficult bottles; each had a metal rim around the edge of the glass lip, which had to be broken. Avril had to be careful not to spill. When she was done, she placed the open bottles on her new plastic tray. And then she stepped into the bathtub for the first time in thirty years.

Later, Avril's lawyer, who found her dead at 6:40 that evening, would confirm that her body was clean and dry, as she had hoped it would be.

Weeks before, Avril had wondered how she would feel while lying there, in the tub. She thought she would "try to feel as little as possible. What I want to avoid is taking a last look around the garden or having a long look at my beautiful pottery. That would just make it difficult and it would only hurt and it would serve no purpose." Avril said she would remind herself that death was inevitable anyway. She did not think she would be afraid. "How can I be scared if I don't exist?" she asked. "Simple logic. I shall know nothing. There will be nothing."

3

Body

Because she had once been a filmmaker, Maia Calloway sometimes imagined what a documentary film about the end of her life would look like. In the first scene, she would be outside in her wheelchair, racing as fast as she could toward the Rio Grande gorge. There would be snow on the ground, lining the dirt path, and the low-lying desert brush would be every shade of dried-out brown. Maia's long, straight hair would blow in the wind behind her, and she would look younger than her thirty-nine years, clear-eyed and flushed.

Tevye, who had once been her lover but was now more like a brother (or a friend, or a mother, or a caretaker; it depended on the day) would be walking alongside her. He'd have his Tilley hat fastened around his chin and a fresh joint in his pocket and he'd be grooving in the New Mexico sunshine. After a while, though, Tevye would step out of the frame, because, after all, this was meant to be Maia's film. Her voice-over would come in, over the crunch of the tires on the dirt. "I'm in hell," Maia would say. "Let me out."

At the end of the scene, she would arrive at the gorge and, maybe, if she was feeling up to it, would rise from her wheelchair and take a few shuffling steps toward the edge, to peer over. The metaphor of the whole thing, Maia acknowledged, might be a bit heavy-handed: the dying woman literally staring into the abyss. But when someone is dying, people make accommodations for cliché, don't they? At film school in New York City, Maia had read the work of Joseph Campbell, a mythologist who studied "hero's journey" narratives. She liked Campbell's idea that heroic tales could be broken down into common constituent parts: the hero venturing forth into the world; the hero encountering strange and supernatural things; the atonement; the reconciliation with the father character; and then, in the end, the acquisition of freedom. Maia wanted her story to be told that way. "It's absolutely a hero's journey," she said. "And one of the things I'm conquering is the fear. And the guilt." Her quest, of course, was to find not the freedom to live, as per Campbell's formulation, but instead the freedom to die.

For the film to be authentic, it would have to show the bad stuff, too. Maybe the camera could capture the aftermath of the gorge scene: the way Maia's eyes became watery and vacant after she exerted herself too much in the wheelchair. Another scene could show her getting out of bed at 3 a.m., as she often did, limping down the narrow hallway in the dark, with her thin arms pressed into the wall for support, and then blinking into the yellow light of the refrigerator as she searched for her pain pills. The film could show her fighting with Tevye in the kitchen about God knows what. All the screaming and all the sulking. In another voice-over, Maia could explain what multiple sclerosis (MS) had done to her body at the cellular level: the way her immune system had malfunctioned, so that her body attacked its own central nervous system. The way the disease had eaten away at the fatty protective coating surrounding her cranial and spinal cord nerves, so that the tips of the nerves frayed outward, like the scales of a pinecone, and so were exposed to damage and ruin.

The final scene would be easy to script. It would take place in a small apartment in Basel, Switzerland, at Lifecircle, one of Switzerland's now famous suicide clinics, where even foreigners can die with the help of a Swiss doctor. In her final moments, Maia thought, she would need to coax herself forward, reminding herself that it was better to die early than to die slowly of the disease. "I can't be childish and falter and say, 'Oh no, I'm scared of dying, I'm scared of dying,'" she told me. "I can't do that. . . . I have to have courage."

Maia said she would die soon. Soon, she would set the date. The administrators at the clinic in Switzerland were ready for her, and Maia had already paid part of the fee up front: $3,300, with another $7,000 to be paid at the time of her death, to cover the medical care and the drugs and the cremation. She just needed to book the ticket and get on the plane. Why did the idea of it seem so weird? "I have canceled two flights, now," Maia told me in March 2018. "What I find myself doing is wavering."

IN JANUARY 2016, a lawmaker in Colorado, where Maia was living, introduced a bill in the state legislature called the Colorado End-of-Life Options Act, which aimed to legalize aid in dying across the state. Maia heard about the proposal on the news and then found the text of the draft law online. She read it through carefully. Right away, it was clear that she would not meet the law's eligibility criteria. Maia felt that she was dying, but under the eyes of the proposed law she wasn't dying enough—or, at least, she wasn't near enough to death. The legislation said that qualified patients had to be within six months of their natural ending, but Maia's doctors told her that she could live for years and maybe decades, inching slowly toward paralysis.

Maia started researching online, and soon she came across a BBC documentary called *Choosing to Die*. It was about a seventy-one-year-old British hotelier named Peter Smedley who had motor neuron disease and who traveled from Britain to Zurich, to a clinic called Dignitas, for what Swiss authorities called an assisted voluntary death, or AVD. "I could do this," she thought. Maia learned that assisted death has been legal in Switzerland since the 1940s, by a kind of legislative omission. According to Article 115 of the Swiss Federal Criminal Code, assisting a suicide is illegal only if the person giving assistance does so out of "selfish motives." By logical extension, assisted death is permitted if those motives are unselfish. What exactly constitutes a selfish or unselfish motive is left undefined in the criminal code, but Swiss authorities have since interpreted the law to mean that assisting is OK as long as the assister does not profit financially from the death.

Over the years, several nonprofit euthanasia clinics have opened up in the country, each with eligibility criteria that go beyond the vaguely worded Swiss law. The clinics require that their patients be suffering; that they have given due consideration to their choice; that they be free from coercion; that they be cognizant at the time of their deaths; and that they be physically capable of administering the lethal drugs themselves. However, they do not require that patients be terminally ill. And unlike in every other jurisdiction where assisted death is legal, the Swiss authorities impose no requirements of citizenship or residency. This means that foreigners can fly into Zurich, be examined by Swiss doctors, and die a few days later.

By 2016, people from around the world were traveling regularly to Switzerland to die. It was so commonplace that locals began to speak, drolly, of a "suicide tourism" industry. According to one study from the University of Zurich, 611 "tourists" traveled to the country for assisted deaths between 2008 and 2012, though annual numbers have likely increased. Maia liked the idea that in Switzerland, people took for granted that assistance in death was a human right. "It's interesting," she said, "because in America we will kill people who are on death row, but we won't allow someone to die peacefully in many states. . . . It's a reverse mentality."

Watching people die in Switzerland, via documentary news film, had also become a kind of global pastime. The 2011 premiere of the BBC's *Choosing to Die* was watched by 1.6 million people in Britain, nearly 7 percent of the country's entire television audience. Since then, variations of the "Grandfather goes to Dignitas" film have appeared on a number of national networks and been uploaded to YouTube, together forming a new kind of documentary genre with its own stock narrative arc: the diagnosis; the treatment failure; the patient's weighty realization that he must travel to Switzerland to get the dignified death he desires; the agonized choice; the resigned acceptance of family members who will be left to wonder if they should have done *something* different; the final words; the strange death in the strange foreign clinic. These films, it seemed to Maia, were framed as heroes' journeys. Still, there was something that felt false about them. The characters came across as gutsy and likable, but also self-edited. They didn't seem to struggle like she struggled.

Maia read news articles about the Dignitas clinic. She liked its slogan, "To live with dignity, to die with dignity." She liked that its founder, the lawyer Ludwig Minelli, referred to assisted dying as "the last human right." But other things bothered her. Maia thought that in television interviews, Minelli came across as emotionally detached and a bit full of himself. She read that he had once been chastised by Swiss authorities for his improper disposal of cremated remains, after locals complained of human ashes washing up on the shore of Lake Zurich. Maia preferred the look of another clinic in Basel, called Lifecircle. "Lifecircle is committed to the dignity of mankind," its website read. With an assisted voluntary death, "no one ever goes alone and lonely." The clinic's founder, Dr. Erika Preisig, said she would accept foreign patients who weren't imminently dying but whose "medical problems have resulted in an unacceptably low quality of life." Maia decided that she would apply and that if she were accepted, she would use the small inheritance she received after her mother's death to buy a plane ticket to Switzerland, travel around Europe for a while, and then die at Lifecircle.

"This is my formal request for Assisted Voluntary Death with Dignity," she wrote in a letter to the clinic in February 2016.

*I suffer from a severe form of progressive multiple sclerosis with
the burden of my disease in my spinal cord and brain stem. . . .
The symptoms that I suffer from on a daily basis range from the
loss of control of my torso, legs, severe intractable pain as if my
organs are falling in on themselves, profound fatigue, loss of function, loss of bladder function, severe dysfunction of my autonomic
nervous system, pain when moving my breathing muscles, and a
host of memory and cognitive problems that prevent me from having the intellect I once had. . . . Much to my sadness, the treatments
that will bring people out of severe disability involving myelin
repair and stem cells are still years away from being available in
a clinical setting.*

She ended the letter with a plea. "As a person of faith and deep spirituality, I believe the soul travels on and wants to be free from this prison
that has become my body. I have fought this devastating illness tirelessly
for fifteen years and I want to be free."

Afterward, Maia sent in medical records and spoke to the clinic's directors over Skype. She thought the process might take a while, but it didn't;
within a few weeks, she was formally accepted as a Lifecircle patient.
Then she booked a one-way ticket from Denver to Zurich. Maia wasn't
speaking much to her father, Larry, by then, but she sent him an email
saying that she was moving to Mexico, where things were cheaper—and
that he shouldn't expect to see her for a while. Later, it would be hard
to recall exactly why she lied to him. Was it an avoidance thing? Did she
think that he would judge and shame her, like he always did, and that she
would lose her courage? Whatever he had to say, Maia was uninterested
in hearing it. At her little cottage in Colorado, she packed a suitcase with
clothing and some mementos from her dead mother's house and then
asked her caregiver to drive her to the airport. In her first-class seat on
the plane, Maia asked the flight attendant for champagne. She thought,
Wow, this is a trip.

Ruedi Habegger, who worked as a coordinator with a Lifecircle sister organization called Eternal Spirit, met Maia at the airport, with his big beard and a boxer dog skipping at his feet. They drove straight to a hotel room in Zurich, where Maia lay on a stiff bed and was examined by a gentlemanly doctor in his eighties. He was one of two Swiss physicians, Ruedi explained, who would need to approve Maia's assisted death request. It was surreal, Maia thought, to be lying on that unfamiliar bed while people touched her and spoke in a language she didn't know. After the medical examination, Ruedi drove her to a psychiatrist's office. The Lifecircle physician, Dr. Preisig, had seen in Maia's medical records that she was being treated for anxiety and depression—and that one doctor, years earlier, had diagnosed her with a personality disorder. Preisig said she needed professional confirmation of Maia's sanity, proof that Maia was thinking rationally about her choice. The appointment was brief. Maia said the Swiss psychiatrist told her what she already knew: that she was indeed depressed, but not in an unbounded and irrational way. "It's a reactive depression," Maia told me. A sadness triggered by her sickness and her situation. "There's no psychic distortion about my wanting to die."

At Lifecircle, Maia met with Dr. Preisig, who was delicate and pretty, her thick gray hair braided and then wound around itself in a bun. Preisig told Maia how things would be scheduled on the day of her death. The AVD would take place in an apartment outside Basel. Maia would be asked to state her name, her date of birth, her hometown, and why she wanted to die. Then Dr. Preisig would insert an IV line into her arm. The whole thing would be filmed, as proof to authorities, should they later request it, that Maia's death had been voluntary. When Maia was ready, she would open a valve attached to the line and start the flow of lethal medication into her bloodstream. She would fall asleep in less than a minute. After her heart stopped beating, the clinic would call the police and report an "extraordinary death." An official or two would arrive to review documents, and then they would dismiss the case. When everything was cleared, the clinic would call the funeral home to arrange for the cremation. The ashes could be sent back to Colorado.

Maia liked Dr. Preisig. She was tiny and sharp and she seemed "very, very brave." At the end of their conversation, Preisig leaned in toward her and said, gently, "It's difficult to leave the planet, isn't it?"

"Yes," Maia said. "It's so difficult to leave the planet."

Because she wasn't ready to die just yet—because she wanted to see Europe first—Ruedi found Maia a caregiver in Ticino, near the border with Italy. The woman had a little stone house by a lake, with windows that looked out at the Swiss mountains. When Maia saw the house, she thought it was nothing fancy but that it would be "the perfect place to die." She agreed to pay the woman $6,000 a month to house and feed and care for her. Over the next weeks, Maia and the caregiver went on trips to Rome and Venice. They went for slow walks around Ticino—Maia leaning on her cane—and drives through the mountains, where the air was thick and wet. Once, Maia took confession with the local priest. "I don't have peace in my heart," she told him, "and I don't want to die with all this anger." The priest told Maia to read the Bible: Corinthians, some lines about love and forgiveness. Maia said she would, but she didn't think that it would help. She wasn't good at letting go of things. Sometimes, she looked up old friends on Facebook and let herself wallow in a secondhand nostalgia—a bitter, almost frenzied longing for a life she never had but still missed. Or was that just how envy felt? Maia kept mental records of all the people who'd wronged her and all the ways they had. Old friends. Old partners. Her father. People who stopped calling. Doctors who should have found a way to help her before she got so sick. Over the years, she had felt herself grow crabbed and resentful, trapped in an impossible past conditional of what should have been done and what could have been.

Sometimes, Maia imagined what her father would tell her if he knew where she was. "Oh, you're going to commit suicide on us," he might say, looking just the way he had when she first got sick and he didn't believe her, back when he thought his blue-eyed daughter was going crazy.

"That's not what this is!" Maia would protest. It wasn't that she was killing herself. She was being killed. This was just how the murder was playing out. It was obscene, in a way, but wasn't it more natural than fighting a disease she couldn't beat?

Maia had been raised as a Catholic by her mother, and sometimes she feared that it was sinful to end her life before her God-given moment. Other times her guilt was Buddhist in tone, because Larry had studied Buddhism and taught his daughter its principles. Maia wondered if multiple sclerosis was her karma: a punishment for some wrongdoing in some previous life. Had she been a bad person? Almost all the time, she felt guilty about leaving her father alone and childless. "I think I'm firm in my resolve," Maia said of her coming death. "Then I digress." She started having dreams about swallowing lethal medication and then throwing it up.

Maia grew restless. Sometimes, she spoke on the phone with Ruedi, and one day she told him softly that she missed her little kitten in Colorado and wished that she could see her again. In this way, Ruedi came to understand that Maia was not mentally prepared to die. Maia felt it, too. In the little mountain house in Ticino, she had become overwhelmed by a psychic sense of incompleteness, a feeling that she owed the universe a course of suffering that she hadn't yet completed. "You haven't suffered enough," she told herself. "You've got to go back and suffer a little more and earn the right to do this." Surely, if she spent a bit more time suffering, she would figure out what this whole multiple sclerosis thing was about. It couldn't just be random, genetic bad luck. Painful, illegible nonsense. There had to be a meaning, or at least a reason.

Maia bought a plane ticket back to Colorado. She told Ruedi that she would return soon, when she was ready. This time, Maia flew economy class because she had spent a lot of money in Switzerland and didn't have much left. She did not order champagne. Instead, she closed her eyes and told herself over and over that she was right to be going home. She thought about Larry and how sad it would have been to die without forgiving him, all the way in Switzerland. In the archetypal hero's journey stories that Maia admired, the heroes always reconciled with their fathers.

MAIA HAD BEEN A serious child with a tight emotional grip on her household. Her moods were turbulent. When she was happy, everyone was allowed happiness. When she was not happy, the world was her hostage. She was raised in Santa Fe, where she and her older sister, Lara, spent days watching movies and reenacting them, often *Planet of the Apes*. Maia's father, Larry, was a journalist who drank six-packs of beer in the evenings. Her mother, Tova, worked as a parole officer and was forever running out the door to save someone from jail. Later, Tova volunteered with Amnesty International in Guatemala and El Salvador and Peru, leaving Maia and Lara for weeks at a time and then returning home with stacks of photographs to show them of all the terrible things she had seen. Maia was clever and sensitive and quick to blame. When she was four years old, Larry took her for a walk to tell her that her dog had died. "I'm just four years old and I've never done anything wrong in my life," Maia told him. "Why did this happen?" Larry thought his daughter had a premature understanding of injustice in the universe.

She studied creative writing in Iowa and then moved to New York City for film school. When she finished the program, she moved to LA and picked up research and production gigs. Maia found the sprawling city to be cold and clannish, but she loved working in movies and dreamed of adapting her favorite novels into Hollywood films. Big, important novels like *Blood Meridian* by Cormac McCarthy. In the evenings, Maia worked boring jobs for money. Once, she did quality control for a reality TV show: making sure that swear words were covered with bleeps and stray nipples were cropped out of the frame. Then, in 2012, Maia lost control of her left leg.

For a decade, at least, she had known that something was wrong. In 2002, Maia woke up to find that she could not see out of her left eye. Larry brought her to a doctor, who did a spinal tap and an MRI. The spinal tap looked normal. The MRI showed a small lesion, but doctors told her that it was inconclusive. She might have MS or she might not. The blindness cleared up quickly, and one doctor thought it might just have been a hangover from a recent sinus infection. After the appointments, Maia and Larry talked through their options. They could wait and see how things developed, or Maia could start regular injections of interferon, which doctors used to treat the first stages of MS. Larry thought the drugs sounded dangerous and toxic and that they might send Maia down a path she shouldn't be on. He also worried that if Maia was formally diagnosed with something serious, she wouldn't be able to get good health insurance later, and where would that leave her? Larry thought his daughter should just move on with her life. She was feeling normal now, wasn't she? Maia declined the treatment. When she moved to New York City for her master's, she thought about seeing more specialists and getting more MRIs, but she didn't, mostly because she was a freelancer and she didn't have health insurance. MRIs were expensive and the hospitals asked for cash up front if you were uninsured. She felt OK. Her dad thought she was OK. She didn't want to be sick.

The symptoms left her for a while, but then they came back. Once, her left hand went numb and she lost sensation in her arm. Once, when she was leaning against her boyfriend's shoulder, a muscle in her leg started twitching so forcefully that they could see it bouncing up against her pale skin. "What the hell is that?" her boyfriend asked, but Maia didn't know. Sometimes, she had the feeling that she was being electrocuted or that her torso was missing. Maia went to see doctors in New York and then LA. She spent hours calling former doctors and arranging for them to mail her thick stacks of medical records, to pass on to newer doctors. Sometimes, when she was scared, she went to hospital emergency rooms, and some-times she shouted at the doctors there. She said she couldn't breathe or walk. That she was suffocating and crippled. Maia felt like a nineteenth-century madwoman, spastic and hysterical. Along the way, she picked up a handful of diagnoses: depression, anxiety, serotonin syndrome, a Cluster B personality disorder, and fibromyalgia. One doctor took Larry aside and told him that his daughter was "just getting all of this stuff off of the Internet." Larry could believe it, especially as Maia's supposed symptoms grew wilder. Meanwhile, Maia took Effexor and Lexapro and Pristiq and Prozac. By 2012, she was so tired that on some days she could barely get out of bed to go to the bathroom. She would turn up the volume on the TV in her room and then lie facedown on the floor.

When her leg gave way that year, Maia's friend drove her to a nearby hospital in LA, but the hospital sent her away because she didn't have insurance. Then they drove to a nonprofit hospital that agreed to take her in. The doctors there were kind and they told Maia that she definitely had MS. There were MS lesions in her brain, but also on her upper and lower spinal cord. She had probably been sick since she was a teenager or in her early twenties. The weird tingling and the paralysis were symptoms. Also the extreme tiredness and the depression, which researchers had linked to MS inflammation. Maia learned that most people with MS have a relapsing and remitting form of the disease. This, doctors said, accounted for the years when she had felt more or less fine, followed by short, acute spells of disability and pain. Some people with MS lived almost normal life spans. Medication, the doctors hoped, would slow the disease progression, but nothing would stop it or reverse it. Maia said that when she called to tell her father the news—to say that after all those years, she had been right all along—he only said, "Don't do this to me."

Maia gave up the lease on her LA apartment and put her belongings into storage. She needed the storage unit, she said, because she would be back soon. Back to LA, back to work. It couldn't be that she had spent her life accumulating potential only to have it end this way. Then she flew to

Colorado and drove to Larry's house in Crestone, a tiny town where he had moved after finding Buddhism and separating from Maia's mother, who took the house in Santa Fe. Crestone sat at the foot of the Sangre de Cristo Mountains, which glowed red when the sun set, and had become known for its spiritual pilgrims. Though it had only a few hundred permanent residents, the town was home to several religious centers, a cluster of Buddhist monasteries, a Hindu ashram, a Zen center, a Carmelite monastery, an American Indian sanctuary, and a smattering of New Age healers. "Throw a brick and you'll hit a psychic," residents sometimes said. Larry rented Maia a little house down the road, which made her feel like she lived on the old frontier. She guessed that she should be grateful for the house, but she resented that Larry was paying for it. As the months went by, Maia acquired what doctors called "a wide-based gait" and had to start using a cane and then a walker. She felt more pain. Each day, she willed herself to surrender to her illness, to need her body less so that she couldn't be terrorized by it. From across town, Larry watched his daughter slowing down. He wondered why Maia sometimes walked funny, dragging her feet behind her, but sometimes seemed to walk just fine.

Late that year, doctors in Crestone sent Maia for more tests in Denver. Maia had told them that she was losing feeling in her body parts. One limb after the next, gone and gone. Why was she getting so much worse and so quickly? The specialists at the University of Colorado Hospital admitted her, gave her some medication, and did some more MRIs. They asked a lot of questions. One young physician said he thought that Maia might have somatization disorder, a mental disorder that causes physical pain. She was sure that she didn't—that this wasn't all in her head—but the doctor wrote it down in her medical notes anyway. When it was over, Maia went back to her hotel room, at the nice hotel that Larry was paying for, and called her mother to say that the whole situation was hopeless. The doctors had done nothing. Her limbs were still busted. "I can't even stand on my own legs in the shower to wash my hair," she said.

A few minutes after Maia hung up, a nice female police officer knocked on the hotel room door. She said that Maia's mother had called the health center, frightened by her daughter's despair, and the nurse who answered the phone had identified Maia as a suicide risk. And would she like to go to a behavioral health unit for a while? "I had so much confusion about what I was," Maia told me later. "I'm thinking, wait a minute, am I depressed?" She agreed to be admitted. "Now I'm surrounded by people who have set themselves on fire. Who have marks all over their necks and wrists. Self-mutilation. People with severe bipolar disorder. This is not where I belonged. At night, the nurses would come in. And it's, like, *Cuckoo's Nest* stuff. You had to take your antidepressant. . . . They put a flashlight under your tongue to make sure you did." A week later, Maia was discharged. On the bus back to Crestone, she felt a new sense of conviction: She was not mentally ill. The system had tried to tell her that she was, but the system was wrong. "Now I'm very clear," she told herself.

Maia's mother, Tova, died in 2014 from complications related to her opioid addiction. She had started taking pills for headaches and had never been able to stop, and she and her daughters had grown distant over time. Maia's sister, Lara—her "sweet, sweet sister"—died a year later of an undiagnosed heart condition while she was studying for her art school exams. At the funeral, Larry gave a eulogy, but instead of saying Lara's name, he accidentally named his younger daughter. "When Maia died . . . ," he told the mourners. Larry thought that Maia might try to kill herself, as she sometimes said she would. He told Maia that he didn't want to lose another daughter. He said he didn't want to be a pallbearer at her funeral.

"Then don't be," Maia said.

Maia stopped speaking to her friends. Or maybe they stopped speaking to her. It was hard to say, really. It was tiring, Maia thought, for healthy people to be around sick people. Healthy people seemed to deflate in her presence, as if she were leeching the life right out of them. Maybe when they looked at her, they thought about death, so maybe they just didn't want to look at her. When Maia met Tevye at a Crestone pizza restaurant, she was drawn to him in part because he seemed fearless around her body. Tevye was older, around fifty, with a long, matted ponytail that he wore tucked into the back of his collared shirt and small, squinting eyes behind wire-rimmed glasses. Soon Maia and Tevye were lovers and living together. Later, they stopped being lovers but stayed loving each other.

Maia applied for Social Security disability and was rejected, so she hired a lawyer to appeal it. At her hearing, she said, she was interrogated by lawyers and accused of trying to milk the system. It was "the most demoralizing thing I've ever been through," she said. While she waited for the outcome of the decision, she took money from Larry every month and felt like a loser. She stayed indoors and read news articles online about how expensive and bankrupting MS could be. There were an estimated 400,000 MS patients across the country; many of them weren't able to work, and some were prescribed treatments that cost tens of thousands of dollars a year. According to US Census data, MS patients were about 50 percent more likely to be poor than the average American. Maia imagined living in poverty forever and the thought of it made her want to die.

The news articles explained that sometimes, insurance companies did not let doctors prescribe the newest and mostly costly MS drugs until their patients had tried older, less effective drugs and had them fail. This meant that the best treatments were sometimes delayed. "Insurance is a *huge* problem for us. It's stupidity," Dr. Douglas Goodin, a neurologist and MS expert at the University of California, San Francisco, told me when I called to ask him about the articles that Maia was finding and sending me. Goodin said that in addition to treating patients, he spent a lot of time fighting insurance companies to get patients on the medications that he thought would work best for them. While the fights were happening, he would watch his patients relapse and become more disabled. The insurance companies, Goodin said, didn't even seem to understand the disease. Some of his patients weren't able to work because of their extreme fatigue—one of MS's most debilitating symptoms—but when they tried to qualify for disability payments, the insurance companies would send private detectives to their homes to stalk them and photograph them whenever they managed to drag themselves out of bed to run an errand. "This is absurd," Goodin would tell agents on the phone. "She has overwhelming fatigue. You can't *see* fatigue."

When Maia was finally approved for Social Security, she was surprised by how little it all came to, about $750 a month, plus food stamps. Because she was so young and hadn't been paying into the system for decades, the payments were less than older patients got. Maia used the money to cover rent on a little house that she shared with Tevye, who became her full-time caregiver. Tevye observed that Maia could seem sharp and "PhD-level intelligent" at some moments, but almost blurry at others, ill-defined and incoherent and not quite there. He never knew, for sure, whether she was distracted by pain, or foggy from the drugs, or just losing the thread. Some days, Maia could seem innocent and overly sensitive: too permeable to the world around her, like a little girl. It was as if she had been frozen in time, emotionally, when she first got sick.

Maia tried to read MS blogs, but she found them obnoxious in their optimism. "They show you all these pictures of people in wheelchairs, smiling with these lives." Each photo seemed to taunt her: "So-and-so is worse than you and yet he finds meaning in life." She preferred to read articles about all the ways that MS might kill her. At some point down the line, she would stop getting out of bed and would lose weight, which would leave her susceptible to skin breakdown infections and urinary tract infections. With her already compromised immune system, either of those things could trigger what doctors sometimes call a "failure cascade": one node in a body system breaking down and, in turn, causing the breakdown of another, and on and on. She read that an infected bedsore could sink down into the skin until it exposed tissue and muscle and tendon and bone. Another possibility was that she would have trouble swallowing and would die of aspiration pneumonia. Sometimes, Maia told Tevye that she wanted to end her life sooner—like, now—but that she wasn't sure how to do it properly. She told Larry the same. To Larry, Maia's admission felt less like a plan and more like a reproach or a manipulation. A way to take out her anger and regret on someone other than herself. "She's got to blame somebody, somewhere," he said.

Larry thought his daughter was making her diagnosis bigger than it was. "Stop living in the future. . . . Enjoy your life while you're healthy," he told her. "We're all going to die, but don't get obsessed about it." She could still walk around. She could still read. She could still talk and make connections with people. Hadn't the doctors said that some people with MS live almost normal life spans? Over and over, Larry told Maia about Jimmie Heuga: the American skier and Olympian who, after being diagnosed with MS, became famous for his can-do attitude. Every day, Heuga would set himself small physical and psychological goals and then accomplish them. Larry told Maia that he admired Heuga's optimism. Maia thought that Heuga's can-do approach was jockish and dishonest. Why shouldn't she be obsessed with her disease and the premature death that would end it? It was a miracle that she wasn't always screaming. But even Maia's doctor thought her hypervigilance—the way she constantly audited her body for signs of weakness and pain—was sometimes making the MS seem worse than it was. She needed to exercise more, the doctors wrote in Maia's charts.

It was around this time that Maia and I started speaking—and emailing and texting and talking on Skype, sometimes for hours. In between calls, she sent me links to articles. Some were about the financial cost of chronic illness. Another was a *New York Times* profile about a lonely man who died alone in his apartment and was only found days later, after his neighbor, "sniffing a fetid odor" in the hallway, called 911. "A good read," she wrote. Maia, I understood, both longed to end her life alone and also thought it would be terrible to die alone. On the phone, she asked if I had spoken to other people like her. "Have you seen that there's a large patient population that's not being helped?" she wanted to know. "You've heard other stories like this? Are they young people?" Mostly, though, she wanted to talk about the right-to-die debate. She had, she said, become obsessed. "Why don't I have the ability to just call my family physician and say, 'Hey, I think it's time.' You know?"

When Maia looked for information online, she sometimes found herself on the websites and blogs of small disability rights groups, who have in recent decades become the most strident opponents of aid-in-dying legislation in the country, more outspoken, even, than the Catholic Church. Some websites recounted the early histories of the American right-to-die movement. Maia learned that at points in the early and mid-twentieth century, it was difficult to separate support for euthanasia from support for eugenics. Some campaigners had advocated for a right to die in the same breath that they called for the mercy killing of "genetic inferiors"— and commended the forcible sterilization of thousands of Americans with mental illnesses and disabilities. Some disability rights activists warned that the two movements were fatefully tangled and that aid-in-dying laws were disastrous for people with atypical bodies, even if they theoretically only applied to terminally ill people.

Maia started messaging with some of the activists on Facebook and reading their blogs. We both read articles by members of Not Dead Yet, a national disability rights group that opposes physician-assisted death. Some of the writers observed that in states where assisted death is legal, patients often choose it for reasons that have little to do with physical pain. They want to die because they fear losing autonomy and because they don't want to be physically dependent on other people—or because they dread the perceived indignity of, one day, needing a spouse or child or paid professional to help them in the bathroom. Well, weren't those things all common conditions of disability? And given that, weren't states like Oregon literally helping people die so that they wouldn't become disabled?

"That's a warrant that has been used against disabled people," Not Dead Yet's regional director, John Kelly, told me when I contacted him after speaking to Maia. "We disabled people have lots of stories of being in the hospital, in extremis, and having people of the mindset that we would be better off dead. That it would be for the best." Death with dignity laws, in Kelly's view, endorse and codify that "better dead than disabled" mindset—and they recruit doctors to take part in the project. In turn, the laws pose an implicit challenge to disabled people: *Why are you still here? Still burdening us by living?* Kelly told me that as aid in dying becomes more common, what is now a choice to die will be transformed into an obligation: if not through the force of law, then by the coercive pressures of medical expectation and resource scarcity and social disdain. A 2019 report by the National Council on Disability, which has long opposed medical aid in dying, said much the same: "When assisted suicide is legalized in the context of the US healthcare system, it immediately becomes the cheapest treatment. Direct coercion is not necessary. If insurers deny, or even simply delay, the approval of expensive life-sustaining treatment, patients can be steered toward hastening their deaths." The disability community becomes Death with Dignity's collateral damage.

"When you create a medical treatment for feeling like a burden, there is no way to keep it limited to an arbitrarily defined group of people," Kelly added. Anyone could claim to feel anything, and the law would have to expand to accommodate it. Kelly said that if people wanted to kill themselves on their own, because of their physical condition, he wouldn't try to stop them. But he would always resist the formal intervention of the medical system.

In recent years, aid-in-dying supporters—generally unenthused by the prospect of debating disability-rights activists on public stages—have tried to assuage these fears. They repeat publicly that the law is limited to terminally ill people who are going to die within six months. They note that multiple doctors are involved in each assisted death, and that these doctors work to safeguard the limits of the law. In a 2007 peer-reviewed study published in the *Journal of Medical Ethics* and drawing on data from Oregon, researchers concluded that there was "no current evidence for the claim that legalized physician-assisted suicide or euthanasia will have disproportionate impact on patients in vulnerable groups." In 2016, Disability Rights Oregon testified that it had never received "a complaint of exploitation or coercion of an individual with disabilities in the use of Oregon's Death with Dignity Act." But when I raised these objections with John Kelly, he brushed them off. Historically, he said, physicians and courts and insurance companies had been untrustworthy guardians of disabled bodies.

Maia cried when she read the articles on Not Dead Yet's website. By then she had come to see herself as a person with a disability. She had also noticed the way that people seemed scared of her cane and her loopy gait. "There's terrible discrimination," she told me. "And it made me feel guilty."

"Like maybe you're a self-hating disabled person?" I asked.

"Yeah," she said. "I worried that somehow being involved was saying that disabled people are less. I cried about that. I don't feel that way at all." In the end, Maia said, she had to interrogate herself, "to make sure that my desire to exit is not about my not wanting to be a disabled person." She decided that it wasn't. Anyway, Maia thought that her MS was different. There was no specific disability for her to adapt to, only a wily disease with an ever-enlarging path of destruction.

When Maia learned about the clinics in Switzerland, she told Tevye that she wanted to die at one of them. It would be better than taking her own life at home, she said, because there would be doctors to help her so that nothing could go wrong. Afterward, Tevye wondered if Maia's fascination with Switzerland reflected poorly on him. "I'm not so grandiose to think that it's all about me and that if I do a *really* good job and *really* make her comfortable all the time, she won't do it, and that if she does do it, how could I have done more? But there's a teeny itty bit of that." Tevye said it was Maia, not him, who thought it would be indecent for him to help her eat and get dressed—and, eventually, go to the bathroom. He said it wouldn't bother him. He had worked as a professional caregiver before, for someone with advanced-stage MS, and sometimes he had used his fingers to disimpact the woman's bowels when they became blocked. He could do that for Maia. He would do it over and over, if it meant that she would stay. He was strong enough to take it. And still, Maia said that she would rather die than let him. How weird was that? She would die, in part, to spare him, when he didn't need sparing. Maia guessed that she should be grateful to Tevye, this former lover who now annoyed her like a brother. Other sick people, she thought, felt more gratitude for things. But Maia didn't want to need him.

When Maia told me this, I thought of an essay that the bioethicist Ezekiel Emanuel published in the *Atlantic* in 1997, arguing that "America should think again" before moving forward with legalized physician-assisted death. In it, Emanuel made a point about suffering that had stayed with me. "Broad legalization of physician-assisted suicide and euthanasia would have the paradoxical effect of making patients seem to be responsible for their own suffering," he wrote. "Rather than being seen primarily as the victims of pain and suffering caused by disease, patients would be seen as having the power to end their suffering by agreeing to an injection or taking some pills; refusing would mean that living through the pain was the patient's decision, the patient's responsibility." In this view, the existence of the choice would inherently burden anyone within reach of it—making them feel as if they had chosen to suffer, because they had not chosen not to. For Maia, Switzerland beckoned.

In November 2016, Colorado voters passed the End-of-Life Options Act by a two-to-one margin, and physician-assisted death became legal across the state. Maia's doctors explained what she already knew: that she didn't meet the law's eligibility criteria. Because MS patients often die by infection, it would be hard for a doctor to say at any one moment, with any certainty, that she had just six months to live. Some people in states like Oregon did qualify for aid in dying because of neurological disorders, but they usually had ALS, which moves much faster than MS and has a more predictable disease course. Maia concluded that, at best, she might be able to use the law "when I'm almost dead." But she did not want to ever be almost dead. She wanted to "exit."

Maia read that in Canada, her situation would have been different. Under Canada's Bill C-14, aid-in-dying patients did not have to be terminally ill, in the immediate sense, as long as their suffering was "grievous and irremediable" and their deaths had "become reasonably foreseeable." A patient was considered to be suffering grievously and irremediably if her condition was serious and incurable and her pain was unbearable—and if there was no available treatment that she found acceptable. The law did not specifically define "reasonably foreseeable" but instead left the judgment up to doctors. According to case law, the term could apply to deaths that were up to ten years away and maybe more. Later, in 2019, a Canadian provincial court ruled that even this time limit was unconstitutional, demanding that the federal government do away with it.

In America, however, MS patients can qualify only when they are in the very late stages of their disease. It's hard to find precise data on how many do. Only some states publish detailed records showing the underlying illnesses of aid-in-dying patients. Oregon data shows that in 2019, 19 out of 188 patients who ingested lethal drugs under the Death with Dignity Act had ALS and 7 had "other neurological diseases." That same year in Colorado, 1 out of a total of 170 patients who were prescribed medication under the End-of-Life Options Act had multiple sclerosis. Many doctors told me that people with MS almost never qualify. One told me that, given the increased risk of depression associated with MS, he would be anxious to even consider such a patient.

Still, some American doctors did, on occasion, approve people in the late stages of the disease. One was Dr. Devon Webster, an oncologist in Oregon who worked near the coast. In March 2019, Webster visited the house of a woman in her late sixties who wanted to die under the law and who asked Webster to be the second, consulting physician on her case. The woman lived in Sweet Home, near the Cascade Mountains, in a dark bedroom that reeked of cigarettes. When Webster walked in, she saw her patient lying still, her bedside table cluttered with ChapStick and lotions and pill bottles. Beside her bed was a garbage bin with a plastic liner that she was using as an ashtray. The woman smiled and said hello in a voice that was slurred by decades of MS deterioration.

Webster spent an hour and a half examining the patient, whose husband and son lingered near the doorway. She was emaciated. It was most obvious in her hands; the woman had lost so much muscle that, in between her fingers, the skin sloped downward into valleys of bone. They looked more like animal claws than human parts. When Webster lifted the blanket covering the bed, she saw that the woman's right foot was pointed downward like a ballerina's and fixed in a muscle spasm. She was taking medications that were meant to release the spasm, but her leg stayed frozen that way. The woman had bedsores on her heels and her back and her buttocks. She had difficulty swallowing and often choked. Webster could see that she wasn't taking in enough calories to sustain her body for much longer. Soon, one of those bedsores would get infected and take her away. Webster agreed to sign the aid-in-dying paperwork. Before she left, she reminded the woman that the Oregon law required her to swallow the medication on her own. She would need to act quickly, before she lost the ability to swallow.

After the appointment, Webster told me that if the woman "had *every* medical intervention that technology could give her"—feeding tubes in her stomach, an IV line to feed her veins, hospital nurses to dress her sores and turn her over every two hours—it was possible, and maybe even probable, that she would live longer than six months. But short of that, she wouldn't. Webster said that the six-month prognosis needed to be measured against where a patient was, not where the outer bounds of life-sustaining technology could theoretically bring her. She also told me that this was an important case for her, personally, because she also had MS and as a result of her symptoms would soon be retiring from medicine. "So I'm very sensitive to the idea of respecting each person's autonomy." When it was time to say goodbye, I wanted to ask Webster what she plans to do when her own final stretch of infirmity is before her, but then I lost my courage.

WHEN MAIA RETURNED from Switzerland in 2016, she started having dreams about travel. "I'm being ushered onto the plane and I'm saying, 'No, I'm not ready. I'm not ready.' The symbolism of going down the plane tunnel, you know?" At some point in the dream, the pilot would turn to her and say, "It's OK. It's going to be a good flight." She told Tevye it was time for them to get out of Crestone. The town was bloated with boomer hippies and moneyed spiritual seekers, and now everything was expensive. Also, she needed change. Also, she wanted to be alone. Some people in town had found out about her trip to Basel and were gossiping about what Maia had planned to do but hadn't done. Her father was flustered and ashamed.

Maia watched while Tevye packed up the house and the two cats and the dog. They drove south on Route 285, through the San Luis Valley and across the border into New Mexico. When they got to Taos, they found a little red house at the end of a long, unpaved road lined with leafless trees. They filled it with Maia's Native American posters and her smiling Buddha statue, and with Tevye's kitschy oil paintings of Jewish religious scenes. In the early spring, the neighborhood seemed like a forsaken place. From her new bedroom on the ground floor, Maia could hear coyotes. She listened to them sometimes while she was having seizures and tremors, after she took her medicine and lay down to wait until her body stilled. When the seizures came, she preferred to be alone. If Tevye were there, he might try to hold down her limbs so that she wouldn't hurt herself, and she, in turn, might get frenzied and angry. She might scratch his face or pull his hair or drool on the blankets.

"Each day disappears into the next," Maia told me. "It's almost like *Groundhog Day*." In the mornings, Tevye woke her up around 10. "Babe," he would call from the top of the stairs. "Wakey, wakey." While she adjusted to the morning, he would make her tea and cut up some fruit and feed the cats. She would lie around for a bit. Tevye might prop her up with pillows so that she could watch a documentary on her laptop, her eyes still clouded from sleep. For a while, Maia had played only *Frontline* PBS news films. Lately, though, she had been watching historical programs about Jesus. She wanted to learn from his suffering and to think about "why God is punishing me with progressive MS at such a young age." Sometimes, Maia read for a few minutes, too. She read *Man's Search for Meaning*, the famous memoir by Holocaust survivor Dr. Viktor Frankl, and thought it was excellent. "Man is ready to suffer," Frankl wrote, "on the condition, to be sure, that his suffering has a meaning."

When it was time to get dressed, Tevye would help Maia pick out a sweater and he would brush out her long brown hair with a flat wooden comb. Maia would wash her face by herself, though this was already getting harder, because of the pain in her neck. She would bend down a little, toward the sink, and then use her cupped hands to splash water onto her forehead and cheeks. As a final step, Tevye would lay her down on the hardwood floor so that he could stretch out her arms and hips and legs. Sometimes, he would play jungle sounds on his phone, so that the room would be filled with the artificial buzz of birds and crickets. Maia would stare absently at the ceiling. Next would be breakfast. After Maia finished her fruit bowl and kissed the little painting of St. Anthony that hung by the kitchen counter, Tevye would ask her what she felt like doing that day. Maybe a walk with Bella, the dog. Maybe a walk around town, past all the adobe-front shops selling soy candles and dream catchers. Maybe a hot chocolate at the café where a cashier once asked Maia what was wrong with her. "We can go to the bridge," he said once, "if you promise not to jump."

One morning in January 2018, I sat with Maia in her living room while Tevye cut flowers and arranged them in tiny vases. "How long will they last?" Maia asked.

"They'll last forever, as long as I take care of them," Tevye said.

Maia looked away and frowned. She said that she was bored in Taos. She said it like it hadn't been her own idea to move away in the first place: like her exile was a banishment and not a choice. I asked her how much pain she was in, on a scale of 1 to 10, and she said she was at an 8. Did she want to stop talking? No, she was OK. Most days, "there is no lust for life," Maia said. "My soul has died." Then she giggled a little and looked up at me expectantly, like she often did after saying something earnest.

When Tevye left the room, Maia told me that she was growing ambivalent toward him. In the new house, he had taken the upstairs bedroom and left her the one on the ground floor. His moods were erratic, she said. He could be volatile or sulky or rapturous. Recently, he had forced her to become a vegetarian and now he wouldn't let her eat meat, even when she craved it. Even at restaurants. She was confused by his attention. It didn't make sense, Maia said, for Tevye to be putting time and energy into a relationship that was going to end with her premature death. "This is valuable time in his life to cultivate relationships with people that have a future," she said. "In a way, I'm stealing that from him." Sometimes, Maia spoke coolly of their life together as an unequal transaction of services—or a bad investment that wouldn't pay off for Tevye. Tevye should be free, she said. When I suggested that Tevye must love her very much, she looked insulted. He gained from her, too, she said. She gave him money and a place to stay and a sense of purpose, none of which he had without her. And he was no saint. Sometimes, when he felt oppressed by the smallness of their lives, he would lash out at her. It was messed up, Maia said, the way they required and restricted each other.

For the rest of my time in New Mexico, I was aware of a kind of stiffness in the house—an affectedness in the way that Maia and Tevye moved around each other. It was as if they were both on their best behavior, presumably because I was there and because I was watching, and because neither wanted to throw a temper tantrum, as each accused the other of being prone to. Or maybe they were stiff inside their own endowed roles: the tender caregiver, the anguished patient. Given everything, neither could perform the act with total authenticity. I wanted to speak alone with Tevye.

Late in the afternoon, one early winter evening, I asked if we could talk under the cottonwood trees. He sat on a brown wooden bench and I sat across from him, on a smooth gray stone. He looked washed out. Strands of wiry hair twisted up and out of his long braid. As we spoke, Tevye rubbed a twig between his hands. "She is getting younger," he said carefully. He had seen this before, in much older people—in elderly people, in their final years. They sometimes grew childlike as their sense of the external world softened and dulled. They grew selfish, too. Tevye thought that Maia's mental faculties were deteriorating but also that she was losing her connection to things. Over the last few months, he said, their conversations had acquired a lag. Tevye would make a comment or joke and watch as it took Maia five or ten seconds to register it. "As if she is just somewhere else," he said. "She is not here. Or she's losing that foundation, *here*." Was she distracted by her pain and her fear? Was it the MS lesions, doing their damage? On the National MS Society website, it said that "more than half of all people with MS will develop problems with cognition," with common symptoms including memory lapses, distraction, difficulty planning, difficulty prioritizing, difficulty with "information processing."

As we spoke, it grew darker around us, until I could see only a silhouetted outline of Tevye's body against the gray sky. He told me that I looked cold and asked if we should go inside, but I said that we should stay out for a few minutes longer. Tevye said he was doing OK. He was managing OK. Only, it was hard because he would have liked to find another job—maybe something at one of the art galleries in town—but as it was, he couldn't. They didn't have enough money to afford a full-time caregiver to replace him, and Maia was afraid of being alone. If he were honest, he was feeling restless. Pretty restless, actually. Most days, Tevye did not think that Maia would really go back to Switzerland.

The doctors said that her MS had advanced. Maia's disease seemed to have moved past its relapsing-remitting phase and into a secondary progressive phase, as it did eventually for most MS patients. This meant that she would no longer have acute attacks that were separated by long stretches of relief. Instead, she would get progressively worse over time. The nerve damage, caused by previous immune attacks, had acquired a critical mass and its own destructive momentum. Earlier damage begets new damage. Damage upon damage. "Once they cross over that threshold," one doctor who treated Maia told me, "it's hard for us to preserve that neurological function." She might lose her ability to move. Already, the MS made her feel like her body was being cut into pieces. Or being squeezed by a violent hug. Or drowning.

Maia took medicines for spasticity and pain, and she received infusion therapy every six months, even though infusion drugs weren't known to help very much at the secondary progressive stage. "In effect, they are carpet-bombing the immune system," Maia said. "Which is ridiculous." It was hard to know how fast things would fall apart. MRIs weren't always good predictors. To Maia, the sadness and the heaviness of waiting started to feel the same. It was like the C. S. Lewis quote: "I am beginning to understand why grief feels like suspense." To Tevye, Maia's progression looked like Darwinian evolution in reverse: her strong, straight body became more hunched and beastlike with each new treatment.

At the insistence of her New Mexico doctors, Maia also agreed to take an antidepressant, even though she hated the idea of psychiatric drugs. She figured that since she was going back to Switzerland soon anyway—possibly in just a few months—she might as well feel better in the meantime. Maia thought that other MS patients were probably handling things better. "They probably have more grace than I do, going through it."

"Why do you say that?" I asked.

"I whine and cry out a lot and I stomp my hands and I throw tantrums because I can't move my body. I probably do act like a little child. There are women who can't move at all and they're not crying and screaming. They are just being very calm."

"Maybe you don't know that," I said.

"Yes," Maia agreed. But other sick people always seemed so brave.

"Do you think you've been . . . unbrave?"

"Yes." But that would change, because soon she would decide on a date to die. It would be in 2018.

Some of the questions around timing, Maia admitted, would be answered by money, which she now had very little of. That year, she finally qualified for Medicare, something that all Americans are automatically eligible for when they receive Social Security disability payments, but only after a two-year wait. Even then, things weren't free. Her MS medicines alone cost around $65,000 a year, and while insurance covered most of it, she still sometimes spent hundreds of dollars a month on premiums and co-pays. She called the National Multiple Sclerosis Society, to ask if she was doing something wrong—if she was missing some insurance trick—but she was told that she wasn't. This was just the lot of a young person who got sick. One study from 2007 showed that while 90 percent of MS patients in the United States are insured, 70 percent still struggle to pay for healthcare, and 21 percent report spending less on food, heat, and necessities because of healthcare costs. Eventually, Maia's savings dipped below $2,000 and she also qualified for Medicaid, the state-run program for "needy persons." Even then, there were costs. Maia was surprised to learn that Medicaid subsidized only a few hours of at-home caregiving each week, most of it by barely trained, minimum-wage workers who probably meant well but who showed up late and didn't seem to care.

Maia started a crowdsourcing campaign on a website called GoGet-Funding and titled it "Medical Fund for Maia." On her home page, she listed her fund-raising target as $100,000 and posted pictures of herself on her walker, in a maroon sweater. "I want to continue to press on with some quality of life," she wrote, "but I must generate funds for my care (holistic medicine, my infusions, medicinal foods, caregiving and special wheel chair). . . . Any contribution to my fund and struggle with Multiple Sclerosis is so valuable. Blessings." Maia hoped the campaign would go viral, but it did not and she raised only $120.

I spoke with Bari Talente, a patient advocate at the National MS Society, and she told me that Maia's story sounded familiar. The first disease-modifying MS treatment came onto the market in 1993 and it cost $11,500. The same medication today costs nearly $100,000. Talente said that drug companies, with their year-on-year price increases, were to blame. Now, because the medications are so expensive, many private insurance companies put them on a specialty tier and charge policyholders a percentage of their cost, sometimes 20 percent or 40 percent, rather than a flat co-pay, as is typical for most other drugs. This can mean hundreds or thousands of dollars a month for just one of several medications that an MS patient is likely to need. In recent years, insult had been added to injury, as many big employers shifted to high-deductible insurance plans, which require people to pay a large amount out of pocket before insurance coverage even kicks in. Today, some patients end up with more than $10,000 worth of bills in just the first few months of a calendar year. Even elderly people on Medicare can be left with unaffordable out-of-pocket costs.

It seemed to Maia that without family to take care of her or money to hire specialized caregivers, she would end up in a nursing home, in a Medicaid-subsidized bed. It would be especially awful because she would be so much younger than everyone else. "I know the system is designed to put me there," she said, "but I don't want to go." Maia imagined sitting in a wheelchair, just staring at the wall for hours, her mind sharp, but her body unable to move. Rolled out for breakfast. Rolled out for lunch. Rolled out for dinner. Rolled around the garden. "This is really one of the reasons why I want to exit," she told me. "It's the pure socioeconomics of MS. It's just very depressing. I hate to say that, but I'll just be frank. The actual time that I choose to self-determine is affected by my dwindling resources."

Maia read that when some nursing home residents are at the very ends of their lives, and already very weak, they choose to stop eating and drinking, to speed things up. There was even a medical term for it: voluntarily stopping eating and drinking, or VSED. The idea of it got under Maia's skin. It enraged her to think that doctors and nurses could legally help her to starve herself to death, over weeks—carefully applying pain patches, monitoring vital signs, and holding ice chips against her dried-out lips—but could not give her medication to end things quickly, in a chosen instant. She imagined what it would be like to starve. And, no. She couldn't.

I wondered, as I read through a file of Maia's paperwork—applications for income assistance, Medicaid rejection letters, descriptions of her growing disability—whether money had more to do with things than aid-in-dying proponents wanted to admit or even understood. In 2016, the lobby group Compassion & Choices published a pamphlet that addressed financial matters, and in particular the "myth" that "profit-driven health insurers and HMOs will encourage medical aid in dying to save money." It read, "There is no financial incentive to pressure patients. . . . This myth is further dispelled by the fact that 92% of people in Oregon who choose medical aid in dying are enrolled in hospice care and not receiving expensive or intensive treatment. Therefore, there is no financial incentive to encourage people to accelerate their deaths." The point seemed reasonable, in its assessment of insurance company motivations, but it did not address the many ways that financial stress can drive patients.

Even the fact that most aid-in-dying recipients are getting state-funded hospice care is not categorical evidence of anything. It reveals nothing about the choices that people made before they hit the six-months-or-less prognosis mark for hospice eligibility. It's possible, for instance, that a patient might have turned down expensive treatment early on in his disease, because of money problems or because he wanted to save his family the expense—and that this made him sicker. Or even that he got so sick, in the first place, because of years of patchy medical access. Money guides plenty of decisions about healthcare in America, so why wouldn't it affect this? The difference is only in the enormity of the choice. The Compassion & Choices pamphlet concluded that "in a combined 30 years of medical aid in dying practice there has not been a single incidence of duress or abuse." Maybe so. But how could DC lobbyists or state agencies possibly know that, especially in cases when "duress" is not physical or personal, but instead a mistier kind of force, expressed in chronic poverty and accruing financial hardship and misfortune?

Many aid-in-dying proponents point to Oregon when dismissing concerns about money. In that state, they note, it is mostly moneyed, educated white people who choose assisted death, not members of marginalized groups whom authorities need to be particularly anxious about. According to 2019 Oregon Death with Dignity data, published by the Oregon Health Authority, 7.4 percent of aid-in-dying patients are concerned about the "financial implications of treatment" at the time of their death, up from an average of 3.7 percent between 1998 and 2017. And even that number might not capture everything. After all, the 7.4 percent figure does not come from patient interviews or surveys, but instead from paperwork that doctors fill out, sometimes weeks after a patient's assisted death. Sometimes by doctors who barely know the patients at all. In some cases, the doctors' responses are informed by conversations, but in others they are just best guesses—by physicians who have, in all likelihood, not had comprehensive conversations with their patients about delicate and possibly humiliating financial matters. Because who talks with a doctor about that?

THE HOME HEALTH NURSE assigned to Maia was named Jonathan. He was a sturdy-set man in his mid-forties, and he thought Maia should try to look at the bright side of things. He arrived at her house in a gray T-shirt with a stethoscope around his neck, his face smooth save for a scrap of beard left abandoned at the bottom of his chin. When Jonathan wasn't working as a nurse, he said, he was writing a science fiction novel set in Pennsylvania. Jonathan told Maia that he was there to monitor her health and fill her prescriptions, but also to help her figure things out, inside the system. It could sometimes take years, Jonathan said, for sick people to get a grasp on everything: what benefits they were entitled to and how to get them.

Jonathan asked Maia if she had fallen lately (no), if she had any dizziness or vertigo (yes), if she was getting enough to eat (yes, but she didn't taste her food very much), if her nose was blocked (yes), if she had any problems "eliminating" (yes), if she had pain (yes, severe), and how her breathing was (a little shallow). Maia told Jonathan about the seizure she'd had the day before, and how she had become furious when Tevye tried to help her. She had banged her head on the counter and scared the cats. Was that the MS? Was that just her being angry? Jonathan told Maia that her seizures were made worse by stress. She and Tevye might want to have a safe word that either of them could use if it seemed like Maia was getting spun up into an outburst, as a reminder that she should slow down and breathe. Jonathan suggested "kumquat." Jonathan said that Maia's anger was understandable. "With any rapidly progressing disease, I feel like people start to have a breakdown of the self and of purpose. They see themselves as being interrupted. . . . They had dreams and aspirations and now everything seems to be cut off or fallen short." Maia needed to find a way to rethink herself.

Maia asked Jonathan to tell her about his other patients. Were there people who were terminally ill but who "were holding on to life in a positive and inspiring way?" Jonathan said that there were. For instance, one of his patients referred to her cancerous tumor as "my teacher," because it taught her to be tolerant of uncertainty and to appreciate things as they were. Gratitude was key, Jonathan said, because if you got depressed and didn't act grateful, it could cause tensions in your relationships. A lack of gratitude might come across as entitlement, which might in turn cause issues with the people who care for you, making them less willing to care for you. "An attitude of gratitude is important," he said again. Maia nodded.

No gratitude could be summoned for her father. On his birthday, Maia had not gone to visit Larry and he had not asked her to. She had sent a card. Same thing when he was sick with pneumonia. Most of the time, they weren't in touch at all, though sometimes Maia would lose her grip on things and, even though she really tried not to, she would send him long emails. Her messages were always frothy with rage. They accused Larry of being tight with his financial help, of being embarrassed of her. They reminded him of when she first got sick and he hadn't believed her symptoms. "Ultimately I'm the one who didn't take the medicine, and my doctors are the ones that didn't prescribe it," Maia told me. "But he had a part to play and he won't admit it. I feel like I can't forgive him." Sometimes, in the emails, Maia included links to TV reports and documentary films about people dying in Switzerland. Larry's girlfriend told him to stop responding. She thought Maia was a bully, a woman of almost forty who couldn't own her own decisions. Larry was too old to absorb that kind of rage.

Maia thought constantly about Switzerland. "You're going to have to have the courage to go forward," she told herself, "because the loss of abilities and the loss of dignity is just increasing." Sometimes she told Tevye about her thoughts, but mostly she didn't. "Tevye threatens that when I start packing to go, he will run off into the woods. He says he can't say goodbye. No, no. He will run off into the wilderness for a week. It's very immature, the way he acts."

When I Skyped with Maia from New York, I sometimes thought about a line from the writer Julian Barnes, who observed that people tend to fear either dying (the process) or death (the state) and that "almost everyone fears one to the exclusion of the other; it's as if there isn't enough room for the mind to contain both." Barnes feared the state of being dead, as do I. But most people, he argued, were the former type; they feared the drawn-out process of life's abrogation but didn't dwell much on what it would mean to not exist. That seemed to describe Maia, who ruminated over the details of her future infirmity but was hazy when I asked what she thought would come after, if anything. "I'm not really afraid now," she said. Still, I wondered. Maia told that me she sometimes woke up in the middle of the night to find herself screaming.

Maia started speaking again to the managers at Lifecircle, in Switzerland. Ruedi told Maia that she didn't need to feel guilty about anything. Death was her right and her choice; she didn't need Larry's permission. Ruedi also told Maia that if Tevye refused to travel with her, then he would fly to Colorado to pick her up. He did that sometimes, he said, for patients without any loved ones.

"Do you worry about Maia's indecision?" I asked Ruedi once.

"She's typical," he said. "We are telling her, 'You must do exactly what you think. You can waver. That's fine.'"

The only thing that would change her plans, Maia said, would be a legal change in the United States. In July 2018, Maia sent me a link to an article in the *Washington Post* with the headline, "In Oregon, Pushing to Give Patients with Degenerative Diseases the Right to Die." The article talked about a legislative effort to expand the state's Death with Dignity law, to include people with Alzheimer's, Parkinson's, Huntington's, multiple sclerosis, and a host of other degenerative illnesses. Campaigners wanted to get rid of the state's six-months-or-less prognosis requirement and to redefine "terminal illness." Maia thought the effort would probably fail. But what if it didn't? If it passed, she and Tevye could pack up everything and move to Oregon, and she could die in a way that didn't feel forbidden and weird. "On an idealistic level," Maia said, "I'm *obsessed* with dying in my own country." Either way, she would die soon, if not in 2018, then at the start of 2019. Of this, she was sure. It would be a relief, she said, to turn on the TV, on New Year's Eve, and watch Anderson Cooper do the countdown on CNN, and know that she would never see another new year. There would be a sweetness in that.

One day, when I was in Taos, Maia asked me if I wanted to come to an appointment with her. It was with a shaman named Carly whom she had met on Craigslist. Maia, I knew, had a way of attracting freelance healers and sages. There had been the retired pathologist in Colorado, the Christian chaplain in Taos, the "hokey medicine woman," the death doula in Los Angeles, and the death doula in Australia whom Maia sometimes talked with on Skype. Before that, there was the high school friend's mother, who thought that Maia was energetically damaged but could be saved. All of them had different interpretations of her disease and the purpose of it. All of them had stories to tell her about her suffering. Maia thought it was a bit cheesy to shop around, spiritually, but it always felt true in the moment. She was flexing her devotional muscles in preparation for a leap.

We drove out of town, through central Taos and then its outskirts, past a few sleepy Mexican restaurants and a juice bar and an e-cigarette café. Then we drove out farther, until everything was brown and dead and desert. We turned down a dirt road and drove past a broken-down school bus and a statue of a green elephant. Carly met us outside, near her teepee. She was tall and beautiful and looked sort of dirty, with a messy blond ponytail and an old brown cowboy hat and flowing red polyester pants. Her feet were bare, even though it was cold out, and she had a dog that looked like a wolf.

Inside her house it smelled sharp, like unwashed bodies. Plants and strings of seashells hung from the ceiling. On the counter, there were jars of castor oil, a set of bongo drums, a candle with an image of the Virgin Mary, and a stack of books: Jung, Nietzsche, Deepak Chopra, the Dalai Lama. Carly and Maia sat facing each other on a patterned rug covered in dog hair. They talked for a while, mostly about Maia's mother and how much Maia missed her, even though Tova's addiction had made their last years together so hard. Maia was sorry that they had fought so much. That she hadn't seen how hugely her mother was hurting, because of the opioids, but also because of the way she soaked up everyone else's pain. When Tova died, Maia had gone to clean out her apartment and had found boxes filled with yellow newspaper clippings, all of them about atrocities in faraway places. Indigenous people being killed in Central America. Sex workers disappearing from street corners. Pretty villages wrecked by ravenous business interests. I hadn't heard Maia speak much about her mother before. Carly told Maia that people carry ancestral damage with them—unresolved shame and guilt from previous generations—and that the damage can live inside them and weigh them down. Maybe Maia had inherited guilt that didn't even belong to her. Sometimes, guilt disguised itself as shame.

When they were done speaking, Carly helped Maia lie down on the soft couch, with her socked toes pressing into the armrest. They were going to clear space and move energy. Energy, Carly said, was neither good nor bad; it was only moving or stagnant, and you wanted it to move. Maia closed her eyes and Carly placed a hand on her collarbone, pressing her fingers into the skin and flesh of Maia's chest, like a potter kneading clay. She slapped Maia's shins and thighs. She blew into her face. She held a small drum over her head and struck it over and over. When it was finished, Maia looked stunned. "Cathartic relief," she whispered. Maia told Carly a story from when she was a little girl, on vacation in Hawaii with her father. She had gone swimming on the beach and "the ocean pulled me back and threw me on the floor." Maia had struggled to swim to the surface, against the tide. When she got out, cold and frightened, she told Larry what had happened. "Again, I wasn't believed."

"Tune in to that feeling," Carly said.

"I think I see the mistake I made," said Maia. "I should have just believed myself."

"HELLO KATIE, I AM really melting like a candle," Maia texted me in the summer of 2018. Sometimes, her legs gave way when she was at the grocery store. Sometimes, she lost control of her bladder. When Tevye or Carly drove her into town, she needed to wear a body brace, and even then, the bumps on the road made her feel like her spinal cord was breaking. The doctors wrote in Maia's charts that her cervical spine showed "a considerable amount of degenerative disc disease." They gave her fentanyl patches, which helped things but also left her weak and constipated. They prescribed her tramadol for the chronic pain in her neck. Maia asked all of the doctors the same question: Was her MS as severe as it was now because it wasn't diagnosed and treated earlier, because of all the people who hadn't believed her? They always said maybe. But they couldn't say for sure.

Her daily life, Maia said, had largely been reduced to a slow-motion migration from bed to couch. Bed, couch, bed, physical therapy, back to couch. She watched hours of television. "I don't like conspiracy theories, but I'm starting to believe that it really is all set up to keep the illness in a chronic state and just keep making money and never curing anything," she said. How did it make sense that there were all these expensive medications and still none of them could fix her? Maia decided that she would stop seeing her doctors. She would go for infusion therapy twice a year, but she would have nothing more to do with specialists. "Big Pharma, the whole medical-industrial-complex empire . . . It's more and more money being made and nobody's getting better," said Maia. "That's the thing." She refused to feel any more hope. "Don't feed me this bullshit. 'Oh, there are drugs coming down the pipeline. And stem cells.' It's false hope and we get hooked on it. . . . Stem cells? They are still working on mice!"

She would explain it all to Larry when she saw him. Maia and her father had started speaking again in the spring, after Maia sent him links to some videos about a British woman named Debbie Purdy who was also young and also had multiple sclerosis and who had also been accepted to die at a Swiss clinic. In 2008, Debbie had become a celebrity figure in Britain, after launching a legal challenge against the British government and its 1961 Suicide Act. Specifically, Debbie wanted the Parliament to clarify whether her husband could be prosecuted under the act for bringing her to Switzerland—whether just helping her onto the plane constituted "aiding, abetting, counseling or procuring the suicide of another," which was punishable with up to fourteen years in jail.

In news interviews, Debbie explained that if her husband could possibly be charged for traveling with her, then she would travel alone. However, if she had to travel alone, she would need to die earlier than she wanted to, while she was still physically capable of making the journey independently. Debbie's lawyer argued that the state was infringing on her human rights by failing to clarify the breadth of the Suicide Act and its possible enforcement. In 2009, Debbie won her case and Britain issued new guidelines stating that decisions about whether to prosecute a family member would take into account "the motivation of the subject." In other words, a loving spouse or child was unlikely to face charges—although anything was still possible. In an interview after the decision, a grinning Debbie said that she wanted "to live my life to the full, but I don't want to suffer unnecessarily."

Larry had connected with the videos of Debbie Purdy. In other reports that Maia sent him, the people had come across "a little bit suicidal" and also immodest. But Debbie was different. She was smart and well adjusted, and she loved her husband—and she had tried her best to live. She didn't have that impulse to self-destruction that annoyed him about the other sick people whom Maia looked up to. Larry watched the videos. He thought about things. And then he agreed to visit Maia in Taos and to come to a therapy appointment with her.

I asked Maia what she expected of the meeting. "It's hard," I added. "Like, you build something up and expect a kind of catharsis. . . ."

"Yeah, we think it's like the movies," Maia agreed. "That you're going to get a resolution. But sometimes you don't."

On the first visit, Larry stayed three days. The therapy appointment lasted an hour and a half and was the hardest part. He and Maia sat side by side in big armchairs, in an office filled with spiritual ornaments and knickknacks from South Asia and little teddy bears, which the therapist kept on hand for her child patients. Maia stared hard at a painting of a

Native American man who seemed to be meditating in front of a roaring fire. She went over the usual chronology of blame: her father's dismissal of her symptoms when she was young, his disbelief at her diagnosis, his initial counsel not to pursue treatment, his whitewashing of her symptoms. Larry repeated over and over that he didn't recollect things that way. "That's not what I recall." After the appointment, they went to a nice restaurant in Taos and talked about religion and guilt and death. Maia thought her father wasn't committed to the conversation. Larry wished they could talk about anything but her dying. Why couldn't they just have one normal interaction? Why did everything have to come back to fundamentals? He felt berated and accused by his daughter's pain, and also drained by her emotional needs; the way Maia demanded a specific kind of empathy from the people around her; the way she forced people to feel sorry for her in precise and insistent ways. Larry told Maia that he liked spending time with her and that he would come back to Taos, and that he would help her out with rent payments in the meantime. But he warned her that he would never be able to care for her full time. He was too old for that. Just before leaving Taos to drive home, Larry told Carly that his daughter was "a hard person to love."

Soon, Larry was visiting Taos every few weeks. He came back to the therapist's office, too, which was good, Maia thought, except it sometimes seemed like the appointments were getting harder over time instead of easier. Some days, Maia raged at her father in front of the therapist. If he had done more to help her, "maybe I would still be working part-time in the media," she said. Maia wanted Larry to say that it must be hard for her, to be so young and to have lost her life. She wanted him to wallow in regret, to bend over himself in apology. Mostly, though, she wanted his pity, because if he pitied her, the pity would be its own kind of vindication. But Larry just repeated, again and again, "That's not what I recall." At one session, he told the therapist that he didn't want to be with Maia at the Switzerland clinic for the same reason that he had refused to cover death-row cases while working as a journalist: He had no interest in watching an execution.

Other times, seated in the big armchair, Maia would look over at Larry and be startled by his eighty-year-old face and how old it looked: crumpled and pinched like a sweet old raisin. *Oh God*, she would think, *I can't do this to him. . . . I have to go on for my dad. I have to live longer.*

"Maia," I asked her once, "did you tell him why you came back from Switzerland? That it had to do with him?"

"No," she said. "I didn't."

After I had known Maia for nearly two years, Larry agreed to speak with me on the phone. He was polite, but our conversation was brief and starchy. Larry wanted to know my intentions in speaking to his daughter. He had worked as a reporter for decades. He knew how these things worked. What was my angle? Larry told me that Maia "should not feel that she has to die to give you a story. There could be a quiet, implicit pressure," he said. I agreed that there could be and said I hoped there wasn't. "I don't want her to be a martyr for the cause," Larry said.

A few months later, we spoke again. Larry sat in his living room, which was bright, with yellow knotted wood covering the walls and ceilings. He wore wire-rimmed glasses on a long, rectangular face that looked like his daughter's. Larry said that therapy was helping him to understand some things, among them that he had been wrong to doubt Maia. He should have trusted her instead of the doctors—and despite everything. Therapy had also helped him to see "that people who seek medical aid in dying are not suicidal." Still, he wasn't sure how he should behave around his daughter now. "It's a very difficult conundrum," he told me. "If you buy into the hopelessness of someone with MS like Maia who sees nothing in the future but more pain . . . If you buy into that, then you're encouraging their suffering. If you oppose that, if you say, 'No, it's not that bad! It hasn't happened yet!' then you're not supporting your own child. It's a conflict that I've never been able to resolve." He paused. "I don't believe suffering is a virtue. I don't believe in original sin or, in fact, all of those Christian concepts that relate to suffering. I don't believe that." But then, how to explain his sense, however weak and ill defined, that a certain amount of suffering should be endured rather than evaded? How to deal with the fact that she wasn't *that* sick yet?

There it was, I thought. There were the two of them, father and daughter, both convinced in their own ways that Maia had not suffered enough yet. That she owed something, or someone, or herself, a course of suffering that she hadn't yet completed. I wondered if they had spotted the rhythm in their own quivering conclusions.

Larry asked me if I'd heard about the horses. I said I hadn't. He told me that a few months earlier, Maia had noticed some horses standing by the road near her house. They looked like they were starving. Their ribs pushed out through the patchy skin on their shrunken bellies. "Suddenly," Larry said, "she decided to save them." Maia collected money from her neighbors and used it to buy oats and hay, which she started feeding to the horses in the dark of night. She also tracked down the owner and learned that he had given up on caring for the animals because he could not afford the food. Maia called the state inspector and got the horses taken to an animal refuge. "She was very pleased that they were OK," Larry said. "This is not the activity of a suicidal person, I think."

For her fortieth birthday, Maia drove with Carly to Mexico. It was a difficult ride. Maia was tired—doctors thought she might have sleep apnea—and whenever she stood up, at a rest stop or a gas station, her heart seemed to beat too fast. She was always very cold or too hot. Along the way, Carly asked Maia if she had any regrets. Maia said she wished that she hadn't withdrawn from the world when she got sick, that she had been less self-conscious about her disease. Less vain.

"You can have regrets and also be a beautiful human being right now," Carly said. "They don't need to be separate from each other." Carly told Maia that it was OK if she didn't resolve all her guilt and bitterness before she died. Not everything gets resolved. The important thing, Carly said, was that Maia try to sing something on the day of her death. Maia told Carly that at Lifecircle, in Switzerland, everyone picks a song to die to.

In early 2019, Maia texted me to say that a proposed aid-in-dying bill had not passed the New Mexico legislature. The proposed criteria expansion in Oregon, which might have opened up the law to earlier-stage MS patients, had failed, too. Maia said she cried when she heard the news. People didn't understand, she said, "that there are some illnesses whose fate is *worse* than death. And that is where my illness falls." Now there was only Switzerland. In the end, her hero's journey wouldn't be about defeating MS or helping to change the law, as she had once hoped it might be. Her heroic quest would just be to accept things as they were. "I wanted to sue everyone at some point in my life," Maia said. Now she just wanted peace. It was a tragic story only because she had tried so hard to make it otherwise. Maia said she would return to Switzerland soon, just as she had been telling me every month or so for the last three years. All she had to do was buy the plane ticket.

In the meantime, Maia's therapist thought she should start preparing herself to die. She should start thinking about spiritual matters and the possibility of an afterlife. She should start weaning herself off life. But it was difficult. These days, Maia confessed, she was spending a lot of time binge-watching broadcast TV: news about Russian election interference and the Mueller report. "I watch hours and hours of the Mueller report," she told me, laughing a little. Maia thought Roger Stone would flip. She thought that Donald Trump would resign before he could be impeached. She hoped she would be alive to see him charged for his crimes. "My therapist is like, 'You don't want to spend your final months watching coverage of the Mueller report!'" Maia promised that she would stop. But then again, why should she? That was the thing about suffering and dying. In the end, it didn't mean anything at all. It had to mean everything or nothing, and it meant nothing. All this time, Maia had been trying to find significance in her pain. But there was "no meaning, just endless, endless days."

4

Memory

It was the start of January 2018 when Debra Koosed started working on her taxes. Or was it mid-January? She knew it was January. She knew that she would get confused and would need the extra time. Months, even. Soon, Debra was spending several hours a day bent over the paperwork, her soft body in the heavy wheelchair, pulled up to the round kitchen table that looked out at the Oregon coastline.

Brian, Debra's "exit guide," wanted to know why she was so intent on filing her taxes anyway, given what she planned to do?

Because she wanted her affairs to be in order. Because she did not want things left unfinished. "I am tying up loose ends," she said. But when Debra looked down at the tax forms, it was as if the pages lost their outer borders and the words danced away.

Her small home was quiet, save for the beeps and vibrations coming from her late husband David's cell phone: alarms reminding her when to eat, when to take her medications, when to water the plants. In the mornings and evenings, there were alarms to open and close the curtains in the living room, and, at regular intervals throughout the day, alarms prompting her to use the bathroom, because she did not always remember to go and would sometimes have accidents. Debra imagined that David's cell phone was David himself, re-embodied a year after his death, and ministering to the needs of her failing body and mind. "I used to be a Maserati," she liked to say. "Now I'm a clunker."

The neuropsychologist had used another word, which was "dementia." At Debra's appointment a few months earlier, he had told her what she already knew: things were not all right. MRIs showed that the frontal and parietal lobes of Debra's brain had atrophied, *were* atrophying. The atrophy was already at a moderate stage. During the appointment, Debra could recite the alphabet and count to twenty, but she could not recall the day of the week or where exactly she was. She was sixty-five. When he delivered the news, the doctor was nonchalant. "Here are your results."

After the appointment, Debra started having visions of life in a nursing home, lost and unglued. Doctors would ignore her, and nurses wouldn't know how to position her in just the right way so that she wouldn't be in pain. She would forget how to think. She would forget how to chew and swallow. The other patients would cry and moan, each nudging the next into ever-more hysterical and demented states. It would not be a nice facility, because Debra could not afford a nice facility. In Debra's vision, things would be worst at night. "Strangers are touching me . . . touching me in a way that might be inappropriate." If it happened in some locked-door nursing home, would she even know that she was being hurt?

Debra said that if she were a dog, someone would have put her down long ago. Debra had euthanized sick dogs before, dogs she loved, and even as a child she had understood the act to be merciful. "I thought, wow, this is such a wonderful thing, that I am able to ease the suffering and pain of my beloved." When Debra watched her grandmother die, she thought, "I wish there was something we could do for humans."

Sometimes the question was *if*. Usually, though, it was *when*. Debra said that she would kill herself before she lost herself completely. She would wait for as long as she could, because she did not want to die, but she wouldn't wait too long. "I have to be cognizant in order to do it," she told me. Brian would show her what she needed to know, but he couldn't help. "No one can help me, because that's murder. I have to do this on my own, so I have to go at a time when I still feel I know what I'm doing." For the moment, there were still good days and bad days. Soon, though, a bad day would stay a bad day, and then she would vanish.

BRIAN RUDER READ through the application package slowly from his home in Portland. He had worked with clients like this before, people with fresh diagnoses of dementia, but never someone so young. "I'm writing this letter to request the services of the Final Exit Network in hastening my death," the applicant, Debra Koosed, wrote in her introductory letter. "I'm hoping you can help me . . . before my brain robs me of ALL my dignity." Not every would-be client was as circumspect. Sometimes, people got scrappy in their pleas for help, in an "If you don't help me, I'll blow my brains out" kind of way.

Brian, now seventy-seven, was born to a German Catholic family in Kansas. He was raised to fear God and to believe that the taking of one's life was a mortal sin, a degradation so complete that it fell beyond the bounds of his mercy. As he grew older, though, Brian shed his faith and acquired in its place a rigid devotion to the secular tenets of personal autonomy, especially as it concerned the end of life. "I don't believe in letting doctors decide when I should die," he told me. Now that he had lost his God, there was no redemption to be found in anguish, no transcendence in pain. There was no purpose to pain at all. "I don't believe in suffering." When Brian left his corporate job in Portland, he started volunteering with Compassion & Choices, the national nonprofit group that lobbies state legislatures to legalize physician-assisted death.

But the more he volunteered, the more Brian heard about patients whom the Oregon Death with Dignity law didn't reach. People with MS who might live for years but didn't want to. People with chronic pain who weren't terminally ill. People with dementia. By the time a dementia patient is within six months of death, Brian learned, she will likely be too far gone to consent to much of anything—and so won't qualify. Brian thought the law was too narrow and that activists should fight to expand it, but the people at Compassion & Choices didn't seem to think that way. "They were not very interested in moving things along." In 2015, while researching online, Brian found out about the Final Exit Network (FEN), a group of volunteers who teach people how to kill themselves and then sit with them when they do it, so they won't be alone. He had never heard of anything like it.

Brian read that FEN had grown out of the Hemlock Society, a right-to-die advocacy group formed in 1980 in California and named after the poison that Socrates drank before weeping disciples in ancient Athens. Its founder was an offbeat British newspaperman named Derek Humphry, who in 1975 had helped his forty-two-year-old wife, Jean, to kill herself after she was diagnosed with terminal breast cancer, sourcing barbiturate sleeping pills and then mixing them in a large mug with coffee, sugar, and codeine. Humphry wanted his new organization to be an agent of mainstream political change. Through Hemlock and its political arm, Americans Against Human Suffering, he and his followers would raise money and fund Death with Dignity ballot initiatives in a handful of target states. They would get laws passed. Ideally, Humphry told a *New York Times* reporter, in an article titled "Some Elderly Choose Suicide over Lonely, Dependent Life," the new laws would not allow "Hitler-style forced euthanasia of the elderly and mentally deficient," while at the same time responding to "a groundswell of public opinion which feels the time has come for thoughtful, planned, justified voluntary euthanasia for the dying."

"My God," one of Hemlock's first members declared at a July 1980 founding meeting. "They firebomb the houses of pro-abortion people. . . . What do you think they'll do to us?"

Ten years later, Hemlock claimed to have 50,000 paying members who attended meetings at ninety local chapters, coordinated by thirteen paid employees. Still, in all that time, none of Hemlock's political initiatives had amounted to anything. Physician-assisted death was still illegal in every state. And Humphry, in turn, had grown impatient with his own creation. It wasn't just that Hemlock was politically impotent; it was that the group's aspirations, which had been Humphry's own aspirations, didn't seem to match those of its rank-and-file members. At chapter meetings, many held in tiny Unitarian Universalist church basements, people ostensibly gathered to talk about Hemlock's upcoming legislative efforts, but in practice they asked a lot of questions about how to die better. They wanted to know what dying was like and how to talk to their doctors about it—and how to make sure they never ended up as mindless vegetables, kept alive by hospital machines. Also, they wanted to know how to coax physicians into prescribing enough sleeping pills to overdose on. The AIDS patients especially wanted specific instructions: What pills? How many?

In 1991, Humphry offered a direct response to their searching, in the form of a self-published book called *Final Exit: The Practicalities of Self-Deliverance and Assisted Suicide for the Dying*, which was effectively a step-by-step death manual, one that Humphry printed himself because he couldn't find a willing publisher. The book considered different means of self-murder and promised straight-up "instructions for a perfect death, with no mess, no autopsy, no post-mortem." One chapter explained how to die with pills and a plastic bag. Another explained death by self-starvation and dehydration. There were chapters on "The Cyanide Enigma" and "Life Insurance." And there were spirited entreaties from Humphry, who urged his readers to open their eyes and confront the certainty of human expiration. "You are terminally ill, all medical treatments available to you have been exhausted, and the suffering in its different forms is unbearable," he wrote. "The dilemma is awesome. But it has to be faced. Should you battle on, take the pain, endure the indignity, and await the inevitable end, which may be days, weeks, or months away? Or should you take control of the situation . . . ?" In Humphry's language, obtaining the physical means to a peaceful death was not just personally shrewd, but morally venerable as well. Absolute control at the end of life was its own form of heroism.

In the beginning, so few people were interested in the book that Humphry would hand out free copies to his fringe activist friends at Hemlock events. But then, to pretty much everyone's surprise, the book started selling—and eventually sold so well that it ended up on the *New York Times* best-seller list for fourteen weeks. The newspaper called it "one of the most unlikely success stories in publishing history," noting that "numerous Hollywood producers have even sought the film rights—apparently without bothering to read the book, which has no characters, scenes or dialogue." Dr. Arthur Caplan, the preeminent bioethicist, called the book "a shot across the bow. It is the loudest statement of protest of how medicine is dealing with terminal illness and the dying."

Humphry left Hemlock soon after the book was published—and shortly after Ann Wickett, his second ex-wife and former Hemlock collaborator, ended her life with barbiturates, leaving behind a suicide note that accused Humphry of pressuring her to die after her cancer diagnosis. *There*, the note read. *You got what you wanted.* The Hemlock Society continued without him, but with an altered mandate. In 1998, the group set up a program called Caring Friends, run by a doctor from Canada. Under the program, volunteers were trained to act as death midwives: guides who would help sick and dying Hemlock members procure an adequate stash of lethal drugs and would then sit with them while they swallowed the pills. Demand for assistance was immediate and the clients came quickly. There was the accomplished global insurance executive whose dog lay silently by her feet while she ate a bowl of barbiturate-laced applesauce. There was the beautiful woman in her thirties with a motor neuron disease, whose family members all flew in from Europe for her death and then took turns feeding her pills, one by one, until they were gone. There was a man with a neurological condition who was so full of rage that Hemlock guides insisted on postponing his death for several months, so that he could work out some issues with his brother and die with a bit more serenity. There were funny deaths, too. One older woman shouted out, midway through drinking her barbiturate solution, "It is really bitter! But I'm going to drink this down, even if it kills me." Then she paused. Then she laughed, delighted by herself. "Even if it kills me," she said again, to her Hemlock guides, before finishing the drink and falling asleep.

In the early 2000s, Hemlock merged with several other right-to-die groups and then underwent a bitter schism. Most members went on to become the Washington, DC–based Compassion & Choices, devoted entirely to above-the-board lobbying efforts, and a much tinier faction reconsolidated as the Final Exit Network. By the time Brian Ruder joined, FEN had evolved into a peculiar sort of organization. The network had a Facebook page, a janky website, a formal hierarchy, and a claim to several thousand paying members. It was a 501(c)(3) registered nonprofit whose donations were tax deductible and, according to FEN's website, "contribute to the advancement of the basic human right of autonomy." On the other hand, its volunteers worked in the shadows, without oversight. Brian made contact with the group and was invited to train as an "exit guide."

At a two-day seminar in San Jose in 2016, Brian was schooled in the FEN protocol. He learned that while FEN guides were there to help people, they couldn't help in the literal sense. The act of assisting a suicide was illegal in most states, including states with physician-assisted-dying laws—and even in places where there weren't specific laws on the books, an exit guide was vulnerable to criminal charges. And so FEN had to work around the law. The rule that the network's leadership came up with—the rule they hoped would keep them free from prosecution—was that exit guides could instruct and advise and sit with but could never touch their clients. FEN lawyer Robert Rivas explained this in a presentation to the new trainees. "The first reflex of a lot of people is, 'Yes, you're just giving us a wink. If there's nobody else in the room, we're going to give him some physical assistance. We're going to put our hands on something. We're going to open the valve. We're going to help him hook up the tubes or whatever,'" Rivas told me. "We, at the very start, have to disabuse them of the idea that we're winking or nodding." Under no circumstances could an exit guide "help." To avoid confusion, it was best to avoid the verb entirely when discussing network business.

Rivas had closely studied the subject and had found that in around forty states, there are laws that explicitly criminalize the assistance of suicide, though the laws themselves vary broadly. In some states, a person has to commit a "physical act" of assistance to be prosecuted; in others, it is enough to verbally encourage someone to die. In a handful of states—these, the most dangerous places for FEN to operate—merely educating someone on how to suicide is a chargeable offense. As it was, FEN had already been the subject of a multistate undercover sting operation, and its volunteers had been charged on three separate occasions: once, after the death of a fifty-eight-year-old woman named Jana Van Voorhis, who, it turns out, was not physically sick at all but had fabricated pathologies on her FEN application because she was depressed and delusional and believed that insects were eating her body. Jana's sister said later that if FEN hadn't been around to take Jana seriously, and if its guides had not indulged her hypochondriac fantasies, she never would have killed herself.

In 2015, the network received a felony conviction in Minnesota for assisting in the suicide of a fifty-seven-year-old woman with chronic pain—after the Supreme Court of Minnesota, in a separate case, defined the word "assistance" to include "speech" that "enables" a suicide. FEN was fined $33,000. It appealed the decision, pointing out that the information shared by its guides was readily available in books and on the Internet. Under the state's interpretation, FEN lawyers argued, a librarian could be convicted just for handing a patron a book about suicide, if that person later killed himself. The appeal was denied.

At the seminar, Brian and the other trainees also watched a demonstration of the network's suicide method: inert gas asphyxiation, using a sturdy plastic bag and a canister of pure nitrogen. Barbara Coombs Lee, the president of Compassion & Choices, had once referred to FEN's plastic-bag hoods as "sort of the end-of-life equivalent of the coat hanger"—and Brian agreed that the whole process was "not very dignified." Still, the network preferred asphyxiation over drugs because the equipment was easy to find and legal to buy. And it was said to be painless. FEN's primary goal, Brian learned, was not to change the law, but to help people who suffered outside it, because they lived in states where assisted dying was illegal or because their symptoms didn't match the law's eligibility criteria. According to FEN rules, clients didn't need to be terminally ill or even dying, in the immediate sense, as long as they were suffering "intolerably" and "unbearably" and were mentally competent at the moment they pulled the plastic bags over their heads and flicked on the nitrogen gas.

There were around fifteen volunteers at the training and Brian liked them all. Most were younger than he was, in their forties or fifties, but they slipped into an easy fellowship. There was Peter, whose sister had died by suicide when he was young. There was John, an Episcopal priest who had fallen out with organized faith. Many FEN volunteers shared a belief in free will that seemed to verge on dogma, and many had joined the organization after seeing terrible deaths. Some of the deaths they described were blood spattered and spectacular, but others were just awful in the usual way: slow and confusing. A few of the volunteers had found themselves searching for an organization just like FEN, without even knowing that it existed—and then, after finding the network online, had felt an incredible relief. *There it is.* Within six months of the training, Brian attended his first "exit." The client was a man whose partner kissed and embraced him before leaving the room, because he could not bear to watch.

When I first made contact with the network and started meeting its guides, I was reminded of the Jane Collective: the underground women's service in Chicago that provided abortions in the years before *Roe v. Wade*, when the procedure was still illegal. By some estimates, the anonymous "Janes" helped to terminate more than 10,000 pregnancies between 1969 and 1973. FEN, it seemed to me, was a kind of end-of-life equivalent. But other FEN members, I learned, preferred grander historical parallels— one of which made me wince. "In pre–Civil War, you had abolitionists who spoke out for the abolition of slavery," Janis Landis, FEN's then president and a former IRS bureaucrat, told me when we met over a coffee in Manhattan. "Without the heroism involved, we operate more along the nature of the Underground Railroad—which is to say, that until the law is passed, we have to deal with the people who are suffering now. We have to show them a path that brings them out of harm's way."

DEBRA LEARNED ABOUT FEN on the Internet. One day, while she was researching ways to die, she found a site that listed all the normal methods of suicide and explained why each one was problematic: the cramps, the mess, the awkwardness. The possibility of incompletion. Debra had thought about using the little handgun holstered to the side of her wheelchair, but the website said that suicide by bullet was risky. "You can miss, shooting yourself," she told me. "You can become a veg . . . you know what I mean." It was harder to kill yourself than Debra had imagined. One Internet search led to the next until, eventually, she came across the Final Exit Network. *Son of a bitch*, she thought.

When Debra called FEN in the fall of 2017 and said that she had dementia, she was put in touch with a woman named Janet Grossman, who told Debra that she would serve as the coordinator on her case. Debra learned that she would have to submit medical records showing proof of her diagnosis and a specific account of how her pathologies made her suffer. A panel of volunteer doctors would then review the application and decide whether Debra could be helped; whether she was truly sick and whether her suffering met FEN's criteria for "incurable" and "unbearable." If she met the criteria, they could move forward with what Janet called, slipping into FEN vernacular, Debra's exit.

Debra told Janet about the forgetting and losing herself. She talked about her father, who had plunged into Alzheimer's in his seventies. He had been a bad Alzheimer's patient, Debra said: not the doddering, childlike kind, but the paranoid and nasty kind. As parts of his mind disconnected, he convinced himself that his wife was cheating on him. He stalked her when she went to the grocery store. In the end, he died in a care home, tied down to a hospital bed. He weighed just 130 pounds, a stretch of skin and flesh across his once imposing frame, because he could not remember how to chew and swallow.

Janet was sympathetic. Her late father had suffered from congestive heart failure and her mother from dementia. In 2015, Janet's father had stepped outside the independent living home that he shared with Janet's mother and placed a plastic sheet on the concrete surface of the parking lot and brought his wife to lie on it. He had called 911 and told the paramedics to expect gunshots and that he wanted his body donated to science. He had then shot his wife of sixty-four years and shot himself. He died instantly; she died a little later. As it happens, Janet learned, these sorts of deaths are not uncommon: elderly couples dying in suicide pacts to escape Alzheimer's or men killing their demented wives of many years, because the women are losing their memories and want to die, or because their husbands assume they *would* want to die, if only they could remember to want it. Sometimes the men are prosecuted afterward and sometimes the judges forgive them—because, they say, the men acted out of mercy.

In late 2017, Janet called Debra to tell her that she had been approved, and Debra wept on the line. "It meant everything," she said. Sometimes, Debra had allowed herself to wonder whether things were really as bad as the diagnosis made them seem, but now she wouldn't have to. The FEN doctors had read the paperwork and thought that things were very bad indeed. On the phone, Janet told Debra that she should be careful about whom she told. If the wrong person found out, Debra could find herself under lockdown suicide watch. It had happened to clients before. Debra also needed to understand that she had a "window of opportunity." She should live as long as she liked, but if she waited too long to act, she might lose the ability or the will to die and then FEN would have to drop her case.

"The problem that we run into with me is, right now, I don't have a disease that has a clock to it and we don't know when my brain is going to turn on me," Debra told me the first time we spoke. "I don't know what faculties I'm going to lose, when I'm going to lose them, and how I'm going to lose them. Is there a list of what you lose first? . . . I don't think there's a list anywhere that says what you lose first." It was just that one day, she would forget to take her dinner out of the microwave and then she'd never remember again. Debra promised herself that she would not wait too long and that she would not miss her chance. Except it was hard to know if her malfunctioning mind would even recognize when the clock was winding down.

"It looks like she can enjoy many more months of a pretty decent life, and she may," said Brian, who was assigned to be one of Debra's two exit guides. We had met at a bar in downtown Portland one Saturday night to discuss Debra's case.

By then, I had spent months interviewing dozens of people associated with the Final Exit Network: guides, administrators, past administrators, volunteer physicians, current clients, and the family members of long-ago clients. One conversation led to the next and most lasted hours. Sometimes I called people who lived across the country. Other times, I met them in person. I interviewed one former volunteer at the Metropolitan Museum of Art in New York City, and we whispered to each other about gas canisters and eligibility criteria while wandering between Rembrandts. Of everyone I spoke to, I was most interested in the exit guides, who risked so much to sit with strangers while they died. Most of all, I was interested in Brian, who always spoke freely and who described himself on LinkedIn as a "Chief Happiness Officer."

At the bar, Brian told me that he was hearing more and more from people with dementia. That made sense to him; the population was growing and aging, and the ranks of the dementia sufferers were swelling. "They are living for the sake of living and it's costing more," Brian said. "And their quality of life is crap." By 2030, nearly 10 million elderly baby boomers were expected to have dementia. Researchers were already warning of a Generation Alzheimer's, or a Dementia Tsunami that America's healthcare systems were unprepared to weather. In Brian's civilian life, he heard people say all the time that if they got dementia, they would kill themselves or get someone else to kill them. That they were *not going there*. OK then, he would think, so what is your plan? People were scared, and there was nobody to hold their hands and help them find a way out.

But didn't Debra still seem OK? I asked him.

"It's her choice," he said slowly.

In addition to working as an exit guide, Brian volunteered at a suicide prevention hotline, trying to keep strangers alive for a few more hours, until the crisis passed and "usually they realize that they don't want to die." Those death wishes were different, Brian said, because they weren't about control; they were about chaos. Disturbed minds. Minds that had shifted off-kilter. Brian knew how to talk a person out of it—and, in fact, many people needed to be talked out of it. Debra, however, was clear in what she wanted. She had thought things through. So who were we to judge whether her cognitive decline was sufficiently severe? Who were we to say that it needed to be severe anyway, for the exit to be, what, worth it? "She doesn't want to lose her selfhood," Brian said. "She sees it happening." Brian believed that nobody wants to die, only sometimes they can't live a certain way.

. . .

DEBRA GREW UP IN a spiritually unmoored home, in a known-for-nothing town in California. When she was small, she was baptized as a Catholic and then a few years later, when her father changed his mind, rebaptized as a Protestant. He changed his mind again, and the family stopped going to church altogether. It was an unhappy household. Debra's father drank himself stupid at night and yelled a lot. Sometimes, after he was done yelling, he came into Debra's bedroom and sexually abused her, and she would lie still and try her best not to breathe. It would be many years before she could admit to herself what he had done. For all of her girlhood, Debra imagined that it was a tall monster who made the nighttime visits. When her parents divorced, Debra moved in with her mother, who took up ballroom dancing. She retained a certain unease around strangers. She told herself that she would never have a child of her own.

Debra had wanted to go to college, but she didn't have any money, so instead she got a job at a phone company, first as a typist and then as a manager. She rose as high as a person could without a college degree, which was pretty high, she thought, for a woman. She was the point of contact for hundreds of people. "I set up everything," she said. Debra did not consider herself to be especially clever, but she was good at her job and was proud of how hard she could work. On Friday and Saturday nights, she and some of the other company girls would go out to TGI Fridays and hang out by the bar. They'd spend hours swaggering around the place with their fresh, eighties, second-wave boldness: all acrylic nails and hair combed up into Q-tip puffs.

Her mother died when she was thirty and that changed things. The two women had planned to meet for lunch, but Debra's mother never showed up. On the way, a drunk driver had crossed over the painted line of his lane and into hers. Medical workers attempted to resuscitate her: first by doing CPR and then by cracking her chest open and trying to massage her heart back into life. They broke so many bones, but she died anyway. Debra took a leave of absence from the phone company. Then she stopped sleeping and went on Zoloft. When she came back to work, she excused herself from the nights out with the company girls.

When Debra met David—who had red hair and a big, earnest mustache—she told him that she was no Betty Crocker. But David was not like the jerks at work who sometimes grabbed at Debra or the old boyfriend who urged her to turn down a promotion because he thought the job of secretary suited her just fine. David supported her. He would ask to hear stories about the phone company, and he would repeat them at parties, to Debra's astonishment. "My wife is the only person in the company who does this," he would boast. "She designed this!" David had been an antiques trader before going into construction, and his house was filled with old things: objects that, Debra would agree, were definitely not junk, as some people thought, but were precious and wonderful. Sometimes, Debra and David imagined that they had known each other in the Victorian era but that their relationship had been cut short for reasons they didn't know and that God had sent them back to earth to meet again.

In 2000, Debra suggested that they move to Pacific City, on Oregon's central coast, where people said there were more cows than humans. Things were cheaper there. Neither had close family. Neither thought they needed anyone but the other. In Oregon, they could start their lives anew and build a house by the water, with walls made out of cedar. When they did, they filled it with things they loved: crystal figurines, bouquets of plastic flowers from their wedding at Disneyland, old biscuit tins, imitation Tiffany lamps, and bookshelves lined with hardback thrillers, arranged alphabetically by author. They pasted vintage posters of Kellogg's cereal and Cadbury powdered chocolate in the kitchen and hung David's collection of old fedoras and pageboy caps on the living room wall. They made it perfect.

It was a few years later that, in Debra's telling, she died. "I was in a catastrophic, deadly accident in 2008," she told me. She wouldn't remember much, except that she was going into the city to do some Christmas shopping and had just steered the van around the crest of a mountain when things went dark. Debra's car hit a tree at around sixty miles an hour, throwing her body into the dashboard, ripping out her knee implants, and, somehow, tangling the bones of her foot around the gas pedal. She remembered waking up, briefly, to think: *This car is going to catch on fire and I will burn to death*.

Debra said that when she died, she crossed over into a place of brilliant light where she was free from pain and where her mother was waiting for her. The women stood together, but when Debra tried to walk farther into the light, her mother barred the way. She needed to go back, for David. "The next minute I'm awake, and I'm in a helicopter. . . . Someone is pressing on me." Paramedics had performed CPR and resuscitated her. Most of the major bones in Debra's body were broken, and doctors told her that she would have to use a wheelchair from then on. She learned later that a truck driver had spotted her car, folded up like an accordion against the tree, and had called 911. That had saved her life. But the driver had also stolen her purse.

The thing about near-death experiences, at least as they play out in fiction, is that they tend to demystify death. Someone almost dies, and when he doesn't, he comes to see how close he is to death—indeed how close he has always been to it. His mortality becomes present and material. As it does, the man stops trying to ignore death or to evade it. He grows resigned to his own finitude and maybe even comes to accept it. Or to learn something from it. But this is not how almost dying felt to Debra. As her body repaired itself, Debra found that her godless idea of death had been remystified: made enchanted and otherworldly—lush, where it had once been spiritually parched. Debra thought constantly about the bright, beautiful place in the sky and knew that she was not afraid to return.

After the crash, Debra and David spent more time taking care of each other. They went out less. They saw fewer people. David helped Debra with her pain pills: the Vicodin and morphine for pain, the Oxycodone for breakthrough pain, the muscle relaxer and the Xanax for PTSD, because of what her father had done to her. David swore that the wheelchair didn't bother him one bit. He became Debra's arms and legs. In turn, Debra tended to David through blood clots and heart surgery and cancer treatment. When David was out building fences or doing odd jobs, Debra spent hours researching his various maladies. Each time she presented David's doctors with a new suggestion for a new treatment, she felt certain that she had saved his life. By then, Debra had acquired a low opinion of the physicians who treated her husband and the medical community behind them. She believed that most doctors were "total arrogant asses," pseudogods who thought they knew what was best for everyone else but also didn't really care. And they were no help when, one day in August 2017, David stopped breathing and dropped dead in the kitchen.

It was only after David died that Debra began to see herself as she was. The dislocations and forgetting, which she had brushed aside, now lay in plain view. It was also after David died that Debra finally read the terms of the reverse mortgage that he had signed to cover their medical bills. Debra was stunned by how little money she had left. She wondered if she would lose her home. But then again, it was hard to think about money because it was getting harder to think in straight lines. Debra's thoughts felt like seeds that never fully germinated but instead sprouted sinuous half thoughts that waved at her distractingly. She forgot things: appointments, words, to eat dinner. Her attention was flighty; her stories lost their narrative threads. Her moods became unpredictable: detached and floating. Sometimes, when Debra was at her computer, she'd come to suddenly and find that she had typed a page of gibberish. "I call them brain farts, for lack of a better description." She said her brain was "bleeding," that it was "oozing something every day." Debra took a memory test online and scored poorly. "Proof I'm worse than I thought," she said. Once, on the phone with me, Debra cried down the line and said that she didn't recognize herself anymore. "I loved my brain."

When she finally saw the neuropsychologist, after putting the appointment off for years, she was almost relieved to hear him say "dementia."

At least the thing had a name. At the appointment, the doctor ran Debra through a battery of memory tests. He found that she was "generally fluent and well-articulated" but noted that her speech was "punctuated with frequent word-finding pauses" and that, during testing, she experienced "several absence episodes" that might be indicative of a seizure disorder. On a Mini–Mental State Examination, she scored 24/30, consistent with mild dementia. On a Global Assessment of Functioning test, she scored 55/100, showing "moderate" overall capacity. The neuropsychologist thought that Debra's coping skills—especially the way she used her late husband's old cell phone to schedule her every waking moment—were "absolutely amazing . . . one in a million." Still, she would get worse. It was hard to say how much or how quickly.

Debra slept all the way home, in the back of the taxi. The next day, she read the doctor's notes through and found herself grow cold. "It is strongly recommended," the note said, "that Ms. Koosed explore possible alternative care environments such as an adult foster home. Until an appropriate care environment is located, Ms. Koosed will require in-home assistance on a regular basis."

Debra promised the doctor she would start looking at nursing homes—because she worried that, if she didn't, he would report her to local authorities and get her committed to an institution. She knew she wouldn't really. Instead, Debra read blogs about how gross and expensive most long-term-care homes were. She sent me links to articles. "Up to over $97K/year! Ouch! Talk about 'sticker shock,'" she wrote in one email. "Where will the $$come from? I feel sorry for the thousands of Baby Boomers who didn't plan for this." Debra was surprised to learn that Medicare would fund almost none of what she needed—no assisted-living apartments, no at-home caregivers. Wasn't Medicare supposed to take care of old people?

The more she read, the more it seemed to Debra that her only option was to spend down whatever savings she had until almost everything was gone and she could qualify for state assistance—and then find a facility that would take Medicaid and Social Security checks. "This is where the neuropsychologist wants me to live. Yuck!" Debra wrote me in another email, linking to an article with information about adult foster care. "And for what?" Debra hated the idea of wasting her money on some depressing institution. When she died, she wanted her savings to go to the Oregon Humane Society, to help dogs, like all the ones she had loved over the years. She had saved her whole life to help those dogs. Debra did not want her final legacy, however small, to line the pockets of the medical establishment.

Later, I asked the neuropsychologist who assessed Debra what his responsibility was, in instances when he was worried about the safety of an elderly patient living alone. "Oregon has a mandatory reporting law," he said. That meant he was obliged to report concerning cases to the Department of Human Services (DHS). But, he said, "it doesn't always make things better."

"People get taken from their homes?"

"No. I think the more general rule is *nothing* happens. Someone goes out and talks to them. They say, 'Well, there's some food in the fridge. Whatever.' The bar to intervene is pretty darn high. . . . The joke in healthcare is that you might have to call DHS, but don't expect them to help."

"With someone like Debra," I asked, "would her symptoms have been serious enough for that?" Would the state have intervened?

He paused. Maybe a local service provider would have driven out to meet with her, he said, but in the end, the county would likely not have offered much. There weren't many professional caregivers in Debra's area, and it was expensive to bring them in from nearby cities.

"That must be difficult," I said. "You see a situation and you think, 'This isn't sustainable.' But what option is there?"

"Exactly." The doctor sighed. "It's a difficult process and a lot of people disconnect emotionally. It's easier not to have any emotions. That's the dilemma that a lot of clinicians face."

. . .

IN THE MONTHS AFTER the appointment, Debra became an obsessive student of her own cerebral decline. At her kitchen table, by the window, she wrote up tidy lists of her symptoms: signs of a growing rupture between body and mind.

- Inability to plan a sequence of complex movements needed to complete multi-tasked steps, such as making coffee
- Inability to focus on a task
- Changes in personality
- Inability to express language (Broca's aphasia)
- Problems with reading
- Difficulty in distinguishing left from right

"More 'mystery' pains frm damaged brain interfering w/Life," she texted me.

Once, I asked Debra what she thought it would be like to be demented—this thing she would rather die than experience. But Debra didn't seem to know. She wasn't sure if she would feel anxious and depressed, or if she would forget to feel either of those things. She didn't know if she would even feel. Maybe the disease would be its own kind of numbing agent. "The existential experience of dementia is almost completely ignored," the writer and nurse Sallie Tisdale has observed. "Vanishingly few studies have considered what it is like to *be* demented." Debra did wonder if she would find the state of dementia to be undignified. She thought she probably wouldn't, that she would have no self-respect left by then to offend. But still, she believed that some part of her would continue to hurt from all the small indignities of life in an institution where nobody loved her.

Skeptics of physician-assisted death sometimes argue that our focus should be on facilitating good lives, not curating good deaths. This, they contend, is because there are no good deaths, or because the quality of our death is largely out of our hands, or because our quixotic preoccupation with engineering the perfect final hour is a disproportionate use of our efforts, which would be better spent on improving life. But Debra believed that her ending mattered. She would have to live her ending, after all. Also, endings had a way of bending back on themselves and changing the way a person's whole life was remembered. Debra did not want a bad ending. With FEN's help, she thought, she could script her life story all the way to her final breath.

In early February, Debra called Brian to say that she was ready for the next step. She had ordered the supplies that she needed: the canister of nitrogen gas and the plastic tubing. The postman who delivered the gas tank had once been friends with David, but he dropped off the package without asking questions. Debra didn't need to order large plastic bags because she already had some, left over from when David used to cook Thanksgiving turkeys. A few weeks later, Brian and Lowrey Brown, the other exit guide assigned to Debra's case, drove west from Portland to Pacific City.

Lowrey, who was forty-five, had joined FEN the same year as Brian, after she "watched some ugly endings. Like so many people at FEN, I looked at these situations and said, 'Never.'" As an exit guide, Lowrey had worked with dementia clients before. The last had been a firecracker of a woman who wasn't exactly ready to die, but who took her life anyway so that she wouldn't forget to do it. "We take people with even mild cognitive impairment," Lowrey told me. "When it comes to dementia, we do require that they have a diagnosis, but we don't try to measure where they are." Some people killed themselves early, out of caution. Others waited until they hit more of a gray zone. Brian's last dementia client had definitely been in the gray zone. He had been "pretty far along" and Brian had been troubled by the situation. "I convinced myself, as did the other guides, that the person understood what they were doing," he told me, "but it was a lot further than I would have liked to see."

When Brian and Lowrey entered Debra's home, they almost gasped aloud. In front of and all around them were immense quantities of very neatly organized junk: dozens of figurines and knickknacks, arranged in polished-glass cabinets and along windowsills. On the kitchen countertop, they saw a sea of pill and vitamin bottles, which Debra left out so that she would remember to take them. Before they started, Brian asked Debra to sign a piece of paper acknowledging that she had explored all her medical options and that she still wanted to proceed. Then Lowrey went through the standard FEN demonstration, using her own equipment, which she had brought from Portland so that she wouldn't have to touch Debra's supplies. It didn't take long, fifteen minutes maybe. It wasn't, as the guides told Debra, and Debra agreed, "rocket science." Lowrey showed Debra how to fashion a hood out of the plastic bag; how to attach the plastic tubing to the gas canister; how to snake the tubing up the bag. Debra practiced pulling the bag over her head and, just for a second, releasing the gas valve. The exit guides wanted her to see that breathing inert gas wouldn't feel like suffocating or drowning. It would just feel like normal breathing until, after a minute or so, she wouldn't feel anything at all.

In their training, Brian and Lowrey had learned that there were options when it came to dealing with suicide equipment after an exit. If the client was very sick and close to death, the exit guides might agree to dispose of the gas tank and tubing—usually in industrial dumpsters, some distance from the client's home—so that the death would look natural. If this were the case, family members should be advised on how to report the death to authorities. They might want to leave the house and go to a shop to buy something, making sure to pick up a receipt, in case they later needed an alibi—and then return home, drop the receipt on the counter, and call 911. They should say something along the lines of, "I just came home from the store and my mom is not breathing." Or, "She's cold! She's blue!" The police and the fire department would arrive quickly. The officers might look around for a while, but they probably wouldn't stay long. The family members should remain calm and remember that nitrogen gas is not detectable in typical autopsies.

When a natural death was not imminent, exit guides were meant to leave the equipment in place, so that the death would look like a suicide. That way, nobody would get in trouble. Ideally, the client would leave a suicide note: *After careful thought and deliberation, I have made a choice to end my life.* In these situations, family members should definitely have alibis. And they should wait a few hours before calling the police. Dementia cases like Debra's fell into this category. If Debra chose to exit, authorities would find her body with the plastic bag still over her head.

When Lowrey finished the demonstration, Debra said she felt great. She loved Brian and she especially loved Lowrey. They were such nice people! The guides chatted with her for a while and looked at some old photographs of David. They remarked on her beautiful view. But they didn't stay long. That wasn't the point. On their way out, the guides reminded Debra that she needed to come up with a plan for the discovery of her body. "That's part of what we do," Lowrey told me. "We don't want somebody accidentally stumbling across a death scene that they're not expecting." The exit guides could close the curtains before they left the house, but they could not be the ones to alert the authorities.

In most FEN deaths, clients had a loved one or two to help them along: a spouse or child or friend who could be present throughout the planning process and who could call the police—sometimes in feigned panic—to report the suicide. In recent years, exit guides had started to insist on this, in part because it was nicer for the client to have emotional support, but also as a way of insulating the network from the legal wrath of aggrieved family members. When FEN had gotten in trouble in the past, clients had killed themselves without telling those they loved, or without their approval. "People certainly don't need the permission of their family to do this," one senior guide told me, "but we have to know that the family knows of their decision and will not try to stop them." But Debra had no one to tell.

Debra's scattering of acquaintances had not reacted to her diagnosis in the way she supposed they would. They didn't seem to feel that bad for her. Her friend Dean thought she still seemed "very sharp to me, with language and all that." Robin also thought she sounded normal. They were all getting older, weren't they? They all forgot things. Robin thought that Debra's opioid painkillers, which she'd started taking after the car accident, were slowing down her mind as much as the dementia was. She also thought that Debra had lost the will to live when David died.

Her friends' incredulity enraged Debra and tended to provoke frenzied diatribes about the many cognitive screw-ups that she experienced in the course of a day. There were the lost hours. The lost words. The time she dropped the bottle of balsamic vinegar because she forgot that she was holding it. The time she forgot how to apply eye shadow and needed to watch a YouTube makeup tutorial to learn again. The time she forgot how to swallow. The taxes! They used to take days and were now taking weeks. And how was she supposed to prove anything, anyway? How could Debra show evidence of the small holes appearing in her consciousness? She *knew* the holes existed, because she felt them, but she couldn't recall exactly how they had once been filled—and with what mental material. "It's not like I've lost a leg and you can see that I've lost a leg," Debra jeered. "They can't even tell how bad my disease is until I'm dead and then they can slice my brain open. . . . I would never lie. I don't like people who lie in the first place. Why would you lie about your medical condition? That's so stupid. . . . I'm not lying. I just choose not to let people see the bad side of me. The broken side." Debra didn't tell her friends about the exit guides or what she was planning, though she started leaving hints. She told Robin how she had put down her dog in February, because the dog was suffering, and didn't Robin agree that when you love somebody, you can't just watch her suffer?

One morning in mid-March, Debra and I sat at her kitchen table eating breakfast burritos. She had moved the tax forms out of the way, but the surface was cluttered with tablecloths and decorative crocheted

coverings and patterned napkins. Debra faced the window, looking out
at the water, in a gray tracksuit and dangly silver earrings, her swollen
legs propped up on a footstool next to my chair. When her phone beeped,
Debra glanced at it briefly and then took two pills from a plastic pillbox
in her handbag. She had called early that morning to warn me that she
wouldn't be wearing makeup when I arrived. "Au naturel!" she said.
She looked older without her painted-on eyebrows. She asked me to get
the green taco sauce from the fridge.

The night before, Debra said, it had occurred to her that I was writing
a sort of biography of her life. It made sense, now, why I had asked so
many questions about her childhood and her mother. Debra asked if she
was going to be a chapter in my book and I said that she might. I asked
if that was OK, and she said that it was. Then she told me that she had
worked out a plan for the post-exit discovery of her body. It went like
this: Debra would tell Robin that she was feeling unsteady and was worried about falling, and she would ask her friend to start checking in on
her every day, by phone. If Debra didn't answer the phone or the doorbell, Robin should know that something was wrong and she should call
the police. "I don't want my body lying around here for hours on end,"
Debra said. "I think of decomposing."

I asked Debra how she thought her friends and faraway cousins
would feel after she was dead. Some would be disappointed, she granted.
But she wasn't close to them anyway. They would understand or they
wouldn't. If they didn't, "it's not my problem."

After breakfast, Debra said there was something she wanted to show
me, and she slipped an old tape into her VCR and turned on the kitchen
television. On the screen, an image of a younger, more made-up Debra
appeared. She was in her early thirties and had just been promoted at the
phone company and had enrolled in a public speaking course, which was
taped for instructional purposes. In the video, off-screen teachers called
out tips to "Debbie." Smile more, they said. As the videotape Debbie began her mock sales pitch, real-life Debra shook her head at the kitchen

table beside me. "The first thing I'm doing wrong is I have my hands in my pockets," she scoffed.

Debra watched the video all the way through, her face turned up toward the screen. "Cheesy," she whispered whenever thirty-something Debbie said something hackneyed or cute. I watched Debra, watching Debbie, and said nothing.

Before I left, Debra showed me the spot by the living room window where she planned to kill herself: overlooking the beach and the waves. On the phone, Brian had told her that she should start thinking about her final hours in more detail. What kind of music did she want playing? What about a last meal? But all Debra wanted was to have a photo of David beside her and for her last sight to be of the water. Already, Debra was checking the weather forecasts every day and praying for clear skies. But the weeks ahead were filled with rain.

No American state has seriously considered the idea of extending aid in dying to dementia patients, and no major American lobby group is advocating for it. Compassion & Choices CEO Kim Callinan told me that her organization has no interest in expanding the Death with Dignity Act's eligibility criteria. This is largely a matter of philosophy; Callinan does not think that a person with compromised mental capacity should be helped to die, though she does think that people with dementia should be empowered to refuse, in advance, aggressive medical treatment. But it's also a matter of tactics. "Politically, it's hard enough to get laws passed that have *these* requirements," she said. Compassion & Choices is committed to the enormous task of passing Death with Dignity laws in the states where they do not exist, and in Callinan's view, this means replicating the tried-and-tested Oregon model. Here, the Final Network Exit is not always helpful. "Talking about death is already hard, so when you start talking about death with gas tanks and plastic bags . . ."

In states like Oregon, elderly residents are sometimes confused about the law's limitations. They know, in a vague sort of way, that assisted dying is legal in their state, and to the extent that they ever think about it, they assume it can be used to stop dementia. They're distraught when they learn otherwise. FEN's former president Janis Landis has written about this misplaced faith on the network's website. "If you can't obtain the benefit, then the law is worse than useless: it promises a feeling of 'our work is done' when the reality could not be further from the truth."

But advocates also know that any expansion of Oregon's eligibility criteria to include dementia patients will fulfill the darkest prophecies of right-to-die opponents, who warn that after Death with Dignity laws are passed, they will inevitably be expanded to include more kinds of patients, starting with the most vulnerable and least self-assured—until a narrow right to physician-assisted death for terminally ill people becomes a near obligation to die for anyone who is dependent on others for care. Or at least, in this case, the normal and expected thing for someone with dementia to do. Wouldn't greedy or distressed family members encourage it? Even if they didn't, wouldn't the selfless patient feel bound to choose death, before she drained the people she loved of more money and time and patience?

In 2015, when an Oregon legislator named Mitch Greenlick introduced a bill to amend the Death with Dignity Act—extending the terminal prognosis requirement from six months to twelve months—Compassion & Choices lobbied against it. The bill went nowhere. In January 2019, Greenlick introduced another bill that would have broadened the law's definition of "terminal disease" in a way that, he hoped, would qualify people with dementia. Compassion & Choices opposed this proposal, too. It also failed. Senator Greenlick told me that his efforts were inspired by the suicide of an esteemed Oregon lobbyist. "He got a diagnosis of Alzheimer's. Then he went down to the nearest police station and shot himself in the bushes. And that just horrified me. That it was the only way he could deal with the situation."

In Belgium and the Netherlands, an early-stage dementia patient can qualify under the country's assisted-dying law, provided that her request is "voluntary" and "well considered" and that she is mentally competent at the time of her death. Dr. Peter De Deyn, a Belgian neurologist at the University of Antwerp, told me that when one of his patients is interested in assisted dying, he will meet with her at regular intervals to make sure that she is "still capable of making decisions." Dr. De Deyn promises to say "when the moment is getting doubtful. . . . But of course, it's not an on-off switch. Demented or not demented. It's a process." How close an individual person is willing to cut it will depend on temperament and circumstance. A patient can miss her chance if she waits too long, but once she is approved there is no such thing, legally, as too soon—and it is not the job of any doctor or bureaucrat to insist that there is still plenty of good time left. There are only more finite questions: How demented is too demented? Is she lucid enough?

Between 2002 and 2013, sixty-two Belgians with dementia diagnoses died this way: "preventatively," to quote medical reports. But these patients ask something difficult of their doctors. Physicians are, after all, taught to treat symptoms. When the dementia patients ask to die, however, they are often not suffering physically at all—or, not much. If they can be said to suffer, it is from fear of future suffering. According to a 2016 report on early-stage dementia sufferers in Belgium and the Netherlands published in the *Journal of Neurology*, "the loss of dignity, the knowledge that the lasting memory of their loved ones will be of the decomposed version of oneself, causes them to suffer now. This is definitely the main reason for those who opt for euthanasia in the early stage of the disease." These patients are hedging their bets: making guesses about how and when their future selves will hurt. Those who opt for euthanasia are betting that they will fare poorly—that their future selves will not accommodate to things. But some doctors, even ones who largely approve of physician-assisted death, have said that they want nothing to do with this sort of prophylactic medicine.

In the Netherlands, where euthanasia now accounts for more than 4 percent of total deaths in the country, the law goes further. There, a patient with very advanced dementia can be euthanized at an agreed-upon moment, if he has left written instructions in an advance healthcare directive—and if he appears, to his physician, to be "suffering unbearably" at the time of his death. The moment might vary from patient to patient: when he has lost the ability to speak, say, or when he does not recognize his wife. Dutch doctors are allowed to euthanize a patient by injection, even if he is "no longer able to communicate." According to the Dutch euthanasia review committee's code of practice guide, a doctor in this situation must "interpret the patient's behavior and utterances" and watch for any physical signs "that the patient no longer wishes his life to be terminated."

In fact, many physicians have refused to carry out these preordered deaths: some because they can't imagine filling a syringe with lethal drugs and then pushing it into a patient who is awake but has no idea what is happening. In 2017, more than two hundred doctors took out an advertisement in a Dutch newspaper to declare themselves opposed to the practice. "Our moral reluctance to end the life of a defenseless human being is too big," they wrote. Some object to the law in principle; they question what constitutes "suffering" in a state of profound cognitive loss. Do deeply demented patients really suffer? What about the ones who seem oblivious but happy? Even Jacob Kohnstamm, head of the country's euthanasia review committee, appears equivocal. "The unbearable suffering can often not be identified in these patients," he has said. Kohnstamm urges would-be euthanasia recipients to act early, before they lose themselves and must rely wholly on ambivalent physicians. "Decide for yourself five minutes before midnight, rather than five minutes after midnight." In 2018, 146 dementia patients received euthanasia in the country, but only 2 of them were in the late stages of the disease.

The Dutch Association for Voluntary Ending of Life (Nederlandse Vereniging voor een Vrijwillig Levenseinde; NVVE) has referred to this widespread reticence among the country's medical practitioners as a tragedy and a fundamental dishonesty. "People sign such [advance declarations] with conviction," said Robert Schurink, NVVE's director. "They think that it is settled. But as soon as they pass the time of mental competence, doctors suddenly don't want to anymore." The law is rendered meaningless by doctors who make big promises to their patients but then don't want to get their hands dirty.

On the ground in Amsterdam, the working through of these competing moral impulses has been taxing. One landmark case, later investigated by authorities, involved a seventy-four-year-old woman who lived in a nursing facility where, according to medical reports, she spent her days fitfully: wandering the halls, angry and restless and missing her husband. She was so demented that she could not recognize her own reflection in a mirror. In an imprecisely worded living will, the woman had written that she wanted to make use of the country's euthanasia law "whenever I think the time is right" and "at the time when the quality of my life has become so poor." Later, though, as her dementia progressed, she seemed to grow disinterested in the prospect. When the patient was asked if she still wanted to die, she responded, "It's not so bad yet."

Still, a euthanasia was scheduled, and on the planned date, the woman's doctor agreed to go forward with the procedure. She began by drugging the patient: furtively slipping a sedative into her coffee without her knowledge. Then she prepared the lethal injection—only, when she moved to administer it, the patient recoiled, as if she were trying to get up. The doctor asked the woman's husband and child to restrain her and then completed the injection. The woman died. Afterward, authorities from the euthanasia review committee judged that the physician had "crossed a line" by failing to stop the euthanasia when the patient pulled away, though they acknowledged that the woman's movements may simply have been an automatic response to the prick of the needle. A childlike wince.

For her part, the doctor said she was simply carrying out the patient's written request. She also said that she didn't find the patient's behavior on the day of her death to be particularly relevant anyway—since it was the living will, written when the woman was still lucid, that mattered most and was most expressive of her true preferences. "Even if the patient had said at that moment: 'I don't want to die,' the physician would have continued," the review committee determined. She would have continued even if the patient had been smiling. (The physician was initially charged but in 2019 was acquitted.)

Whether or not the doctor's actions were justified depends, in part, on how "the patient" in the story is defined. Was she the spaced-out woman who seemed, at best, indifferent to her death, on the day she pulled away from the lethal injection? Or was she the same woman as she had existed years earlier: the clear-minded author of the advance directive? Critics of the Dutch law have challenged the idea that a competent patient should be able to assume irrevocable decision-making power over a future, incompetent version of herself, even as she fades away and the new self comes into being. Dutch doctors continue to debate whether these two versions of the patient, the "then-self" before dementia and the "now-self" after dementia, are even the same person. If they are not, then why does one get to dictate choices for the other?

Those in the business of debating such questions usually look for guidance from the late legal scholar Ronald Dworkin and his 1993 book *Life's Dominion*. In the book, Dworkin made a distinction between "experiential" and "critical" interests. An experiential interest, in Dworkin's formulation, was corporal and reactive: the pleasure of a delicious meal or the comfort of a warm bath. A critical interest was more sophisticated and more essential to the personality of the interest holder. It was about how a person wanted his life to play out. His desires, his ambitions, and his estimations of what made life meaningful. In the case of advanced dementia, Dworkin noted, critical interests tend to fade, leaving only the experiential. So the question becomes: Which interests deserve to be honored and, in turn, which version of the patient? The demented person as she is, or as she was? Dworkin argued that critical interests must be respected, because it was those interests that gave human life its intrinsic dignity—that made life "sacred," even in the absence of a spiritual divine. He wrote, "People think it important not just that their lives contain a variety of the right experiences, achievements and connections, but that it have a structure that expresses a coherent choice among these." Human dignity was secured by a kind of narrative consistency.

But some are disturbed by Dworkin's thinking. They accuse him of holding too limited an understanding of meaning. Couldn't the tinier pleasures of experience be sources of deep meaning, even if they aren't part of a sophisticated, critical life plan—even if, a few years earlier, the person in question would have been horrified to draw pleasure from such a tiny thing? Detractors have asked why we should privilege the critical judgments of a being who effectively no longer exists over the expressed desires of a person who is with us here, now. Why not, instead, think of the person with dementia as a new person, unconstrained by the choices of any past self? On a practical level, what authority could the previous version of a patient, long gone, possibly have over her now?

In Canada, lawmakers have debated whether to expand the country's legislation to allow "advance requests for medical assistance in dying." According to a 2016 poll, an overwhelming 80 percent of Canadians agree that people should be able to consent, in advance, to assisted deaths if their medical conditions are very serious: "for example, if a patient has a diagnosis of dementia and requests to have assistance to die when they become bedridden and unable to bathe, shave and toilet themselves." Even in the absence of any formal legal change, some insurgent west coast doctors had gone ahead and adopted a looser reading of the rules—and in particular the definition of a "reasonably foreseeable" death. In 2019, Canadian newspapers reported that several dementia patients in British Columbia had died with the help of their doctors. One was a retired civil servant named Mary Wilson who, in another life, could recite the names and ascension dates of every British monarch dating back to 1066, but at the time of her death forgot two of her three children. When I asked

Shanaaz Gokool, then director of Death with Dignity Canada, whether the tension playing out in Belgium and the Netherlands over the very same issue worried her, she was unwavering. "You do as much as you can with the information you have to mitigate against harm," she said, "but you don't exclude a whole category of patients because there have been some problems in Belgium."

From the start, the Final Exit Network accepted clients with early-stage dementia. "Alzheimer's was always, in my mind, one of the most important areas we could work in. Still is," Faye Girsh, FEN's cofounder, told me. But Girsh admitted that clients with dementia present their own unique challenges: For instance, you can teach them how to use the nitrogen canister, but they might not remember afterward. "They find out everything and then they are ready to go—and they've forgotten what they've learned!"

ONE COOL MORNING IN mid-March, Debra woke up and did not know where she was. "Seconds. The longest seconds that I can imagine." Then she remembered. "And then I went, 'Oh.' Then I went, 'Fuck.' Because you realize what you're forgetting." A friend told Debra that she should write a note and tape it to her bathroom mirror: *DEBRA, YOU ARE DEBRA. THIS IS YOUR HOME. YOU ARE SAFE.*

She said she wasn't wavering. She said she had taken stock of her life as it was and could see only bad omens ahead. Debra started talking to God for the first time in years. "I said, I *really* need a strong message. You know, one way or the other I need to know. Either you put a light at the end of the tunnel that says it's not time for me to go or you point it in the direction that makes me understand that it *is* time."

One Saturday, Debra woke up and felt like she was a decade younger. "I was firing on all cylinders." She could multitask again. She did laundry while she watched television. She started writing goodbye letters to the people she knew. Everything was vivid. But then, the next day, she felt like crap again. "I just went from smart to dumb. I went from eight cylinders down to maybe one. . . . Oh thanks, God." Debra thought that God had given her one last good day so that she could see how far she had fallen. She thought the stars were aligning around her choice. "Aligning. Is that how they word it?" It seemed to me that Debra's faith had become liquid—able to fill whatever hollows of doubt opened up, as the weeks moved forward. God was finding new ways to deliver her messages, and she in turn was finding new ways to receive them. The broken boiler was a sign. The bottle of balsamic vinegar that she dropped on the kitchen floor was a sign. The letters from the mortgage company, addressed to David, which Debra nervously sent on to her estate lawyer, were also signs.

By the end of March, Debra was spending up to six hours a day on her taxes. "I've lost my way," she said. Most mornings found her on the phone with TurboTax, waiting on hold and then, when it was her turn, pleading for customer service help.

Though Debra spoke often of her taxes, it took some time before I could bring myself to ask the obvious question—the one I knew I had to ask but that she wouldn't like. "I guess what I'm asking is, is this a stalling tactic, or . . . ?"

"No." Debra cut me off briskly. Later, she said, "The thing that is keeping me alive, choosing not to exit right now at this moment, is the fact that I am the type of person that will not leave my estate a frigging mess."

Debra was dismissive of the hypotheticals I sometimes lobbed her way, questions about whether she would stay if David were alive or if she had enough money to keep the home. "If I had money and people who I cared about and cared for me, then I would," she said. "But I don't." Another time, she demanded, "How would you feel if you knew that you were no longer going to be you? That you could not write this book? That you couldn't put into words, on paper, what you're thinking in your head because your brain isn't allowing it anymore? It comes down to dignity." Sometimes, Debra said that if she were a dog, she would have been put out of her misery long ago. Once, she asked me: If she were my dog, wouldn't I put her down?

I called Brian because I felt anxious about things. I worried about how much Debra worried about money and the house; about how alone she seemed, and at the same time how certain she was that she would meet David again in the afterlife. How much she looked forward to that. "She is doing this because she doesn't want to lose herself," Brian said firmly. "It took her eight weeks to do her taxes, whereas it usually takes two days." Anyway, he said, it wasn't really FEN's business if other factors pushed and pulled at an exit decision. "I think loneliness *is* a big factor. Not wanting to be a burden is a big factor. There are a lot of factors that weigh in, and I think it's easy to assume that one of those is playing a bigger role than another. I try not to get into that."

"What kind of society do we live in to make people feel like burdens?" I asked faintly.

"I think the argument about being a burden is easy to talk about intellectually, until the time comes when it's *you* that is there, and feels like your kids are going to have to spend their money, their time—or that you are going to live in some tiny nursing home and have people come and wipe your ass." Brian paused. "Tell me this: Why would anybody who is seventy-five or eighty-five years old want to live in pain? Or suffer? . . . Why would any rational person?"

"Financial stuff comes up. It's all part of the picture," Lowrey agreed when I called her. "One hates to have that be a complicating factor, but, I mean, illness and financial trouble go together. It's not uncommon." What else could she do but accept that? What would the alternative even be? "If somebody qualifies, I'm not going to say, 'No, I'm not going to help you because you're not financially sound.'" The answer to the problem, Lowrey said, was not to give poor people fewer options. "People don't want to be moved into state housing. We want to stay in our homes and that is a strong component of dignity that people really value. . . . Whether one is going to lose one's house because one's mind is going or whether one is going to lose one's house because one's finances are going, those are actually similar life indignities."

But what about how sad Debra sometimes seemed? Lowrey spoke carefully. "We don't accept clients on a mental health basis alone," she said. "But it's normal to see a bit of depression."

IN A SAFE NEAR THE front of her house, Debra had stashed several months' worth of medication; pain pills that she and David hoarded over many years, by skipping a pill here and there or by refilling a prescription a few days early, when the pharmacist wasn't keeping track. It had been David's idea. If there was some kind of national emergency, he said, they could live off their stockpile. Now Debra had enough medication to keep her going, which meant that she could stop seeing her doctor. This was important, because Debra didn't want anyone noticing how demented she was and calling the authorities and forcing her into a facility. When the secretary at the doctor's office called to remind Debra that she was due for an appointment, she did not return the call.

She started shredding documents and old photographs, deleting emails and text messages. From her friends. From FEN. From me. She didn't want strangers rifling through her business when she was gone. She didn't want anyone to get into trouble. Debra had planned to write goodbye letters to the people she knew, but she soon gave up. It was too tiring. She also stopped watching the news in the evenings. Once, she and David had watched television side by side; she always irritated him by talking over the broadcasts. But now she didn't care. Anyway, Debra thought the world was hurtling toward Armageddon. Moral corruption. Global destruction. China, Iran, kids killing kids. Did I think the Treasury was capable of paying back America's debts? Did I know that a portion of Africa was running out of water? She had grown afraid of the world, and for the world.

"It's very difficult for people to understand what I'm going through, because what you see and what you hear is not the real me," Debra told me, her voice high and quaking. "You see a fake. I put on a face for you. . . . David was the only one that saw the real me."

"I definitely don't claim to understand at all," I said, wavering a little.

"No, you don't. It's unfortunate. Because you're writing about a subject and . . . What's the word? Being able to step into that person's shoes would be a tremendous benefit. If you could put yourself in my shoes."

At the end of March, Debra said that she was getting worse. "I notice that I'm losing words," she said. "Am I stumbling with words?"

I paused. "No."

"So I am still like I was at the beginning?"

"For as long as I have been talking to you."

ON APRIL 17, DEBRA woke early and ate a carton of coconut-flavored Greek yogurt in the kitchen and then spent some time wheeling around the house, looking at all of her belongings. She looked out the window, too. For weeks, it had been raining, but now the weather was fine. Debra had finished her taxes. "It took weeks," she told me. "Not *a* week. Weeks." Brian and Lowrey had told her to expect a range of emotions in her final hours and she did. "I get panic attacks all the time, so I took a Xanax and said, 'Quiet down.'"

"You took a Xanax today?"

"Oh yeah. I needed to focus. And get the jitters in my hands to stop trembling."

In her final hours, I had expected Debra to be different somehow. Lighter, maybe. But Debra was just ready to go in the same way that she had been ready to go for months. She talked about the mortgage company and how it had "screwed with us." She asked me if I owned a cat. She wondered aloud whether she should strip the data off her iPad, so that she could give it to one of David's old friends, but she wasn't sure how to. "I'm now leaving a complete void," she said.

"I wish you peaceful travels, Debra," I said.

When Brian and Lowrey arrived from Portland around 8 a.m., Debra had already taped letters to the door with Scotch tape. One was addressed to Robin, telling her not to come inside and to call the police, and also thanking her for her friendship. Robin would find it when she came that day to drop off Debra's mail. Another letter was addressed to the authorities.

Inside, the exit guides saw the bag and the gas canister waiting by the living room window, beside a small table that Debra had covered with pictures of David and their dogs. Brian told Debra that she didn't have to go through with it. She could change her mind. They could leave. No big deal. But Debra said, "Let's do this." So Brian and Lowrey each hugged her. Then they knelt down on either side of the wheelchair. Debra did not cry.

That afternoon, the Tillamook County Sheriff's Office received a call from a woman named Robin about a possible suicide in Pacific City. It took the sergeants and one sheriff a half hour to drive to the house. It was 2:01 p.m. when they opened the note from Debra, telling them where to find a key to the front door. When the officers stepped inside, they found yellow Post-it notes on everything. There was a note on the bed frame explaining that Debra had bought it at an estate sale in California. There was a note on the dryer indicating its temperature range. There were notes on some of David's antiques advising that they were valuable. *Don't sell it for nothing.*

Lieutenant Jim Horton observed that this wasn't the kind of thing you run into every day—but then again, he had run into things like this before. After looking through the apartment for several hours, Horton and his colleagues agreed that nothing looked amiss. It seemed obvious that Debra had known what she was doing and that "she had done it completely independently."

Later, Lieutenant Horton told me, there was just one thing he found hard to shake. A strange thing. It was nice out on the day that Debra died, but all the curtains were drawn.

5

Mind

On March 6, 2017, Adam Maier-Clayton logged on to Facebook and pressed the button to go live.

"Can anyone hear me?"

Someone commented that he could hear just fine and Adam adjusted the angle of his laptop. "We're going to have a very important discussion in just one second," he said. "A once-in-a-lifetime opportunity." Adam leaned forward so that his face, which was uncommonly beautiful—angled and severe, like it belonged to a sculpture—was close to the camera. "Up front, I'm going to say you don't have to worry about anything in terms of . . . Uh, you're not going to see anything bad." By this, Adam meant that he would not kill himself on-camera. He worried that if he did, Facebook would take down the video, and he wanted the video to live on after his death and to go viral. Instead, he would kill himself afterward. Adam's hair was pulled back into a ponytail and around his neck he wore a silver pendant; it was a circle with an *A* carved into it, not for "Adam," but for "atheist." Behind him, his Facebook viewers could see light blue walls and a tidy hotel-room bed.

"OK. So yeah. . . . I've planned this out intricately. I've planned everything from the last song to the last meal. I went to Pita Pit. That was so good. . . . But yeah, it's weird to be in this position. I'm twenty-seven years old and I never ever thought that something like this would happen to my life." Adam said that he had ordered poison from China and that it was resting a few inches from his keyboard. That was good, he said, because otherwise he would have had to jump off a building or something. "Something involving gravity and instantaneous demise."

"Adam this is so tragic," wrote one commenter. "<3"

"Did you say this is your last one?" wrote someone named Kyle.

"Yes," someone replied to Kyle. "He said it's his last."

As he often did in his Facebook and YouTube videos, Adam started with a run-through of his afflictions: generalized anxiety disorder, obsession, depression. "OCD is a demon," he said. "Some people are dealt genetic cards that are going to make their existence sheer hell. And I am absolutely one of those people." But soon he shifted to politics, because really, that was the point of the exercise. If he was going to kill himself, his suicide was going to be political.

"This whole idea that mental health should never qualify for medical assistance in dying is simply primitive. It's absolutely primitive," Adam said. "It puts physical illness, especially terminal illness, on a pedestal. And it ignores other illnesses. . . . It's bullshit, OK?" People like him, he said—people with long and tangled histories of mental disorder and psychiatric treatment—had been "screwed over" by the Canadian government when they were excluded from accessing the country's assisted-dying law. Adam said that was wrong. He blamed Prime Minister Justin Trudeau. "It's nonsensical. If someone can't get better, scientifically, and they have been suffering and they want out . . ." He threw up his hands. "What's the issue? It's not *your* life. It's *theirs*. . . . I've said it a gazillion times."

At the start of his livestream, Adam warned that he planned to talk for a while, because he had a lot of concluding things to say. Soon an hour passed, and then a second. Adam said he was in physical pain from speaking so much, and sometimes he rested his head in his hands for a while. Twice he excused himself to go to the bathroom and walked out of the frame. Adam talked about therapy and its failures. He talked about psychiatric science and its failures. He talked about how great it felt to be sharing everything he knew. To be educating society. "Frankly, I wish I would have made more YouTube videos," he said. At times, his voice had a hyper edge to it, but most of the time it was flat and studiously formal. "I'm very, very sick," Adam said. "There's no cure. I have no future. . . . I can't even work at McDonald's. I didn't work my ass off my whole life to live on disability." He had wanted to work at a bank or a hedge fund or a Fortune 500 company. He had wanted to own skyscrapers and be a financial industry baller. But instead, his mind had gone to war with his body—and now here he was.

I was watching the livestream from my apartment, my knees pulled into my chest. I felt sick. *Really pale*, I wrote in my notebook. *Stalling? Or performing.*

"There's so much beauty, even in this room," Adam said, almost two and a half hours in, when his voice was starting to crack. "I mean, look at this light switch. Electricity." After a few minutes, he cried a bit and said he hoped his mom and dad would be OK. He said he didn't want to hurt anyone.

And then Adam signed off.

A nine-hour drive northeast, in Ottawa, Adam's mother, Maggie, sat in front of her laptop, freaking out. She couldn't look away from the screen. "I didn't know if it was real," she told me later. "I didn't know if he was going to do it. . . . When people talk all the time, you think, 'They're not going to do it.' Usually, when people do it, they don't talk. They just go and they do it." Maggie hoped that Adam wouldn't do it. She grabbed her phone and tried to call Adam's father, but he didn't pick up.

Back in Windsor, Graham Clayton was midway through delivering a lecture to his fourth-year economics class at the University of Windsor. When the police officers knocked on the door, Graham told his students that he would be back in just a minute and then stepped into the hallway. "Do you know where your son is?" one officer asked. No. "When was the last time you saw him?" Yesterday. The two cops told Graham that they had traced Adam to London, Ontario, but that they hadn't found him yet. He seemed to be at a hotel. They said something about Facebook. Graham, who speaks with a hard-to-place accent—east coast Canadian, with flecks of British left over from his childhood in the English Midlands—told the officers that he didn't know what Adam was planning to do that day but that he had been threatening "rational suicide" for months on social media. When the officers left, Graham went back into the classroom to finish the last half hour of his class.

"One day," Adam had told him a few months earlier, "you'll get up and I'll be gone."

"When you can't take it any longer," Graham had said, "don't hang in there for me or for anybody else." Graham thought his son had fought for long enough. They were both tired.

By then, Adam had become, in his own words, "the most visible right-to-die activist who stands up and represents mental illness." He was a poster boy: the face of a political push to expand Canada's aid-in-dying law to include patients who suffered from psychiatric disorders but were not terminally ill. In an op-ed in the *Globe and Mail* in May 2016, Adam had written that "physical illness and mental illness can actually induce the same amount of pain. The only difference is the pain in a physical illness has a physical pathology. In a mental illness, the pain is called psychosomatic pain. To the patient, it feels exactly the same." Suffering was suffering, Adam said. Why should mediocre technocrats in Ottawa get to privilege one kind over the other?

After finishing his lecture, Graham waited for his students to leave the classroom and then drove home, away from the unlovely urban campus and along the river separating Windsor from Detroit. He passed tiny parks, where Canada geese gathered in the spring and fall, and low-rise, low-budget apartment complexes, until the streets turned more suburban and he was home. When he walked inside, he found his mother in the living room and told her what had happened. She was nearly ninety and nearly deaf, so he had to shout it at her. Then he poured himself a cup of tea and sat down at the round wooden table in the kitchen and waited under the yellow light.

Eventually the phone rang; it was Adam. The police had found him at the hotel room—and in a panic, Adam had flushed his pentobarbital down the toilet. He had lost his chance. It was over. "So he's OK," said Graham softly, hanging up the phone. His gray mustache twitched and his eyebrows unfurled. "I don't know where we go from here, but anyway . . ." He took a breath. "It's a no-win situation here. It's such a bad situation that there's no winning. I lose my son or I watch my son suffer."

ADAM HAD BEEN A careful baby. When he was a toddler, Maggie wondered if she should cover up the electric outlets in her house with childproof plastic covers, like other mothers did, but she didn't need to. Adam knew not to touch. He was such a good boy that his parents didn't think much of it when, around age four, not long after Maggie and Graham divorced, Adam started making strange noises. They were almost like animal barks. "Adam, why are you doing that?" Graham asked his son. But Adam didn't know.

After a while, Adam stopped barking and started doing things with his hands. He had to maneuver his fingers in certain ways, in certain orders, over and over, because . . . The routines distracted him. *Do this. Do this. Do this.* When Adam started playing soccer competitively, he needed to move his fingers into just the right positions, or else he wouldn't be able to score and his team would lose, but if he moved them too much, he would forget to run after the ball. Adam sometimes taped his fingers together so that they could be still and he could focus on the game. He counted his baseball cards over and over and over.

It took a dozen more years for Adam to be diagnosed with obsessive-compulsive disorder and generalized anxiety disorder and given his first antidepressant. By then, his teenage mind was fizzing with terrible thoughts. At parties and at school, the thoughts told Adam that he had done something wrong. More than that, he had done something wrong on purpose and then forgot about it. Because he was bad. The thoughts said that everyone else knew what he had done and that they were judging him for it. Adam took the pills that the doctor gave him, even though Maggie didn't believe in psychiatric drugs or Big Medicine and she didn't want him to. Adam said the pills didn't help, though he never stayed on any given regimen for very long. He decided that if he wanted to be normal, he would have to beat the compulsions out of himself. He was sick of being "controlled by bullshit." Adam started doing exercises with his brain. When his brain told him to do something, he refused to do it. After a while, the thoughts quieted.

In 2011, Adam moved to Ottawa to start a college degree in business management. In high school he hadn't worked that hard, and he had sometimes been "a dickhead" to other people, but he intended to be different now. Adam wanted to work all the time. To be the kind of person who worked all the time. To be legitimately and also conspicuously obsessed with working. His metamorphosis was quick and deliberate. "I transformed from an ignorant jock," Adam told me. "I became very introspective. I wanted to be a better person." A serious person with a beautiful mind.

"MBA here I come," he wrote on Facebook in September 2011.

"New weekly ritual: one all-nighter a week—just to get that extra 8 hours of efficiency in #focused."

Adam decided that he would become a banker. Or something like a banker: a fund manager, for instance. The details of the dream were still bleary. And never mind that he was only at a second-rate college, studying for a diploma. The point was that, somehow, he would become someone with money and a nice, intelligent wife and adopted children from foreign countries. He would have nice cars, but not too many, because that would be obnoxious and also because he planned to give away tons of money to philanthropic causes. When Adam wasn't in class, he would sometimes drive around downtown Ottawa, past the Rideau Canal and the 1960s office towers, and imagine owning all the buildings he saw. After a while, it felt less like a dream and more like a preview of the future. Adam joined a fraternity and told Maggie—who sometimes worried about how intense her son was becoming but was also very proud of him—that Ronald Reagan was his frat brother.

Things were manageable, everyone would agree, until Adam got high. It was December 2012, at a frat party; Adam was twenty-three. He felt like he had to do it, like the other guys wanted to see what it would be like if uptight Adam, who had never even smoked a cigarette, got a bit messed up. Adam took a hit from someone's bong, and then another. And then it was night and everyone was high and Adam was on the floor, curled up in a fetal position, thinking he was dying.

When he woke the next morning, it seemed to Adam that all his friends were covered in wax. They looked like puppets instead of people, or like fake people masquerading as real ones. When he looked down at a table, it looked like a block of wood with some other blocks of wood. At one level, Adam knew that it was a table, but it did not look quite like one, because all Adam could see were its component parts. Wood. Nails. He felt afloat—not like he was out of his body, but like he was too much in it. "I don't call it sadness," he told me later, of the feeling. "It's a soullessness." Adam didn't believe in souls, per se, but he still felt somehow as if he'd lost his.

"It literally fucked up his brain," Maggie said. When she went to pick up Adam from the party, she felt the strangeness, too. He was so out of it. The next day, it was the same. Maggie brought Adam to an emergency room. And then another. The doctors said he was just high. They said he'd be fine. But in the weeks that followed, the weird feeling stayed and the old obsessions returned. Maggie could feel them in the house. Some days, she said, Adam was "extremely aggressive." Other days, he cried and asked her to hold his hand. Adam met with more doctors, but nobody knew what was wrong with him. One said that he should see a psychiatrist but warned that with an outpatient referral, it could take months to get an appointment. Another told Adam that this was all in his head. It wasn't real. OK, fine, Adam said. So, what's your plan?

Finally, there was a diagnosis. "It's called depersonalization disorder," Adam wrote later on his blog. "It's when a human brain endures a sufficient amount of stress that it says, 'ok soldier, that's enough of that noise, we're taking a break' and dissociates as a defense mechanism. The brain literally pulls out all context, emotion, and feeling from everything you know and you are left feeling empty and foreign to everything you once knew." The diagnosis clicked with Adam. It explained everything. He had a depersonalized mind. On his blog, Adam wrote that a "marijuana induced panic attack" had triggered the onset of symptoms.

Then the awful pain came, and there were other diagnoses too: major depressive disorder, somatic symptom disorder. Adam had never heard of somatic pain before, but he read about it on a website. "According to one theory," the website read, "depression and anxiety are converted into physical symptoms. . . . It becomes almost impossible to tell which came first or where one leaves off and the other begins." To Adam, the order of things didn't really matter because his whole body hurt and his eyes burned, as if a tablespoon of acid was sloshing around in each eye socket. The obsessive thoughts grew louder, and the voices that carried them more brazen. Adam started seeing auras around streetlamps at night. "It's a shame how prevalent mental health issues are in today's society," he wrote on Facebook in October 2013. He thought that he had lost whatever chemical components make up human joy.

Adam started spending more time in Maggie's basement, which he filled with dark furniture and a mini-fridge, even when she begged him to "get out of this dungeon!" He didn't always shower. When he came upstairs for breakfast in the mornings, he no longer talked about what he was studying—the Rockefeller family or the American economy or the steel industry—but instead asked Maggie the same questions over and over. Stupid questions. The point was the repetition, not the answer. Maggie found a private therapist for Adam to see and agreed to pay for it, but Adam thought the therapy was useless. She wondered if she should try to get him admitted into a psychiatric hospital but decided against it. "Because what are they going to do? They are just going to put him on more drugs anyway." Maggie begged her son to try holistic therapies. Years ago, she had used alternative medicine to wean herself off alcohol and believed in its promises. Adam could take supplements to rebalance his physiology and detox his body, she said. She would send him to the best people. But Adam said no. Maggie thought her son had given up, that all he wanted to do "was bitch and complain all the time about how he was feeling." Adam, in turn, blamed Maggie. She was crazy, he said, and she had made him crazy.

Adam managed to graduate from college and get a job at a local bank branch. He liked the work, but in 2014, he quit. He said his physical symptoms—the mysterious aches and the burning and the fogginess— were distracting him from his tasks and that he couldn't focus on the clients in front of him. His fights with Maggie grew worse. One day, Adam took a baseball bat and smashed the furniture in his basement to splintered bits. Maggie sent him home to Windsor to live with his father, Graham, in a brick house that he shared with Adam's grandmother and her dozens of porcelain animal figurines.

He found new work as a bouncer at the Boom Boom Room. At night, he'd break up fights on the sidewalk, a few blocks from the cluster of chain hotels near the Caesars casino. After a while, he was promoted to bartender. He was glad to receive the promotion, even though he worried that the industrial cleaning soaps used by the bar staff were making him sicker. On his Facebook wall, Adam sometimes played himself like a frat guy. He bragged about his long shifts behind the bar. He griped about getting fat. He wished Happy Valentine's Day to his favorite porn site. Other times, he could be arrestingly sincere. "When I was young," he wrote, "I thought the world was more good than bad. However, the more I read, learn and experience, the less I believe that."

In real life, Adam was consumed by his strange sickness. He started seeing a psychiatrist, who started prescribing him drugs—and over many months, Adam took many things. Graham kept a list: Paxil, Zoloft, Ativan, Demerol, hydromorphone, gabapentin, Wellbutrin. Adam tried CBD oil. He tried cognitive behavioral therapy and acceptance and commitment therapy and mindfulness meditation. He tried rest: lying on the couch for hours of his day, watching BBC World Service and reading stuff on the Internet. But nothing made him feel well again. Adam started to wonder if there were some patients who couldn't be helped by modern medicine—and if he was one of those patients. He wondered what doctors would do, if he was. "Dad, as long as I'm alive, the doctors are going to keep trying to find something," Adam said.

"Don't give up. Don't give up," Graham said. "Hang in there. Hang in there. Let them help you."

But Adam's mind was already elsewhere. In June 2014, he logged in to Facebook. "After reading a few things I was curious," he wrote. "What are peoples' opinions on the 'right to die.'"

IN 2015, CANADA'S Supreme Court overturned the country's ban on assisted death, ruling it unconstitutional. The Canadian Parliament was given one year to translate the new judgment into law and to define its practical borders: who would be eligible and who would not. Lawmakers could be as expansive as the court allowed or add additional criteria and safeguards, narrowing the dimensions of access. Adam read the text of the Supreme Court decision closely and was surprised by it. It said that a competent Canadian resident had the right to physician-assisted death if he had a "grievous" and "irremediable" medical condition that caused him to "endure physical or psychological suffering that is intolerable." It said nothing about terminal illness or imminent death. There was no

requirement of a physical pathology at all; psychological suffering was
enough. The Canadian court seemed to care less about the cut-and-dried
particularities of a prognosis—how much life span was left, what part of
the body was diseased or broken—and more about the subjective experience of the patient, who alone could decide whether his suffering was un-
endurable. It seemed to Adam that the Canadian court had theoretically
cleared the way for an assisted-dying law that included him.

Almost immediately, the Parliament and press began debating the
limits of the would-be law, and in particular whether it should include
people whose primary sickness was psychological. The Federal Special
Joint Committee of the House and Senate on Physician-Assisted Dying
heard testimony from both sides. Proponents argued that the law should
be more elastic than its American equivalents in the kinds of suffering
it recognized. They cited reports showing that mental suffering could,
in some cases, be worse than physical pain. A large study of subjective
well-being in Germany, for instance, had found that only end-stage liver
disease was experienced as more severe than some mental disorders.

To the hardest-core advocates, the exclusion of mental illness was
not just overly cautious but also ethically dubious, because it privileged
physical over mental affliction. For years, healthcare officials had been
working to destigmatize mental illness, in part by disputing the notion
that mental illness was the fault of the sufferer or that it was somehow
less than physical pain. Or less real. Advocacy groups had also challenged
the perception that anyone with a mental illness was out of control or
out of his mind, and so unable to recognize his own interests, much less
act on them. They had made progress. But rejecting patients with mental
disorders from an assisted-dying law would seem to communicate, "Your
suffering is absolutely serious and real . . . unless you want to die, in which
case it is not. In that case, we know what's best for you."

In Toronto, Dr. Justine Dembo, a young psychiatrist with pale skin
and dark hair, followed the debate from Sunnybrook Hospital, which
had become famous for treating disabled soldiers after World War II.

Her third-floor office was small and sparse and cold and had a single window overlooking a garden built for the veterans. Its main feature was a glass bowl full of seashells and pebbles that patients could use to ground themselves when they got upset. Early on, Dembo decided that she was open to the broadest formulation of the law and to the possibility of one day helping her patients to die under it.

To Dembo, the idea that doctors should exclude patients with mental illnesses—presumably to protect them from themselves—was born of something even deeper than stigma or fear. It was instead evidence of professional hubris and of the particular obstinacy of psychiatrists, who never seemed willing to admit that some patients just could not be helped. Oncologists and lung specialists were, by contrast, used to surrendering battles: to acknowledging that surgery had failed or that another round of chemotherapy would be pointless. But psychiatrists still believed they could help everyone. There were always more drugs and drug combinations to try, and more therapy techniques to borrow from. And the treatments themselves had no obvious or preordained endpoints. They could go on and on and never end. Or maybe some new drug was just around the corner. Psychiatry, it seemed to Dembo, had lost sight of its own therapeutic limits. Or, at least, doctors were unwilling to acknowledge them and act accordingly.

The thought had come to her a few years earlier, during her residency. One day at the hospital, Dembo was asked to transfer a middle-aged female patient from her room, in the regular hospital ward, to an acute psychiatric unit, where she was being put under 24/7 observation because she had tried to kill herself. The patient had a long, knotted history of refractory depression. Over the course of her illness, she had tried almost every remedy on offer, including electroconvulsive therapy, in which small currents of electricity were passed through her brain to trigger brief seizures. Nothing had worked and now the side effects from all the drugs were getting worse. The woman looked at Dembo and her look was full of betrayal. "I had this feeling of guilt because I could see how desperately she was suffering. So part of me felt really bad about saving her," Dembo told me. "I had come to know her and she had disclosed to me, many times, how desperately she wanted to die—how long she had felt that way, how much she was suffering. It gave me pause. . . . Why are we rescuing people? Why is it an automatic response to intervene in a suicide if we've tried everything we can and someone is still suffering so severely and so chronically?"

Dembo already knew that some patients could search forever and never find anything that worked for long. In the famous Sequenced Treatment Alternatives to Relieve Depression (STAR*D) trial, published in 2006 in the *American Journal of Psychiatry*, researchers found that around 30 percent of people in outpatient care were still symptomatic after four consecutive medication courses. Among those who did respond, 71 percent relapsed within one year. Electroconvulsive therapy (ECT), a neurostimulation technique, was shown to help refractory patients about half of the time, but some people didn't want ECT because it needed to be administered under general anesthesia and could cause retrograde amnesia. Psychotherapy worked for some people and not others. The same was true for inpatient treatment programs and for rarely performed neurosurgical interventions like bilateral cingulotomy, in which surgeons cut or burned part of the patient's brain in a region that connects sensory experience with pleasant or unpleasant memories. Given this, Dembo asked, was it so irrational for some long-term psychiatry patients to conclude that their suffering would never be relieved by science?

The logical leap—that some people should be allowed to die—felt quick and almost traitorous. "In psychiatry," Dembo said, "you really learn that anyone who wants to die is suicidal and should be treated as such and prevented from suicide. In residency training and until very recently, there was no discussion at all about whether a wish to die could ever be a rational response to any illness, let alone a mental illness." Instead, when patients said they wanted to die, their plans were called "suicidal ideation" and taken to be proof of their sickness. Their psychiatrists, in turn, worked to subdue the thinking. That was literally the point of the job: to keep patients alive, to prevent suicide.

In 2010, a few years into her residency, Dembo wrote a searching paper about "treatment futility and assisted suicide in psychiatry." In it, she posed a string of questions: "At what level of probability of no improvement or no cure can we deem treatment 'futile'? Whose role is it to determine what constitutes 'futility' for any specific patient? How many side effects should we expect our patients to tolerate in the name of treatment? And, at what point do we allow our patients to give up on treatment and on life itself? At what point are we, as physicians, entitled to 'give up'?" While researching, Dembo had learned that some countries—Belgium, the Netherlands, Luxembourg, and Switzerland—already considered mental illness as a valid criterion for assisted death, in limited cases. This wasn't a ludicrous idea; there was precedent in Europe. "Is it, then, inconceivable that severe existential pain in the absence of physical illness could ever be a rational reason to consider ending one's life?"

Dembo knew that the vast majority of patients with diagnosed psychiatric disorders were capable of making rational decisions, as measured by standard capacity tests. A central tenet of psychiatry, in fact, is that patients are assumed to have "decisional capability" until and unless their behavior suggests otherwise. Deeply depressed people, for example, can in most cases understand their diagnoses and evaluate the consequences of one choice over another. Even someone in the throes of delusion can show insight and reason when her attention is focused on a specific choice, like whether or not to have knee surgery or undergo chemotherapy after a cancer diagnosis—or whether to buy a car or get married or go on vacation. In psychiatric settings, "capacity" is always judged in the context of a single choice, in a single moment. A person doesn't *have capacity* or *not have capacity*, in a holistic sense; rather, she is *capable* or *incapable* of making a specific decision. By this logic, many of Dembo's sickest patients were already considered capable of making all kinds of healthcare decisions.

Dembo presented her thinking at a grand rounds lecture at Toronto's Centre for Addiction and Mental Health. She wondered aloud what it would look like for psychiatrists to be intellectually open to the idea of assisted dying for incurable mental illness. She asked whether physician-assisted death could ever be considered a form of harm reduction. Some patients were likely to take their own lives; at least this way, they wouldn't die alone and in fear, and maybe in awful pain. After the talk, Dembo thought she might get in trouble for what she'd said. Instead, she was thanked by a few senior psychiatrists. "Don't tell anyone I said this," one whispered, "but I'm really glad you brought this up, because I have patients who I really wonder about."

But beyond the Toronto conference room, some psychiatrists were growing alarmed by the discussions playing out in Canada. Critics argued that patients with the most severe mental illnesses—the ones who were most likely to qualify under an assisted-dying law—were, by virtue of their conditions, not able to make decisions about matters as grave and permanent as death. They noted that the very fact of a severe depression could distort the way that a patient understood his prognosis, making him more likely to anticipate failure and interminable suffering. Because the patient's ability to reason was corrupted, his lethal longings could not be accepted as rational, much less be carried out by an acquiescent physician. They insisted that a patient's despair should never be treated as enlightened thought. Despair, by definition, was blind and reckless.

The most ardent detractors argued that assisting in the death of a psychiatric patient was akin to collaborating in an irrational suicide. To help such a patient, they said, would be to confuse the very symptoms of mental illness—a desire to die, despondence, fear of treatment, a parched sense of meaning—with rational thinking. It would be to recast the existential dread of a sick person into an expression of free will. "How can one distinguish a request for medical aid in dying to relieve the suffering caused by an illness from a symptom of that very illness?"

asked the psychiatrists Mona Gupta and Christian Desmarais in a paper later published in the *Journal of Ethics in Mental Health*. "In other words, how can one be sure that one is not unwittingly colluding with a person's pathology rather than respecting a person's well-considered judgment?"

Some believed that the existence of an expanded law would itself hurt patients. The thinking went that if an already fragile patient was given the option of assisted death, he would give up on life sooner, especially if his own doctors took his request seriously and, in doing so, seemed to validate the fact that his case was utterly hopeless. The very process of evaluating the patient's request could, in other words, influence the course of his mental illness and make it worse. An expression of interest in assisted death could become its own self-fulfilling prophecy. At scale, the effect on an already vulnerable patient group would be enormous. Broadening assisted death to patients with psychiatric conditions "sends a paradoxical societal signal," warned the Dutch physician Theo Boer. "If our citizens want to end their lives, we will try to keep them from doing so. However, when they insist, we will actually help them."

Others condemned the proposal on more practical grounds. They admonished Canadian politicians for even considering such an expansive law, given the state of mental healthcare in the country. "The fact is many mentally ill people live in terrible conditions of poverty and exclusion," wrote the Canadian psychiatrist John Maher in a later paper. "Are we pushing people towards wanting death and then perversely offering a legal path to that end? Shame on us if we are." Some imagined a dystopian future, in which time and resources and expectations were diverted away from mental healthcare and put toward the ultimately less expensive work of helping patients die.

It seemed obvious to Dembo that she could never know with complete certainty that any given patient was incurable. Anyone could be a one-in-a-million outlier, and some seemingly hopeless cases did take a turn for the better. People improved. But what was improvement anyway?

A patient might move up a point or two on a depression scale, in a way that a professional could measure, but still feel dreadful every day. The way it looked to Dembo, many psychiatrists were treating patients who had no reasonable prospect for substantial improvement, while enjoining those same patients not to give up hope that their hideous suffering might end. Was that morally correct? The bioethical consensus in other fields of medicine seemed to be that it was unethical for doctors to offer false hope. But some psychiatrists seemed ambivalent on the point, maybe because they believed that mentally ill patients needed hope in order to get better. That hope had its own therapeutic properties. "We thus find ourselves in a paradox in which hope is vital for recovery but may also lengthen lives of unbearable mental anguish," Dembo wrote in a 2013 paper. "What is an ethical therapist to do?"

Dembo started to imagine ways that her thinking could be converted into professional medical standards. Under her ideal formulation, a patient who was eligible for assisted death would have to demonstrate chronic suicidal thinking, as opposed to fleeting suicidal moods. He would also be subject to a waiting period of several months or even years after his request for death. He would have to have tried a certain number of evidence-based treatments, including medications and therapy, to make certain that his illness was unresponsive to them. The law would require that a patient had *tried*. Still, Dembo thought, no law could demand that a person try everything and anything. Even a patient with a severe psychiatric disorder had the right to say no. To say, enough is enough.

ADAM WAS THE ⁵RST patient to ask Dr. Giovanni Villella, a psychiatrist in Windsor, about assisted dying. It was the end of 2015, and Canadian parliamentarians were still formulating their aid-in-dying law. Adam had met Dr. Villella at the emergency room, where he'd gone in a moment of pain-racked panic, and Villella had agreed to see him in his private practice. Canada's universal healthcare system covered psychiatric care, but the waiting times to see specialists could be long and the visits could be limited, so some patients paid privately instead. Graham said he would pay. One day, Adam asked the doctor whether he thought that assisted dying should be an option for people who were sick like he was, in a mental way.

Dr. Villella, who sat at a large L-shaped desk and often typed into his computer while patients spoke, looked straight at Adam. He knew that he could never physically help a patient to die. He was a religious man and the act went against his faith. But he also didn't think that people who wanted assisted deaths were asking for anything wrong. In Villella's experience, a small fraction of patients—7 or 8 percent, maybe—were largely resistant to treatment. Fundamentally, he agreed with Adam that those patients had the right to a peaceful end. Only, Adam was so young. There were still things to try.

Adam had a low opinion of his psychiatrist. One of the first times we spoke, he told me that Villella seemed like "a very weak man. . . . He doesn't have a backbone. He is nothing like me." Still, Adam followed the doctor's instructions and took all his recommended medications. He tried one drug, and then, when he decided that it wasn't working, he weaned himself off it and tried something else, or had something added to the mix. Adam arranged his pill bottles in neat rows on top of his dresser and sometimes took handfuls of capsules in a single day. The gabapentin, he told me dryly, helped a bit with the psychomotor retardation; with it, he was able to get his mind moving faster in the morning. But overall, he thought the drugs only made him 5 percent better, which wasn't better enough. Later, a psychiatrist to whom I spoke about Adam's symptoms told me that gabapentin, which is sometimes prescribed for neuropathic pain, does not help with psychomotor retardation. She wondered if Adam's academic-sounding descriptions of his medications were "misguided."

Adam told Graham that he wasn't "going to let some psychiatrist take me on a joy ride." He wasn't going to adhere, forever, to a bull-shit "kitchen sink protocol," letting any doctor throw anything down his throat on a whim. And he would die 10,000 times before he tried deep brain stimulation. Adam said he had reviewed clinical studies of DBS and wasn't convinced that the treatment would help his cluster of disorders. He didn't know for sure, but sometimes you didn't need to try something to know that it would fail. Adam said it was like how a tiny country didn't need to declare war on the United States to know that if it did, America would "decimate" it.

The only thing that ever dulled the pain was exercise. As often as he could, Adam would drive to a gym in a nearby strip mall. He would walk through the front entrance quickly, past inspirational inscriptions urging WELLNESS, AMBITION, CHARACTER, INTEGRITY; past the vibrating massage chairs where old people sometimes fell asleep; past the kids' swimming pool; and up the stairs to the weight-lifting floor. There, he would lift heavy things until he could feel nothing but the normal burn that muscles were supposed to feel when they were put to extreme use. The pain from exercise canceled out the other pain, for a while. Sometimes, Adam would look at himself in the mirror and think how wild it was that he could feel as bad as he did without having physical marks on his skin. Sometimes, he would post a selfie on Facebook, something that empha-sized his biceps and chest. How strange that his body revealed no sign of its own treachery. After the gym, Adam would drive home and feel exhausted and would have to limit his conversations with Graham. He was rationing his energy, he said: performing feats of triage on his ebbing life force.

No matter how much he lifted, the pain would find him a few hours later. So would the thoughts. *You hurt that person's feelings. They're going to kill themselves*, the thoughts sometimes said. *After you pet your cat and put him on the ground, you twisted his ankle. You hurt him. You are a terrible person. . . . That bump you hit while you were driving was a pedestrian, but you didn't realize it because you weren't paying attention. Go back to that stretch of road. Go back. Go back.* When the thoughts were in his mind, Adam could act frantic, almost feral. Graham would know not to say a word.

In October 2015, Adam started a blog called *Outpatient Memoirs*. In early posts, he wrote about how hard it was to see people he knew go to work every day and build lives for themselves. He was happy for them, but the happiness was tinged with something jealous and sour. In other posts, he described the business ventures that he had planned to start before he became sick and second-rate. In his narration, they were not frustrated hopes or sidelined dreams, but a stolen future. A golden life that had definitely been coming his way but now wasn't—for reasons that were not his fault. In his posts, Adam didn't dwell on the more material details of his recent past: the business diploma that was not a bachelor's degree, the low-level job at a bank branch. He was more focused on his not-to-be destiny. "A life of mediocrity or worse is not worth living," he wrote. Adam said he didn't understand "how more people aren't suicidal," given how obscure and mediocre their own lives were.

In early 2016, Adam wrote on his blog that he "may one day commit rational suicide." It would just be to stop the pain, he insisted. It wouldn't be an existential thing at all. Or a nihilistic thing. A few years earlier, someone had told Adam about nihilism and he had read about it online, but he hadn't vibed with the philosophy. It was too pessimistic. Also, Adam had no unifying theory of negation. The most important thing to understand, he said, was that when he killed himself, it wouldn't be because "I'm some little pussy who can't deal with life." Around that time, Adam told Graham what he was planning. They were in the parking lot outside a grocery store when Adam said it. He explained that for years, he had hidden just how bad he was feeling. But now he was scared that he would "reach a point where I can't take it anymore." Adam promised Graham that he would keep trying for another twelve months, but after the twelve months were over, he couldn't promise anything. Graham cried.

After the conversation, Graham decided that there was nothing for him to do but support his son. Adam didn't seem depressed in the "down,

down" kind of way. He seemed clearheaded. "Which is more important," Graham asked me, "that you don't give up on having your child with you or that you take mercy on your child?" Adam's mother, Maggie, was less accepting. When Adam told her what he intended to do, she sobbed and begged him to mail out a sample of his hair to have it analyzed at an American lab. Maggie thought Adam's body might contain something toxic that was messing with this mind.

Adam started writing on his blog and on Facebook about the assisted-dying debate. Sometimes, he wrote that if the Canadian law made him eligible for aid in dying, he would definitely choose it. Other times, he wrote that he was "very conflicted. . . . I feel like I'm having some sort of existential crisis or some shit."

"I would be interested in hearing anyone's opinion on the current right to die legislative debate," Adam posted on March 3, 2016. "Specifically should people with chronic non-terminal illness and chronic, refractory mental illness have access . . . Why? Why not?"

A friend commented that he opposed including people who were mentally ill. "Because depression can be helped so it's a pussy move as apposed [sic] to say leukemia where you are actually doomed."

The more Adam posted on Facebook, the more random people friended him. Some sent messages to say that they related to his words and were suffering, too. Those strangers got Adam thinking that maybe he could become a kind of public activist, with a YouTube channel and 10,000 Facebook followers—and then that he could use his influence to lobby on behalf of mentally ill people across the country. He could change the law and then he could die under it. Adam started writing letters to members of Parliament and emailing with right-to-die supporters. He talked on the phone with an older activist in Toronto named Ruth von Fuchs, who had publicly admitted to assisting in several deaths, as a kind of death midwife. Ruth agreed that it was scandalous for psychiatrists to describe Adam's pain as something different from normal pain, just because it originated in his brain instead of elsewhere in his body. "That's so arrogant," she said. "If it's pain, it has to be in your body. Where else could it be, for Christ's sake?"

"I am looking for media contacts," Adam wrote on Facebook in early spring. "I am looking to publicize and discuss all of the realities of my medical situation." In April, he got his first bite. A journalist from the *Globe and Mail* heard about his writing and interviewed him for an as-told-to op-ed titled "As a Person with Mental Illness, Here's Why I Support Medically Assisted Death." The newspaper included a photo of Adam dressed, uncharacteristically, in all black: handsome and squinting at the camera, seated on a set of stairs. "Adam Maier-Clayton was a top athlete and student," the caption read, "until his deteriorating mental health left him in extreme, chronic pain."

In June 2016, the Canadian government finally introduced its aid-in-dying legislation. Bill C-14 was, by all accounts, far more liberal than any equivalent American law, since it did not require that patients be within six months of natural death. Still, when Adam read through the text, he felt wrecked. It would never apply to him. In the end, legislators had excluded mental illness from their eligibility criteria.

Adam sent an email to Dr. Ellen Wiebe, a Vancouver family medicine professor and women's health practitioner who had spoken publicly in support of assisted death, and whom Adam had read about online. He asked her to review his medical files, and she agreed. The two talked on Skype a few times, and Wiebe, who has a pale pixie haircut and large almond-shaped eyes, listened closely. She could see that Adam was sad, but she felt that his sadness was a reasonable reaction to his illness and his situation. "He was so beautiful and so bright, and he was younger than any of my sons," she told me later. "I felt rather maternal."

That summer, after the full text of Bill C-14 was published, Dr. Wiebe told Adam what he already knew: that he was not legally eligible. But even if he had been eligible, she said, she still would not have agreed to help him die, "because I still see you as someone with potential." He was so young. There were still things to try. When Wiebe ended the Skype call, she felt pretty sure that Adam would kill himself on his own, without the help of any doctor. "I knew Adam could do a good job," she told me, as opposed to "your average old lady who is really, really bad at committing suicide."

Adam bought a little camera and started filming lectures for YouTube. He delivered them seated, in front of a bookshelf in Graham's home office, the camera resting on the table in front of him. While filming, Adam wore muscle shirts or tight V-necks. His hair fell in front of his face and he would push it back from his forehead, again and again. To anyone watching, he didn't look sick; he looked like a movie star. Adam warned his viewers that he would probably end up crying a lot on-camera, but he rarely cried, though sometimes he would press his pouty, almost feminine lips together tightly. More often, he got angry, lashing out with manic energy at unnamed haters who allegedly didn't believe that he was sick; or who told him that the nothingness of death would not bring him peace; or who said he owed it to his future self to stay alive. The haters acted like his suicide would be an insult to their existence. In the videos, Adam's voice was sometimes clipped and strange, as if English wasn't his first language and he was translating from some other language in his head, and in translation he became flat and dispassionate. Other times, he was aggressive and snarling. "If I ever kill myself, no one should be feeling like 'Oh my God, if only . . . ,'" Adam said. "No. Stop it. I did what was right for me."

I watched all the videos. In one, a twenty-eight-minute address titled "Approaching What Seems to Be the Conclusion," Adam appeared in a hazy yellow light, not in his father's office, as usual, but in his bedroom. The camera was shaky and soon it became clear to the viewer that Graham was holding it. Adam announced that it was 3:30 a.m. "Dad, would you want to live the way you've seen me living over the last year?" Adam asked.

"No, I wouldn't," Graham replied from off-screen. He sounded weepy.

"Do you think if you were in my shoes, you would be pursuing the right to die or at the very minimum think: 'This is something I deserve'?"

"Yes," said Graham. The film reminded me of a hostage video. Only, in this one, it was the hostage taker, rather than the hostage himself, in front of the camera. Watching on YouTube, I felt the same unease that I felt whenever I spoke to Graham—because he was such a soft-spoken man and because he seemed so afraid, both for his son and of him.

More journalists got in touch, and soon Adam was doing radio and newspaper and TV interviews. "If I kill myself," he told a reporter at the *Toronto Star*, "I'll be proud." In December 2016, VICE Canada described Adam as "the face of mental illness in the ongoing right-to-die debate."

"Some days I feel like I'm Erin Brockovich or some shit," Adam wrote on Facebook. "Goddamn." In another post, he urged "people with mental illnesses [to] stop cowering away in fear and stand up with conviction. . . . Look at the LGBT lobby, look how fucking powerful it is."

"I am wearing out and inclined to believe that my demise will occur within a matter of months," Adam posted in July.

"I'm excited for the future," he wrote a month later. "I often wonder how all of this is going to turn out."

On Facebook, the messages from strangers kept coming. Some of them were deranged. People told Adam that he should "shut up and kill yourself already :) :)." Lots of people wrote to say that he probably had Lyme disease. Adam told them that he had been tested twice and that the tests were clear, but the Lyme people never seemed to let up. A few times, police officers showed up at Graham's house and said they had been tipped off about a possible suicide risk. Each time, Adam told the officers that he appreciated them but that they should leave.

I was one of the reporters who messaged Adam on Facebook. I was anxious the first time we spoke and every time after that. It wasn't just that Adam was sick in the way he said he was, though that was part of it. It was the way he sometimes took my calls: slick and cocky, like he was a professional sick person. He liked these interviews. He had worked hard to get them. He knew that he was good at them and that there was demand for them. When I first called, I wondered if I was playing into something dangerous—or, at the very least, performing an unhelpful role in the Adam show. After we spoke, Adam Googled me and looked at my LinkedIn page and sent me a message to say that he was jealous of my education. "Living the dream, Katie," he wrote.

I asked Adam if I could speak to his father. I said I wanted to introduce myself before the two of us moved forward with more interviews. Adam gave me Graham's number with a shrug. When I got Graham on the phone, I asked him if my communications with his son bothered him or worried him—or if he thought I should stop them. Graham said he wasn't bothered. Adam was his own man and he could do what he liked, of course. Of course. Afterward, I thought that maybe I should never have asked for Graham's permission. Or was it his blessing? I thought I should have trusted Adam when he said he wanted to talk to me. That was kind of the whole point.

But the more news articles and blog posts that appeared about Adam, and the more times he was quoted threatening to drown himself or jump off a skyscraper, the more troubled I felt. It seemed to me that writing about Adam challenged one of the basic tenets of journalism—informal and often contested, but still widely held—that you should not report on suicide. Or at least, that you should not report on suicidal methods, lest your reporting inspire others and have a contagion effect. Simply by telling Adam's story and describing his longing, Canadian journalists seemed to be implying that his case was different: that if and when Adam ended his life in suicide, it wouldn't be *suicide* suicide, but a different, more prudent, more rational kind of self-killing. But was that right? And how did we know? And was it just because Adam told us so?

When I read Adam's Facebook page, I thought of Wolfgang von Goethe's famous eighteenth-century novel *The Sorrows of Young Werther*, about a young and sensitive man who falls in love with an engaged woman who refuses to requite his love, and who eventually shoots himself in the head with a pistol, after declaring that man could take only so much suffering. The book, which was first published in 1774, inspired some of the first reported copycat suicides: young men who dressed up as the book's protagonist before taking their lives with similar pistols. The effect was so startling that authorities in Leipzig, Italy, and Denmark banned the text. Today, social scientists still speak of a "Werther effect" to refer to the way that publicized suicides are sometimes followed by clusters of lookalike deaths, and to dissuade reporters from writing about them. But the Werther effect came into being 250 years ago, when it was reasonable to assume that people might not learn about specific suicidal means unless they happened upon the information in a book or a pamphlet. It was harder to see how it applied in the Internet age, when anyone who was curious about suicide had probably already Googled it and found out everything there was to know. It was harder to see what it meant for Adam's story: for a suicide that hadn't happened yet.

There was already some debate, among academics, about how physician-assisted death impacted broader suicide rates in places where it was legal. The question was whether assisted death made unassisted suicide less likely, because physician assistance was an alternative to suicide for sick people, or more likely via contagion vector. A 2015 paper in the *Southern Medical Journal* used US Centers for Disease Control data to argue that physician-assisted death had increased suicides in Oregon, Washington, Montana, and Vermont—by 6.3 percent. When one kind of deliberate life ending is legalized, the paper suggested, other kinds become more socially acceptable; the collective injunction against suicide is then weakened, leaving space for people who are wobbling on the suicidal brink to move forward with their plans. But when Canadian researchers crunched the same data, controlling for factors like marriage and access to mental health services, they found no evidence of an effect.

As Adam spent more time online, he saw less of his old friends from high school and college. Some of them only learned about his illness from Facebook. "I have tons and tons and tons of friends," Adam told me. "It's

just that I have chosen to strategically isolate myself from them because if
I go out with them, it's going to hurt me." Mostly, in place of old friends,
Adam made new friends on the Internet. He texted on Messenger with
strange girls who offered to hook up with him in Toronto and Hamilton
and Ottawa. He Skyped with a man in Australia who wanted to film his
death, so that his mother could upload the video afterward and make it
go big on YouTube. Sometimes, though, Adam would agree to go driving
with his friend Catrina. They would stop to buy coffees at Tim Hortons
and drink them by the water. They would tell each other weird jokes:
jokes so dark, they decided, that only other dark and sad people would
find them funny. Some days, Catrina talked about the grief she was dealing with, and Adam tried to make her feel better. Other days, Adam said
that he was going to kill himself and Catrina believed him.

"I'm at the stage where I am in the midst of trying to pursue illegal
substances," Adam told me one day in December 2016. He was sitting in
his bedroom in a white T-shirt, with a box of Triscuit crackers. His hair
was greasy and his back hurt. He said he might have to stop talking to
me at any moment, if the pain spiked. He sounded paranoid, and a bit
unhinged. "If any agency tries to interfere and it becomes clear to me that
I have been targeted, I'll just leave a bloodbath," he said. "I'm going to die
one way or another and it's going to be painless." Ideally, the law would
change and a doctor would help him. That would be the most peaceful
way. But if that did not happen, "I'm going to access a skyscraper and
turn myself into Adam pizza." He would call 911 ahead of time and tell
the police to clear the streets, so that he wouldn't hurt anybody.

"Is there any universe you can imagine in which, over the next months,
something starts working for you?" I asked. "To the point that you no
longer think about ending your life?"

He paused. "My hope is surely very little. . . . It's just objective analysis of a lot of clinical and scientific data. We know that if someone has
MDD [major depressive disorder] or OCD and doesn't respond to multiple pharmaceuticals, extensive therapy, et cetera, et cetera, that person

is going to have a bad time." For a while, Adam hoped that ketamine injections could help him, but in October he had tried them three times and said they didn't work. It was clear, Adam said, that no grand pharmaceutical gesture would make the pain go away—or help his obsessive-compulsive mind to slacken. If he did get better, it wouldn't be *better*. It would just be better like being able to talk to a girl for an hour without clenching his jaw because his chest hurt so much. It would be like: If his life was right now a negative 10, it might become a negative 7. It might become slightly less of a joke, but it would still be a joke.

"Hey, Katie," Adam said in January 2017 in a Facebook audio message. "I'm trusting you even telling you this, but I'm doing it out of courtesy and professionalism. I don't know how long I'm going to be alive and kicking."

WHILE THE DEBATE OVER the Canadian law intensified, Dr. Justine Dembo continued her research. She kept coming back to a 2015 *BMJ* research paper, written by a handful of psychiatrists in Belgium, where since 2002 patients with "unbearable" and "incurable" suffering have qualified for assisted death—and where the law is extended to people with mental illness. The report aggregated data from one hundred consecutive patients with psychiatric disorders who asked their doctors for euthanasia. It showed that the typical patient was forty-seven years old—younger than those who requested euthanasia for physical illness—and female. Most had treatment-resistant depression, but others had post-traumatic stress disorder, schizophrenia, eating disorders, personality disorders, and "complicated grief." Almost everyone had multiple diagnoses. According to Belgian law, the patients needed to show a sustained wish to die and have three doctors sign off on the procedure, in a process that often took as long as a year. The conclusions of the research paper were astonishing. Of the one hundred patients who went through the approval process, all were deemed to have decision-making capacity and forty-eight were approved to die. Thirty-five went through with the procedure, with the rest postponing or canceling, or in two cases killing themselves before the euthanasia could be carried out. The authors noted that while all of the approved patients were determined to be suffering unbearably, "the concept of unbearable suffering has not yet been defined adequately" in academic literature. By the time the paper was published, about 3 percent of Belgian euthanasia cases involved people who qualified because of psychiatric symptoms.

Other Belgian doctors admitted to euthanizing patients with more eccentric disorders. One person was approved because of anguish following an unsuccessful gender reassignment surgery. Another, because he could not control his violent sexual urges. Across the Dutch-speaking region of Flanders, in particular, these cases were rarely held up as evidence of a rising dystopia, or a sign that Belgian medicine was veering wildly off course. Instead, they were described as proof of enlightenment. Proof that the Belgians had figured things out. In Belgium, the theory went, secular humanism and freethinking had triumphed over the tyrannical dictates of religious dogma. The country's liberal euthanasia policy was a reflection of that transformation but also an instrument of it. Through euthanasia, Belgian society had invented a new, compassionate morality that was committed to the reduction of human suffering. By 2017, even criticizing the law was considered "sort of bad taste, even something blameworthy," Willem Lemmens, a philosopher at the University of Antwerp, told me. "There was an idea that it was a huge leap forward in ethics."

I read the Belgian paper, too. Then I flew to Brussels and took a train to Ghent, forty miles northwest of the capital, to meet the study's lead author, Dr. Lieve Thienpont. By then, Thienpont had earned a reputation as the psychiatrist who said yes to euthanasia requests when other doctors said no. By some estimates, she had been involved in most of the psychiatric euthanasia cases in the country, though nobody knew for sure. Thienpont had told me that she would be busy that morning and that her partner, Tony Van Loon, a philosopher, would pick me up at the train station, but I had forgotten to look up his picture online. When I arrived in Ghent, I walked through the bicycle-and-padlock-cluttered station, not knowing whom I was searching for until I saw a plump man in round Trotsky glasses and a white scarf, leaning against the side of a car, with a copy of *Mortality* by Christopher Hitchens held inches from his nose. "I think I know you from the book," I said.

We parked on an unremarkable street with a bank and a little supermarket and Tony led me into a house on the corner. Inside, everything was painted white, with accents of lime green. This was Vonkel, the euthanasia nonprofit that Thienpont had founded. Its purpose, Tony said, was to serve as a coming-together place where people could learn more about euthanasia for mental suffering. Inside the house, Thienpont and her colleagues had conducted hundreds of meetings with patients who wanted to die. Some had already asked their own doctors and been turned away. Others lived in Catholic areas and hadn't dared to ask.

Thienpont came downstairs to greet me. She was small and thin, with a silver bob haircut and arching cheekbones. She looked startled. As she set the kettle on the stovetop for tea, she told me that I was younger than she had expected. Why, she wanted to know, was I so interested in the subject?

"Why isn't everyone?" I asked.

"*Voilà*."

That afternoon, Thienpont was going to be presenting to a group of Vonkel volunteers. Already, a handful of people were in the kitchen, arranging bouquets of roses and eating sandwiches. They were mostly older men and women who spent a few hours a week answering phone calls and handing out educational pamphlets. There was a teacher with pink lipstick and a man in a tweed jacket who said he worked at a prison. Thienpont's older sister Andrea was also there, and she told me that her sister had never been afraid of death. When she was very young, the girls' great-uncle had died and tiny Thienpont had asked to see the body.

Nearly every day, Andrea said, someone came to Vonkel for advice. "Yesterday, someone came in and said, 'I want euthanasia. Can you give it to me?'"

"What did you tell him?"

"We said, 'You can have it here. But not like this. There is a process. You need to make an appointment first!'"

The founding of Vonkel had divided Belgian psychiatry and continued to do so. On the one side were Thienpont's supporters, who thought it made sense for complicated psychiatric euthanasia cases to be handled by a small number of specialist doctors. On the other side were critics who had grown wary of the media-friendly psychiatrist. These doctors worried about how many patients Thienpont saw and how young some of them were, in their twenties, even. A Dutch psychiatrist named Joris Vandenberghe told me that Thienpont made it "too easy to grant a euthanasia request. . . . She is not very stringent in requiring that all treatments have been tried." Carine Brochier of the European Institute of Bioethics, which opposes euthanasia, said she thought Thienpont was "a lady cowboy" who takes "all the cases that others don't want." It was Thienpont, several doctors told me, who was responsible for the growing sense abroad that something very strange and very dark was happening in Belgium and that psychiatrists were to blame.

Other doctors worried more about Thienpont's methods. Her stated openness to euthanasia was, they argued, an enticement to vulnerable patients. What if patients thought they should die because Thienpont said they could? Not long after my visit, in February 2017, the Associated Press reported on the existence of a letter written by a group of Belgian physicians who announced that they would no longer consult with Thienpont's euthanasia patients. Dr. Wim Distelmans, an oncologist and one of the country's most outspoken euthanasia supporters, said that Thienpont's patients tended to have "unrealistic expectations" that their requests to die would be approved, and that the weight of these expectations made the patients hard to evaluate.

"I rarely give a negative opinion," Thienpont told me. We were sitting upstairs in the Vonkel conference room with Tony. Thienpont said she preferred not to refuse a euthanasia request outright, even when the patient making the request did not seem to qualify for her assistance. Instead, she liked to keep the door to euthanasia open by putting a request "on hold." Her theory was that this delaying tactic would prevent a rejected patient from withdrawing into discouragement and becoming even more preoccupied with death. A "Yes, but later" instead of a "No" was a way to start a therapeutic process.

Thienpont told me that because Belgium was slow to deinstitutionalize its mental healthcare treatment, many of her patients had spent years in locked psychiatric wards, sometimes in physical restraints. They were broken people. They had been abused or mistreated or raped. They had spent all their money. They had lost or spoiled all the relationships that mattered to them. Some had tried to kill themselves and been stopped and then had tried again, and then had been blamed for not working hard enough to get better. Thienpont found that some of these patients could find solace only in death. But more interesting, she said, were the ones who seemed to come alive again after she approved them to die. "You see often, spontaneously, they start to look again to life."

Perhaps once they were given the option to die, the patients no longer felt trapped in their disease and could put thoughts of death aside for a while. Or maybe the experience of being approved to die made them feel validated, and so more trusting in their doctors and their proposed treatment plans. On a few occasions, patients had decided on the day of their scheduled euthanasia that they wanted to live after all: like brides, Thienpont said, abandoning their would-be grooms at the wedding altar. They had been uncertain all along. Thienpont had simply called their bluff. "Almost everybody wants another life," she said a little wistfully. "Nobody really wants to die, or almost nobody. . . . They want another life. But sometimes we can't give them another life."

After I spoke with Thienpont, she agreed to connect me with a few of

her current and former patients who had at some point asked for euthanasia. Within days, I got an email from a woman named Ann who told
me that she ran a patient-led recovery group at Vonkel and that I should
come to their next meeting. The people in the group had "tremendous
pain," she said. Together, they were helping each other "to be masters in
our own lives. . . . If you want to live, it's ok. If you want to die, it's ok.
But let's look at what makes this life."

It was cold in Ghent on the day I arrived back at Vonkel. I found Ann
in the kitchen, making coffee. She was surrounded by vases of wilting
roses, left over from the annual meeting. I introduced myself. After a few
minutes, a woman named Andy* walked in and dropped her backpack
on the table. "How are you?" I asked.

She looked at me with disinterest. "I could be better," she said, running a hand through her thin, reddish hair. Andy, who was thirty, said
she had once been a PhD student in physics but had since dropped out.
She wanted me to know that she had dropped out because of her illness and not because she wasn't smart enough. In fact, Andy said, her
measured IQ was extremely high. Emily arrived next, with a gray-and-
white Australian shepherd named Spike. In the weeks since their last
group meeting, Emily had taught Spike how to lift up his front paws
so that she could take them into her hands and dance with him. Emily
had adopted Spike a few months earlier, after deciding to postpone her
scheduled euthanasia—because, she said, she had located within herself
a seed of doubt. Emily hoped the dog would make her happier. He did,
at first. Now, less.

Marjorie came last, holding a spongy yellow coffee cake with stewed
apples on top. Marjorie usually cooked for the group: recipes that she had
learned in her cooking class, which she took after the sommelier course
and before the woodworking workshop. She liked adult education classes
because they helped to channel her autism spectrum energy into produc-
tive ends: cakes and cabinets and tasteful wine recommendations. Marjorie, whose pale eyes were a little crooked, told me that she had asked

for euthanasia a few years earlier, after quitting her job on a cruise ship, where she had worked for more than a decade as a massage therapist. Away from the unyielding routine of boat life, she had felt her mind slip off-balance. She spent six months in her apartment, not saying a single word to anyone and peeling her fingernails off at their roots.

She probably would have died, Marjorie said, if she hadn't asked Dr. Thienpont to euthanize her in May 2012, when she was forty. At their first appointment, Thienpont had asked Marjorie to get tested for autism spectrum disorder and then, when the test came back positive, had urged her to get coaching and therapy. The coaching helped. Marjorie learned how to interface with the world: how to follow social rules that she had always been aware of, in an abstract sense, but hadn't been able to see or track or adhere to. "You have to rewire yourself," she said. After she did, Marjorie didn't want to die anymore. Her fingernails grew back, arched and uncommonly shiny.

Ann asked everyone to be seated. It had been a year since the eight women first came together. Some had seriously considered euthanasia in the past. Others were still considering it, and three had already been approved to die under the law. Frauke, who was "almost twenty-six years old" and had a round, girlish face, was the youngest. She had been introduced to the group by Emily, whom she met at an inpatient psychiatric facility a few years earlier. Ann, at fifty, was the oldest and the group leader, and she had trained as a recovery counselor in the Netherlands. The women met every other week, to talk and smoke cigarettes and keep track of one another.

Andy went first. She looked older than she was, with rough skin and sharp features and thick plastic glasses that cast a reddish shadow on her cheeks. When she spoke, she tugged at the sleeves of her sweater, flashing a latticework of scars on her wrists and forearms. Since the last meeting, Andy said, there had been a few good days and a few bad days. More bad than good. She had sprained her wrist and the pain had triggered a memory of when she was a teenager and some psychiatric nurses had shackled her to her bed by her wrists, and she had dissociated mentally to escape the experience. In her memory, the hospital room was freezing cold and had blue-tinged lights. That had been a difficult thing to remember. Andy said that she was experiencing a general sense of—she searched for the English word—"is it *ambivalence*? Still, I tried to say to myself, 'Well, you had the good days.'" On the good days, she had slept well. She had watched random stuff on Netflix. She had also gone shopping for new clothes. Andy hadn't been shopping in years, she said, because "why would you buy clothes if you're not going to wear them anymore because you're going to die?" Now that she had decided to postpone her euthanasia, she needed some new things to wear. She noticed that she had lost a lot of weight. She wondered if she was anorexic.

Andy told me that it was her family doctor who first brought up the possibility of euthanasia. "My GP actually came to me like, 'Did you ever consider euthanasia?' . . . She brought it up because I was thinking about suicide for more than ten years already and she said, 'We can't go on like this. You can't keep feeling like this.'" Andy was referred to Dr. Thienpont, with whom she met many times, over many months, sometimes with her parents. When Thienpont finally told Andy that she was approved to die, Andy wept in her office. "I was so happy that I could do it in that way," she said. But now, months later, she was debating whether or not to go through with it at all. If she did, she would have to find time to meet with all her loved ones and explain herself to them. It would be an exhausting process, but important. Andy wanted to make it easier for people to grieve once she was gone. Maybe that was the difference between euthanasia and suicide, she thought; with euthanasia, you eased yourself out of your relationships, instead of disappearing in a blink.

While Andy was speaking, the rest of the group listened quietly and passively. No sympathetic nods or murmurs. Just practiced, stolid faces: the kind that belonged to women who had sat through many group therapy sessions before. Emily went next. The last few weeks had not been easy weeks, she said. "It's really hard to feel that I'm falling back into the same things as a few months ago." A few months ago, she had been in crisis. She had smashed her head against the walls and the floors, crying and smashing until she gave herself headaches that left her virtually paralyzed for days, but somehow feeling better. Emily, like Andy, had already been approved for euthanasia. "I'm working really hard with my psychiatrist and that is going very well," she said. "But he is going on vacation."

"So you have to be careful," Andy said.

"Yeah," said Emily. "I have to be really careful."

"Can you email him?"

"Yes, I can."

"But it's not the same," said Andy.

"No." Emily would try to focus on the little things, she said: pouring a bath for Spike, noticing the first signs of spring. Still, she was thinking about scheduling her death. She was tired of being a mental patient.

Next, Ann, who had short gray hair and a halting voice, reported that she had fallen in love with someone the week before, but that the woman had not returned her love. "It was very confusing," Ann said. "I thought I would have to go to the hospital, but it's not necessary. But I'm taking a lot of medication."

Frauke was doing better. She said that she had started a new internship at a healthcare facility and was liking it. She thought she might have found her calling. "It's nice connecting with people," she said, "and doing something that makes their day more bearable."

After the meeting, Andy and I went for dinner. Over thick beef stew and French fries, she asked me what I thought of the group, and of her. "What do you think about euthanasia, when you see me?"

"You seem very certain of what you want," I said.

"Do you think I am able to make a valid decision? Or no?" I mumbled something and Andy interrupted. "I can make a valid decision on my own."

"Are you still trying new medications?" I asked. "New therapies?"

"Of course! But you can go on and on and on."

"I'm still struggling through what I think of this," I told Dr. Dirk De Wachter, another Belgian psychiatrist, when I met him at his home in Antwerp the next evening. It was dark when I arrived and De Wachter pushed a glass of red wine into my hand and gestured toward the couch in his library.

"Me, too. . . . I still don't know." He turned toward me and arranged his face so that it was expressionless. Psychiatrists in other countries, he said, can't believe "that little Belgium is doing such wild things." De Wachter had longish hair and thick eyebrows and a bulbous nose: the sort of features that once, in his youth, must have overwhelmed his face, but that he had since aged into. He looked interesting. Surrounding him was a kind of organized intellectual chaos: expensive-looking light installations, paintings, Leonard Cohen CDs, and hardcover philosophy books. Heidegger. *Siddhartha*.

Years ago, De Wachter said, he had been more certain. He had known, absolutely, that he could never sign his name to a euthanasia request. One of his patients had asked him to do it: a woman with borderline personality disorder whom he had treated for more than ten years and who sometimes watched him from across the room without saying anything at all, silent and cruel. When she asked him for euthanasia, her request had felt like a manipulation: "Help me, or else . . ." De Wachter had said no. Then one day in 2004, the woman stepped onto a downtown street, set up a camera to film herself, and then set herself on fire. Her suicide made De Wachter question his opposition to euthanasia, though all these years later, he still thought he was right to refuse that particular patient. He still believed she could have been helped.

"We never know," he said. "For a psychiatrist, rational thinking is not one hundred percent truth. It's an intersubjectivity, which is in the conversation. . . . There is not a scan, or a blood sample or a psychological test with hard evidence to say, 'Here is suffering that is too much' and 'Here, it is not enough.' It doesn't work like that. It is always two people, meeting and trying to understand." After his patient's suicide,

De Wachter had started serving as a consultant psychiatrist on euthanasia cases, though he still declined to give the injections himself.

"Emptiness and nihilism and no sense in life: These are, I think, the core symptoms of Western society," he said, leaning back in his chair. "What is the sense of life when there is no God? . . . We killed God and here we are."

"At the same time," I said, "*you* want life to stay sacred."

"Yes."

"How do you do that if there's no God?"

"I don't know. I just ask questions."

"It's fragile, right?" I asked.

"It is extremely fragile," he agreed.

"Each case of euthanasia is a test. Or a threat."

"Yes," De Wachter said. "That's right."

"You sound uncertain," I said.

"Yes, of course." Before I left, De Wachter told me that his critics sometimes accused him of speaking like a priest. Of sermonizing. He thought the critique was valid. There had been many priests in his family. "'Thou shalt not kill.' That is very crucial and very true," he said. "Humanity is defined by 'Thou shalt not kill.' Let that be clear. The question is: What is the exception?"

IN WINDSOR, CANADA, Adam started seeing a new therapist. At his first meeting with Luke Di Paolo, Adam explained that he had exhausted all treatment options and that nothing was going to work and that he was going to kill himself one day. Di Paolo had never met anyone like him. He found Adam to be intelligent—sad at moments, but not at others. More than anything, the therapist found his patient confusing. Adam claimed to have given up on life, and yet, when Di Paolo gave him homework— emotion journaling or cognitive behavioral therapy techniques—Adam always completed the assignments.

In late December 2016, Adam left me a voice message on Facebook telling me that in our future conversations, he would be speaking more cautiously. "Because I know obviously there would be questions of ethics," he said. "A lot of people would say, 'Well, why did you interview this suicidal individual instead of stopping him and trying to have him institutionalized, et cetera, et cetera?'" Adam said he would be careful not to say anything that would force me to intervene. I listened to the message a few times. He was right, I thought; there would certainly be questions of ethics. But intervene how? His parents knew what he was planning. His friends knew. His therapist knew. His psychiatrist knew. The police knew. Facebook and YouTube knew. Adam told us all not to worry; he was rational.

Graham watched his son move silently around the house. He worried about how many hours Adam spent on Skype and Facebook every day, talking to people across Canada and Asia and Latin America and everywhere else about their problems. Adam tried to respond to everyone, but each day he fell short. "You can't carry the load on your shoulders," Graham said. "It'll break your back."

On January 1, Adam logged on to Facebook and announced that his "insurance policy (a lethal compound) had cleared customs."

"Unwise to post this on FB. But good for you!" someone replied.

He was vague about the particulars. Adam had connected with Exit International, the right-to-die advocacy group, and then met some people online who offered to help him get pentobarbital. He was grateful for the strangers and their help, though he felt the arrangement left room for error. What if one of the purported do-gooders was actually a nefarious person who wanted to poison him with arsenic? A few weeks later, Adam posted a picture of a medicine jar. He claimed that it contained sixteen grams of pentobarbital and that it had come from China. "No noose, no skyscraper, no blood, no traumatizing innocent bystanders, just sleep," he wrote. "#sorrynotsorry, #bitcoin, #illegalimportation, #provocation."

Maggie stopped watching her son's videos. She also stopped reading news articles about him. At first, she had kept newspaper clippings and even allowed herself to be a bit proud of her son's campaign. But now it enraged her. She thought Adam should be spending time getting better, not talking to journalists and obscure people on the Internet.

Around Windsor, people started to recognize Adam on the streets. Once, at Walmart, when he was grocery shopping with Graham, someone stopped him in the aisle and asked if he was the man who wanted to die. "I feel like I'm the voluntary euthanasia guy," Adam told me, sounding pleased. Sometimes in the evenings, he went to a local strip club—just to drink water and take his mind off things, he said—and a couple of the dancers recognized him, too. Once, a girl came up to him and told him that he was very handsome. "Not for very long," Adam said.

But Adam was growing bored of media interviews. It was just the same old thing, over and over. And no matter how many nuanced philosophical points he made, his sound bites were "chopped to shit." He wanted to tell his own story. Adam told me that he had started recording audiotapes for Graham to publish after he died. Already, he said, with the detached interest of a radio producer, he had captured some "pretty heart-wrenching stuff."

DR. JUSTINE DEMBO watched the new aid-in-dying law take effect in Toronto's downtown hospitals. Sometimes, she was asked by oncologists and other doctors to do assessments of patients who requested assisted death and theoretically qualified, on the basis of terminal illness, but who also had complicated histories of depression and mental suffering. In these cases, Dembo's role was to confirm that the patients had "the capacity to understand the nature and consequences of their actions and choices." Under the Canadian formula, a mental illness wasn't disqualifying, as long as the patient met all the other criteria.

The depression assessments were interesting, she said. "I've had patients who have chronic depression, who have had passive suicidal ideation chronically, who have wanted to die consistently for a long time. They had a previous suicide attempt or several, and were still depressed at the time of the MAID request. . . . Then the question becomes: How much, if at all, is the depression creating any disturbance with respect to the person's capacity?" It wasn't enough to identify the existence of depression. Rather, Dembo had to consider its sense of direction. Did the depression exist alongside a request to die, or was it propelling it? Was a person just very sad or did her sadness bear weight on her physical pain, magnifying and distorting it? Dr. Ellen Wiebe, the Vancouver doctor who talked with Adam on Skype, told me that she had once judged a schizophrenic patient to be capable of choosing assisted death. "What she had to say about the FBI did not make any sense, but what she had to say about the quality of her life was very clear."

The point was that each case was different. Some assessments were straightforward, and others were knottier. A patient might lack insight into his mental illness. He might be hazy about the source and character of his suffering. Dembo sometimes suggested that a patient's request to die be put on hold until he had tried another round of antidepressants or a different sort of therapy. That recommendation made sense if the person's natural death was not imminent and there was still time. She paid special attention to patients who had previously attempted to end their lives. Those cases were tricky. But then again, you couldn't deny a patient the right to die just because he had tried to kill himself before.

There was no single, decided-upon protocol for how doctors in Canada should measure mental capacity, so Dembo put together her own guidelines. She relied heavily on the Appelbaum criteria, which test a patient's ability to understand decisions and express choice. Sometimes, if a patient had dementia, she also tested for cognitive impairment. She felt confident in her process. But elsewhere, some Canadian physicians had begun to criticize the use of standard capacity evaluations on assisted-death applicants. Dr. Alec Yarascavitch, a Canadian emergency physician and lawyer, wrote in the *Journal of Ethics in Mental Health* that "the assessments in which assisted dying advocates and courts put their faith are highly subjective and lack rigorous thresholds." He noted that in the Netherlands, physician evaluators often disagreed about whether would-be euthanasia patients were competent or not.

Others looked to the United States and worried about how rarely aid-in-dying patients seemed to be sent to psychiatrists at all, in states where the procedure was legal. Opponents noted that in Oregon, just a tiny fraction of patients who are eventually found eligible for physician-assisted death are sent for psychiatric assessment. This, they argued, was proof of widespread negligence in the state. But that number does not capture all the patients who might have been sent for assessment and then, as a result of screening, been declared ineligible under the law—and never counted by researchers. More persuasively, skeptics cited a 2008 study, published in the *BMJ*, that found that about one in four people in Oregon who requested assisted death met the clinical criteria for depression, and that some of these depressed patients were given lethal drug prescriptions without any mental health evaluation at all. Dr. Linda Ganzini, the lead researcher on the study, told me that when the paper was published, a number of big-time aid-in-dying advocates—national groups that had praised the quality of her research in the past—suddenly became critical of her methods and her awkward conclusions. "The right-to-die people loved my studies until that one," she said.

As Dembo assessed more patients, it struck her that sometimes the line that advocates drew between physical and mental illness—the line they insisted was real and effective at sorting the deserving patients from the undeserving ones—was blurry. Physical pain could cause mental pain, and mental pain could manifest itself physically in the body. Depression caused pain as much as pain was depressing, and both caused suffering. Sometimes, people grew bitter and depressed after learning that they were dying and going to die soon. In other cases, people were mentally ill before they got physically sick. Chronically depressed patients sprouted cancerous tumors. Patients with delusions or drug addictions succumbed to ALS. It seemed obvious that when these patients asked to die, mental illness was part of the calculation. How could it be otherwise?

In Toronto, Dembo read articles about a young man named Adam Maier-Clayton who wanted to expand Canada's aid-in-dying law. Then she watched some of his YouTube videos. In them, Adam described all the therapies that he had attempted and all the drugs that hadn't worked. Still, Dembo wondered about the treatments that Adam hadn't tried yet. There were evidence-based therapies for OCD that could help with severe cases. There was an inpatient program in Toronto, and several in the United States, that Adam had not attended. Also, he was so young. Dembo thought, *He is not the ideal face to put to this particular cause.*

"COPS ALLOVER ME," Adam wrote on Facebook on the day of his thwarted suicide—after police found him in his hotel room and he flushed his supply of Nembutal down the toilet. "Hard to have a dignified death when you're concerned the cops are going to magically track you and arrest you. Absolutely disgraceful . . . I took a risk, I got burned. Next time, there won't be a risk."

By then, I had stopped my occasional talks with Adam. His intentions had simply become too obscure to me. I knew that Adam was in terrible pain—but also that whatever he was doing, whatever *this* was, was not helping him. I didn't want to be part of it anymore. Also, his narcissistic energy had started to frighten me. Still, I followed him closely on Facebook and on YouTube. Fundamentally, I agreed with Dembo: If Adam was a poster boy, he was not an ideal one—though it was hard to say exactly what an ideal poster child for this cause would even look like. There are no perfect patients. No perfect victims.

"What is your interpretation of the word iconoclast," Adam wrote on Facebook. "Would you consider me an iconoclast? Or a heretic?"

Later, my voice wavered when I asked Graham about the torturous three hours that his son spent broadcasting his purported almost death on Facebook. "One of the things we commonly say about suicide is that suicide attempts are . . . pleas for help. Did any part of you think Adam's could have been a plea for help? Maybe, I know it lasted—"

"It wasn't."

"—lasted many hours. Do you think there was a part of him that was—"

"No."

"—hoping to be interrupted?"

"No."

In the days that followed, Maggie tried to stage an intervention from Ottawa. She found a doctor in the United States who she thought could treat Adam's OCD and help him detox from all the poisonous pharmaceutical drugs. She would raise money for the treatment and the trip. "We have to force him. We have to do *something*," she told Graham on the phone. "Put him in the trunk of your car. I don't care." Maggie was a recovered alcoholic and she knew something about interventions. Mostly, she knew that if an intervention was going to be successful, everyone needed to be on the same page. But when Maggie called the house to talk with Graham, Adam picked up and listened down the line.

"How are you going to force me, Mom?" he said coolly.

After the call, Maggie asked herself, "If my son dies by suicide, will I be able to live with the fact that I've done everything in my power to help him?" She decided that the answer was yes. "A lot of parents cannot say that." Maggie told herself that she needed some distance. She needed to be away from her son's tyrannical moods and impulses. She told herself that Adam would never really go through with it. He wouldn't do it. Graham wasn't so sure. One afternoon, Adam went out shopping and came back with a new suit and new dress shoes: to be buried in, Graham thought.

On April 14, 2017, Adam left his house in the middle of the night and drove down the expressway in the dark. Past the Applebee's and the car wash and the Harley-Davidson dealership. Past the sickly patches of grass that lined the streets of downtown Windsor and the enormous bill-boards advertising personal injury lawyers with aggressive smiles. The lights from the cars ahead would have burned his eyes and face. "I am my own savior," he had written on Facebook. "Always have been. Always will be."

When he turned off the freeway, Adam checked himself into one of the cheap motels lining Huron Church Road. There were a bunch of them. Some advertised rooms for $59.99 a night and had space to park a flatbed truck. When he got inside, Adam ate two pieces of raisin bread and a muffin and drank a glass of milk. He left letters by the door. One was addressed to the building manager, and in it, Adam apologized for taking his life in the motel.

When the police arrived at Graham's house to tell him that his son was dead, he did not invite them inside. They spoke on the front porch. Then Graham called Maggie. Neither knew exactly how Adam had gotten the drugs. And now they were childless. In the notice of death that they published online, Graham and Maggie wrote that Adam had "died of rational suicide after suffering from an exotic neurobiological illness with no known cure."

"My son died all alone in a hotel room," Maggie said at the funeral. "My son deserved to die with dignity. With his family and friends beside him, in his own comfy bed." The funeral was held in a chapel that looked like a hotel conference room, with plain walls and gray upholstered chairs and an electric chandelier. As I listened to Maggie cry into the microphone, I thought of the eerily fitting line from Arthur Miller's play *After the Fall*: "A suicide kills two people, Maggie. That's what it's for." Maggie asked an attendant at the funeral home for a lock of Adam's hair, so that she could send it to a lab for heavy-metal testing, but then she got distracted and forgot about it and Adam's body was taken away.

On April 17, Adam's final Facebook post was quoted at the top of an op-ed in the *Globe and Mail* titled "The Mentally Ill Must Be Part of the Assisted-Dying Debate." In another op-ed, published two days later, the journalist Sandra Martin wrote that "Canada's assisted-dying laws must be open to those with mental illness." Online, the CBC ran an article about Adam that included a photo of a teary Graham, wearing a tweed jacket and staring vacantly into the distance. Alongside the text of the article, editors placed a sidebar with the phone numbers of local anti-suicide crisis lines: "Help is available."

"Is there a duty to 'keep living no matter what'? Most of the people seem to think so and I often feel alienated for thinking differently, wondering 'what is wrong with me?'" wrote someone named Fabrice on Adam's Facebook page a year after his death. Adam's page had become a kind of memorial to its fallen curator—and also an emotional dumping ground.

"I think about this guy a lot," wrote someone named Nicole. "I read his story over a year ago and watched his videos online. I felt like I was watching myself talk. It was weird. I felt like I knew this guy, but I never met him once."

Around that time, I traveled to Windsor to speak again with Graham. I flew into Detroit and then drove across the bridge to Canada. I was distracted and jittery. At a tollbooth, I handed the attendant my passport instead of cash. "I need money, sweetheart," he snarled. When I got to Windsor, I drove past the casino and the homely downtown, until the buildings thinned and the streets turned humdrum suburban and I was there.

Graham led me into the living room. He told me that his mother was in the basement. She didn't want me to think that she was being unsocial, but she just couldn't stand to hear us talk about Adam. Graham wore khakis and a dark blue polo shirt and patterned house slippers and sat in an armchair beside a brown cat that blended almost perfectly into the thick brown carpet. Occasionally, he told me, he still got calls about Adam. Strangers would reach him at home or at his office; they called from around the world to say that Adam's videos had been meaningful to them. Some said, "I've got a son that's going through this right now. Your son's stuff helped me understand."

Before his death, Adam gave Graham a list of all his email and social media passwords. In the last few months, Graham had started logging in and sifting through the digital detritus of his son's life. He was starting with the Facebook messages.

"Why?" I asked.

"Well, it's part of his legacy, isn't it?" From what Graham could tell, Adam had spent hours a day corresponding with people who were lost and hurting. What was amazing, Graham said, was how often Adam had urged people to keep trying. To slow down. To stay alive.

6

Freedom

The last time Dr. Philip Nitschke, founder and president of Exit International, tried to run a DIY Death workshop in Ireland, it had gone badly. Only a handful of people showed up; there were more protesters than attendees, and they came with enormous signs. DR. DEATH IS HERE, some posters announced. LOCK UP YOUR GRANNIES, read others—an allusion to the headline that Irish newspapers used to run when the Rolling Stones came to play: "Lock Up Your Daughters." Now, four years later, in May 2015, the streets were quiet as Philip, age sixty-eight, and his wife, Fiona Stewart, hurried into the hotel lobby and down the hall toward the conference room.

Fiona shrugged off her backpack and took out a large purple cloth, which she draped over the wooden lectern at the front of the room. Philip got out his laptop. It had a purple sticker across the front that said, I'D RATHER DIE LIKE A DOG, and Philip gestured at it. "Animals, as many people point out, get treated better than humans do. They say, 'If I kept my dog in *that* state, I'd be prosecuted.' You'd be prosecuted for cruelty! You'd be expected to put your dog down as an act of compassion. Yet if you start talking like that about your close friend or partner . . ."

Philip connected the computer to a small projector and opened his PowerPoint presentation to its first slide:

A peaceful death is everyone's right
Philip Nitschke, MD, PhD

A journalist with stringy hair approached Philip with her hand out. She was here to report on the workshop, she said. Philip nodded. "One of the damning statistics for Ireland," he said, "is that the commonest method that elderly people use to die by their own hand is by hanging. That's a grim and horrible death. And the reason it's numerically the largest method is that you don't have to know anything. And there's no prohibition on rope." Philip told the journalist that he saw his workshops as a form of "harm minimization." Older people were going to try to end their lives anyway; they might as well know what they're doing.

He had dressed for the occasion in clear plastic glasses and a flamboyantly patterned dress shirt, blue and black and shiny. He was expecting a good turnout. His seminars were often full these days, he said, because after all these years people had finally given up on the idea that their governments would pass laws to legalize physician-assisted death anytime soon—and actually, many had stopped caring. "That's a growing sentiment among baby boomers getting to their twilight years," Philip said. "They just want access to lethal drugs."

Earlier that year, my colleagues and I had started meeting with Philip as part of a documentary film project. Whenever I had to describe the film, I would tell people that I was profiling the modern-day Jack Kevorkian, which never felt quite right, but which communicated the essential gist of the story. By 2015, Exit International claimed to have 10,000 members across the world, and Philip was running DIY Death seminars in cities like London and Sydney. He had become a kind of celebrity, described in international newspaper reports as a well-heeled Australian doctor who taught elderly people how to kill themselves with efficiency, to the chagrin of law enforcement officials, who were disturbed by his activities but who could never quite find a criminal offense to charge him with.

People began filling the rows of empty plastic chairs. Some were long-time Exit International members who paid around $100 a year to support the organization. Others had heard about the seminar by word of mouth. Fiona greeted people at the door, entering names into a spreadsheet and asking each person to sign a disclaimer form. "I acknowledge that I am not of suicidal mind, & that none of the information provided in this meeting will be used in any way to advise, counsel, assist in the act of suicide," the paperwork read. "I hereby state that I am not a representative / agent of the Police, or other government agency."

The attendees were mostly in their seventies and eighties. They carried handbags and notebooks. One pale woman in a white sweater held a copy of Philip's how-to suicide manual, *The Peaceful Pill Handbook*, to her chest. In every respect, it was a typical gathering. Exit International seminars were open to people over fifty years old, but the audience tended to skew older than that. "There's no good reason why we selected fifty," Philip conceded, "except we don't want people coming in here who are troubled teens, after having some sort of desultory collapse of their relationship. Seeking some easy answer to their emotional pain. We don't want that." At fifty, he thought, people had sufficient life experience to act in their best interests.

Philip had run his first Exit workshop in 1997, in Melbourne. Almost twenty years later, his presentations followed a standard formula and he spoke with the waxy disposition of someone who has said the same thing a thousand times over. In the first half of the meeting, Philip explained, he would lecture broadly about his activism and his peaceful death philosophy. In the second half, which was open only to Exit members—though nonmembers could enroll with Fiona during the tea break—he would get specific: explaining the pros and cons of various suicide methods and the means of obtaining them.

When everyone was seated and quiet, Philip pulled up an image on a PowerPoint slide. It was of himself in 1996, wearing a tie and a pair of aviator glasses that made him look like the creep character in a Hollywood film. "That's 1996. I was younger then," Philip said. The picture had been taken just after the world's first medical aid-in-dying law came into effect in the Northern Territory of Australia, and after Philip became the first person in the world to legally end a patient's life by physician-administered lethal injection. He explained that Australia had later rescinded the legislation and that he, in response, had founded Exit International. Philip believed that in the absence of the law, he should continue to help terminally ill people—educating them about different ways to peacefully end their lives.

And then Philip told the story that he always told: the one that explained why they were all sitting there, at a suicide seminar. In Philip's telling, he met Lisette Nigot, a seventy-six-year-old French academic living in Australia, at a seminar in Perth in 1998—back when, he said, he still held the "quaint" idea that he should only help very sick and imminently dying people to hasten their deaths. Lisette had approached him after his presentation. "I'm going to die in four years' time," she said, unsmiling. When Philip asked what she was sick with, what strange affliction offered such a predictable and lethal trajectory, she told him that she wasn't sick at all. "But I'll be eighty in four years' time and eighty is the time to die."

"I said, 'Lisette, you're not sick! Go on a world cruise. Write a book.' And she looked at me and said, 'Mind your own business. This has nothing to do with you.'" Lisette told Philip that if the universe had been ordered differently, it would be she who had gone to medical school instead of him and he who was forced to beg her for the technical information he wanted. "What gives you the right to hold that information and dole it out to the people who you think are eligible?" she demanded.

Philip told the Dublin crowd that Lisette's challenge had changed everything. After Lisette, he stopped imagining himself as a noble gate-keeper of medical ways and means. After Lisette, he decided to throw open the gates: to let not just dying people, but old people and sick people have access to his information as well. Because who was he to decide? Sometimes, critics told Philip that this was a despicable thing to do, that it would inspire any number of suicides. "It's a quaint notion," Philip said, "the idea that the only reason any of us are alive is because we haven't figured out how to die."

Four years later, in 2002, Lisette took her life with barbiturates: the kind that Philip had taught her about and told her where to find. "I might as well go while the going is good," she said. She left a suicide note pinned to her bed, in which she thanked Philip, calling him "an inspiration and a crusader."

At Exit workshops, Philip started talking about how the men and women of his generation—people who had fought for civil rights and women's rights and the end to the massacre in Vietnam—shouldn't have to bow and scrape to healthcare bureaucrats in their final years. He started to speak of a "fundamental right" to "a peaceful death at the time of one's choosing." He started telling people that "life is a gift. And gifts can be thrown away. If it can't be thrown away, it's not a gift but a burden." For this, Philip's critics sometimes called him Dr. Death, the title formerly bestowed on the infamous Jack Kevorkian. At first, this annoyed Philip, but he had come to sort of like it. "Sticks and stones et cetera." Also, Dr. Death was better than the other things he was called: dangerous and irresponsible. Sometimes Philip bragged that he was one of only several Dr. Deaths listed on Wikipedia. "I'm the only one on the list who is still practicing," he would say. He wasn't wrong, though he failed to clarify that Wikipedia listed him alongside Dr. Josef Mengele, the infamous Auschwitz doctor; Dr. Harold Shipman, the British GP–cum–serial killer; and an Indian-born physician who was accused of killing patients by "gross negligence." I had become interested in Philip, in part, because I wanted to understand the Dr. Death prototype; the way that, from time to time, men like Kevorkian and Nitschke emerge, both revered and despised, as flawed celebrities of the right-to-die cause.

After the break, Philip announced that it was time to discuss practicalities, and some of the Exit members in the audience took out their
notebooks. Philip often began this part of the workshop by addressing
the obvious question: Why does anyone need his seminars at all? Why
don't people who want to die just kill themselves? He would explain that,
yes, people could make a go of things on their own, but that what he was
offering was a "peaceful, reliable death," and that this required a bit of
know-how and the right equipment. "You're only going to die once,"
Philip liked to say. "Why settle for anything but the best?"

The important thing, Philip told the Dublin crowd, was to plan ahead.
Hope in the face of illness or injury was OK, but hope could also be its
own kind of tyranny if it prevented you from preparing for the worst.
He leaned his weight against the wooden lectern and flipped through
his PowerPoint slides, each displaying a different lethal option. There
was a certain antimalarial drug that in high doses could bring about a
timely death. "Cyanide? What can I say about cyanide? It's quick. It's
very quick." But it could burn. Philip talked about carbon monoxide and
anti-nausea pills and charcoal. But from a technical standpoint, he said,
in what felt like the presentation's grand reveal, the best way to go was
with a fast-acting barbiturate called pentobarbital sodium, or Nembutal.
A person who took enough of it would likely fall asleep quickly, but not
suddenly, and would stop breathing over the course of fifteen or twenty
minutes. A bonus: If a family member threw the bottle away afterward,
the death would look natural. Back in the fifties, Philip said, Nembutal
had been a popular sleeping agent. It had even been advertised in *Wom-
en's Weekly* magazine as a "new improved Nembutal elixir." But by the
sixties it had fallen out of favor because it was so easy to overdose on. Mar-
ilyn Monroe died by Nembutal. In response, pharmaceutical companies
released new drugs, like Valium, which they marketed as safer alternatives. Now pentobarbital was hard to come by, outside of veterinary
offices, where it was used to sedate and euthanize animals.

But here was the silver lining: Nembutal could still be obtained, and

Philip knew how. There were places you could go in Mexico and Peru and Bolivia and Ecuador, veterinary supply stores that weren't fussy about official prescriptions—in part, Philip suspected, because locals were often too poor to afford life-prolonging veterinary care for their pets. Better yet, there was the Internet. Over the last fifteen years, Philip had scoured the globe and connected with a small band of trusted dealers in Mexico and China who would ship the drug internationally to Exit International members. Anyone who joined his organization could apply for access to the group's $85 digital suicide manual, which included the names and email addresses for those dealers, as well as instructions on how to download the Tor anonymous web browser and set up an encrypted email address. People ordered it all the time, Philip said. And after they did, they usually felt a little better, just for having the option.

To many of Philip's detractors, these workshops were their own dystopian visions: rows of white-haired men and women—maybe frightened, maybe alone—being spun a tale about the terrible and painful deaths that awaited them and then offered suicide as a solution, by a silver-tongued Dr. Death who sold suicide manuals for $85 apiece. Who sometimes talked as if Nembutal was the only honest answer to the loss of physical health and youthful vigor. In 2009, one of Philip's oldest allies, Dr. Michael Irwin of Britain's Voluntary Euthanasia Society, had broken off ties with him, on the grounds that Philip's seminars were "totally irresponsible. . . . I am totally opposed to this easy-access Nembutal."

In Philip's seminars, these critics found all the excesses of neoliberalism—radical individualism, a sanctified solipsism, a swollen sense of self, an obsession with personal narrative—carried to a hideous conclusion: a world stripped of existential meaning, in which each individual is bound only by his own preferences and so should take his life whenever he sees fit. Forgetting family and friends. Forgetting obligation. In Philip's formulation, loved ones who resisted a death wish were selfish and greedy. In the stories he told, suicide was stripped of its melodrama and horror. "Exiting" was quick and clean. To others, Philip's logic wasn't dangerous so much as it was incoherent. In his workshops, he emphasized that control at the end of life mattered more than anything. But how could the point of life be to control it?

After everyone left the room, Philip and Fiona and a few Exit members made their way to a nearby pub with blue walls and blue plastic chairs. They ordered coffee. Fiona said they were tired because they had stayed up the previous night to watch the Eurovision Song Contest on the hotel TV. As they sipped their drinks, my colleague asked Philip what it felt like "to take someone's life."

"What does it feel like to kill someone?" Philip asked, with a linguistic pivot that I considered only long after the fact. "You can't help but feel other than being an executioner."

IN THE LATE 1980S, a string of Dr. Deaths appeared in America. It began in 1988, with an article published in the *Journal of the American Medical Association (JAMA)* titled "It's Over, Debbie." In the article, an anonymous author, who revealed himself only as a young gynecology resident, admitted to killing a patient during an early morning shift in a room in a large private hospital. The twenty-year-old patient, who was dying of ovarian cancer, could not sleep. Indeed, she had not slept for days, the anonymous resident wrote, and "her eyes were hollow. . . . It was a gallows scene, a cruel mockery of her youth and unfulfilled potential." When the author walked into the room, the woman looked up at him and said, "Let's get this over with." A second dark-haired woman, who was holding the sick woman's hand, said nothing. A short while later, and without saying a word more, the doctor injected the patient with morphine sulfate. He remained in the room as her breathing slowed and then ceased. He noted the relief on the face of her companion. "It's over, Debbie," he wrote.

Dozens of readers sent letters of protest to the journal, condemning the anonymous young resident. They noted his professional inexperience:

the source, surely, of his naïve certainty that there was no way to ease the woman's suffering, short of killing her. Even though he wasn't a pain specialist. Even though he had never met the patient before. Even though he never asked her, clearly, if this was what she wanted. "*Murder* is the only word for it," wrote Dr. Sherwin Nuland, in his best-selling book *How We Die*. "It pleased [the doctor] to interpret her plea for relief as a plea for death that only he could grant." Others had bigger worries. They wondered what it would mean, for the sanctity of the medical profession, if sick patients came to equate white hospital coats with mercy killings. The editors of *JAMA* wrote a defensive editorial, insisting that they had published the article "to provoke responsible debate within the medical profession and by the public about euthanasia in the United States. . . . Such discussions should not be confined to whispers in doctors' dressing rooms."

That same year, an uncelebrated pathologist with a middling career began advertising "death counseling" services in local Michigan newspapers. His name was Dr. Jack Kevorkian, and for a few years, his strange publicity efforts won him almost no attention at all—and no clients. Then, in 1990, Kevorkian was featured in a series of news stories in which he showed off a homemade suicide device that he called the Thanatron (from the Greek *thanatos*, meaning "death"). The Thanatron was pieced together from spare parts: household tools, toys, an electrical switch, some magnets. "A high school student could do it," Kevorkian said. It had an intravenous needle attached to a drip of saline solution—and a button that a user could push to trigger the consecutive administration of two lethal chemicals. After the news stories were published, a fifty-four-year-old woman named Janet Adkins, who had Alzheimer's disease, called Kevorkian and asked if she could be his first Thanatron patient. According to her husband, Ron, Janet wanted to "err on the side of going too soon rather than too late."

In June 1990, Janet took her life in the back of Kevorkian's beat-up 1968 Volkswagen van. Her last words were reportedly to the doctor:

"Thank you. Thank you." Later, when Kevorkian announced the death publicly, he would insist that while his patient was deeply demented, "she knew enough to know what was coming and to know she didn't want it." He would also account for the unusual suicide venue: a van, in a parking lot beside a county park. It was only because he could not find a willing hotel or homeowner to host the suicide, he said. There was "no room at the inn." The next day, newspapers around the world ran articles on the Thanatron suicide. "The case," wrote the *New York Times* on its front page, "raises the specific legal question of what constitutes assisted suicide and the more general philosophical question of what role, if any, doctors should play in helping their seriously ill patients die."

Kevorkian was brought to trial in Michigan. Because the state did not have a law on the books that explicitly criminalized "assisted suicide," as about half of states did, prosecutors opted for a first-degree murder charge. But in the end, that charge was dismissed, mostly because of the Thanatron, which had allowed Janet to administer the lethal injection herself. In 1991, prosecutors tried again: this time, in a civil case, led by an attorney who said he wanted to stop the doctor from "roaming around the countryside in his van, zapping people." During the hearing, prosecutors compared Kevorkian to Josef Mengele and kept a copy of a book called *The Nazi Doctors* displayed prominently on their table. Kevorkian's defense lawyer, contesting the charges and indulging his client's taste for self-aggrandizement, likened him to the great intellectual martyrs of eras past: to Socrates. At the end of the trial, these charges were also dropped, but not before Kevorkian became a household name and an enduring shorthand for physician-healers who also kill.

People loved him. "We thought patients would be horrified by the rusty van in the parking lot, the unsterile solutions. It sounded so sleazy," Dr. Howard Brody, head of the Michigan State Medical Society ethics committee, said at the time. "Instead, a significant number want to erect a statue to the man. It became clear that many people see doctors as the enemy when it comes to death and dying, and you have to see that as a terrible failing." Kevorkian built a second suicide machine, which he named the Mercitron, or "mercy machine."

In a 1991 essay in *Vanity Fair*, the writer Ron Rosenbaum hypothesized that the public's infatuation with Kevorkian was about more than the man himself: It was about the Thanatron. "There's something about it," Rosenbaum mused, "something about its crude shop-class mechanicalness, that has struck a dark chord in the national imagination." By the early nineties, Americans had grown used to having their deaths mediated by machines: respirators and pacemakers and feeding tubes. Just a few decades earlier, a majority of deaths had occurred at home, but now most Americans died in intensive care units or skilled-nursing facilities, often hooked up to devices. There were even new conditions emerging that were born of technologies meant to stave off death, like prolonged mechanical ventilation (PMV). Patients needing PMV sometimes became permanently dependent on their machines and lost the ability to breathe without them—and also to eat independently and to speak. Some died with their hands tied down, to prevent them from pulling the connecting tubes from their necks or stomachs during sleep or in a moment of panic.

To some, Kevorkian, who went on to assist dozens of people in dying, was a messiah, an undaunted man who was ready to martyr himself in the service of a fledgling patient-autonomy movement. To others, he was a murderer who had taken advantage of a demented woman in the back of his dirty van, after having met her only once before, over dinner. Either way, it didn't matter to Kevorkian. His objective, he would later explain, was not to win over skeptics or to change the law, but "to knock the medical profession into accepting its responsibilities, and those responsibilities include assisting their patients with death." Here he was, a rugged philosopher-frontiersman, just trying to make medicine understand its own hypocrisy.

But even doctors who favored physician-assisted dying were wary of the new Dr. Death, who, it seemed obvious to everyone, was an imperfect flag bearer for the right-to-die cause. Kevorkian was a trained pathologist who had not practiced medicine on a living patient since the 1950s. He was reckless in his interactions. More than that, he was weird. Morbid and excessive. A notorious ascetic, Kevorkian ate little and wore ratty Salvation Army sweaters and spent much of his time writing papers for obscure European academic journals, in a barely furnished apartment above a Detroit flower shop. He reportedly painted with his own blood. The man's professional career had also been confused. Before he unveiled the Thanatron, Kevorkian had advocated for the harvesting of organs from death-row prison inmates and experimented with blood transfusions from corpses, giving himself hepatitis C in the process. ("We were working on a solution for Vietnam. That's why it made sense," his former assistant Neal Nicol later told me. Kevorkian wanted to design a way for wounded soldiers to receive blood transfusions from dead soldiers on the battlefield.) Over his years in the public eye, Dr. Death only grew more outrageous. He acquired a kind of macabre campiness and an affection for ghoulish shtick. Once, he left a corpse in a hospital parking lot.

Proponents of legal physician-assisted death were right to fear him. When, in October 1991, Washington State residents rejected an assisted-dying bill in a statewide ballot, some blamed Kevorkian. Derek Humphry, the founder of the Hemlock Society, wrote that his organization had "spent ten years bringing the medical profession around to accepting its point of view. We believe 60% of doctors are on our side, as long as the law is changed. Now, Dr. Kevorkian has muddied the waters." In Kevorkian's wake, a number of states passed laws that explicitly banned assistance in suicide, in a hurried effort to forestall future Dr. Deaths.

Dr. Timothy Quill, of Rochester, New York, thought of Kevorkian when he published his confession in March 1991. "Diane was feeling tired and had a rash," the forty-one-year-old palliative care physician wrote as the opening line of his essay in the *New England Journal of Medicine*. In the article, Quill explained how he had diagnosed his patient, whom he called Diane, with acute myelomonocytic leukemia, and how Diane, after learning that she had only a 25 percent chance of surviving the cancer with aggressive treatment, had turned down chemotherapy—against Quill's counsel and to his dismay. Diane thought the odds weren't worth the pain. She said she would rather go home to her husband and son and die without a fight. Months later, as Diane was growing weaker, she had called Quill and asked for a prescription for barbiturate sleeping pills—for insomnia, she said—and Quill had immediately understood what she was really asking for. He knew that "pseudo-conversations" between doctors and patients happened all the time. Patients lied to their doctors, claiming they had joint pain or sleeplessness, as a ruse for getting powerful drugs. Doctors, who felt bad for them, joined in on the charade. "Be careful with these," a doctor might say, handing over a prescription. "Too many of these at once can kill you."

Quill was uninterested in playing the role of an obtuse prescription writer. Also, he thought the charades were dishonest. Instead, he asked Diane to come to his office. "In our discussion," he wrote of the meeting, "it became clear that preoccupation with her fear of a lingering death would interfere with Diane's getting the most out of the time she had left." In other words, Diane was so afraid of dying badly that she was finding it hard to live. Quill thought Diane's fear was so great that she might try to kill herself, to cut short the anticipation—and that she might die violently. He tried to reassure her. As a palliative care doctor, he said, he could manage her pain and keep her comfortable through the dying process. But Diane had seen dying people get caught in a purgatory of "relative comfort." She dreaded having to choose between horrible pain and drugged-out sedation.

Even Quill could admit that his abilities—that all doctors' abilities—were limited and often conciliatory. He could lift "bad pain" up to "OK," but he could not promise painlessness. He could engineer the "least bad" death possible, but he could not promise a good one. Quill also knew that while he was equipped to treat pain, he couldn't always palliate the fear of future pain or lessen the symptoms of expectation. Quill considered Diane's request and then decided that he would, "with an uneasy feeling about the boundaries I was exploring," prescribe the sleeping pills. After Diane's drug overdose, he personally drove to her home to view the body. He called the medical examiner and reported her cause of death as "acute leukemia."

Quill had written the Diane article with other physicians in mind, but soon his story was picked up by journalists and replayed in news reports across the country. To his relief, he was widely praised: as an antidote to the anonymous young medical resident who wrote, "It's over, Debbie," and as a correction to the heedless Jack Kevorkian. The *New York Times* ran an editorial lauding Quill's "courageous action." The bioethicist George Annas predicted that, if Quill were prosecuted, the American public would be appalled; "the vast majority of Americans would say, 'I'd like this guy to be *my* doctor.'" Later that year, a grand jury in Monroe County declined to issue an indictment.

In his 1993 book *Death and Dignity*, Quill described his decision to help Diane as a reaction to Dr. Death. Kevorkian, he wrote, had "deeply frightened us [physicians] by the ease with which he helps patients to die, and by his apparent lack of doubt." He had also shamed the profession by exposing a widening chasm between desperate patients who feared painful, drawn-out deaths and the doctors who could not comfort them—or offer an alternative. "I think these cases are as much an indictment of our current medical system as they are of Dr. Kevorkian," Quill told PBS. "Where are these people's doctors?"

Twenty-five years later, Quill told me that he still receives letters about the Diane article. He has received thousands and has kept them all. Quill's theory is that the power of the Diane story was rooted in his mainstream professional credentials. At the time he published his article, he was already a respected physician at the University of Rochester. This meant that he couldn't be dismissed by critics as a rookie or a madman. He had to be listened to. "In a certain way," he told me, "I was more dangerous, from a social change point of view, than Kevorkian."

In the eight years following Janet Adkins's death, Jack Kevorkian reportedly took on 130 patients. Many were people he barely knew. Some had psychiatric histories and, it would turn out later, weren't physically sick at all. Kevorkian, for his part, rarely tried to hide what he was doing. When he helped someone to die, he did it flagrantly. In Michigan, he was sometimes spotted pushing a dead body in a wheelchair toward the medical examiner's office. His flirtation with the media was chancy but effective. In 1993, after Kevorkian was briefly jailed and began a hunger strike, a Harris poll showed that 58 percent of Americans supported his mission. Dr. Death had presented himself as a sacrificial offering—like Gandhi—and the people had embraced him.

It wasn't until 1998 that his transgression stretched too far: when instead of helping a patient to self-administer a lethal dose, Kevorkian injected the drugs himself—and then sent footage of the euthanasia to *60 Minutes*, which ran the tape on its November 22 broadcast, to the amazement of pretty much everyone. Later, people would speculate that Dr. Death had been chasing martyrdom. Or maybe he had just become drunk on his own audacity. Kevorkian was charged with murder and brought to trial in a courtroom so bloated with drama and pageantry that it rivaled the OJ Simpson proceedings. Here, at last brought to answer for his actions, was Jack Kevorkian, with his pinched face and long ears, seated before a gallery of spectators. Here was Dr. Death, insisting that it had been his professional duty to kill. When Judge Jessica Cooper delivered her guilty verdict, she turned to face the condemned man. "This trial was not about the political or moral correctness of euthanasia," she said. "It was all about you, sir." But anyone sitting in the courtroom that day would have known that this wasn't quite right.

The same year of Kevorkian's arrest, the *New England Journal of Medicine* published the results of an anonymous survey, which found that 3.3 percent of American physicians had "written at least one prescription to be used to hasten death" and that 4.7 percent "had administered at least one lethal injection." The clear line between doctor and Dr. Death began to look fuzzier. The *Lancet* medical journal also ran an article about physician assistance in death, which quoted Kevorkian as saying that he had deliberately sought out arrest "to force the debate back into the public eye." Underneath the Kevorkian article, on the same page, was a shorter piece about a lesser-known Kevorkian-like character in Australia: "Australia's own 'Dr. Death' Philip Nitschke."

PHILIP NITSCHKE NEVER planned on becoming a doctor. At university, he studied engineering and then got a PhD in physics. Afterward, he worked as an Aboriginal land rights activist and a park ranger. He only enrolled in medical school, in Sydney, when he was thirty-five years old—and only after a foot injury made it impossible to continue his outdoor work. When he graduated in 1989, at age forty-two, Philip moved to the Northern Territory, a rural expanse that covered one-sixth of Australia but contained fewer than 200,000 people. He liked the area's self-consciously rugged spirit. He liked being alone in the desert and understanding his place in life as a tiny grain of sand.

Philip found work as a medical intern at the Royal Darwin Hospital and very quickly found himself treating the territory's sickest patients. In one of his first rotations, he wrote later, a supervisor asked him to take a blood sample from a man who was terribly ill and nearly dead. "Why?" Philip asked.

"We want to run some tests," the supervisor said.

"Why?"

"What do you mean why?"

"He's dying," Philip said. "Why are we doing tests?"

A few years later, Philip left the hospital and started his own after-hours practice, mostly attending to the sex workers and junkies who hung out near the fishing boats. It wasn't until 1995 that he thought about assisted dying in any coherent way. He had been lying in bed listening to the radio when he heard the Northern Territory's chief minister, Marshall Perron, announce his government's intention to introduce an aid-in-dying bill that would apply to terminally ill patients. *That makes sense*, Philip thought before falling back asleep. He would later say, "There was no 'road to Damascus' moment that transformed my thinking." It wasn't until the Rights of the Terminally Ill Act came into effect in July 1996, and news crews from all over the world descended on Darwin, that the magnitude of the measure became clear to him. Oregon had passed its own Death with Dignity bill in 1994, but the legislation hadn't gone into effect yet. The Netherlands had effectively stopped prosecuting doctors for assistance in the eighties, but it would take until 2002 for the country to pass a law. And so, Australia's Northern Territory became the first place in the world with legalized physician-assisted death. Philip put his name to a list of local doctors who supported the legislation.

Not long after that, Philip got a call from a taxi driver named Max Bell, who was dying 3,000 kilometers away, in a small cottage in a town called Broken Hill. Max told Philip that stomach cancer and surgery had left him unable to consume solid food. He was nauseated all the time and often vomited. He lived alone. "I'm just existing," he said. "I can't see the point anymore. I'm ready for a sweet, long sleep." Max wanted to know if Philip would take him on as a patient and Philip said he would, so Max put his house up for sale and euthanized his dog, and then got into his Hudson Commodore taxi to drive north, across the country.

Six days later, when Max arrived in Darwin, Philip set out to organize everything that he needed to . . . what should he even call it?—administer? oversee? practice? perform?—the assisted death. According to the law, Max would need signatures from two other doctors who confirmed that he was terminally ill and a note from a psychiatrist certifying that he was mentally sound. Philip started making calls and, quickly, things fell apart. There weren't many doctors in the area and, over the course of several weeks, all of them turned Philip away. Philip blamed the territory's chief medical officer, who promised to repeal the law and who hinted that participating doctors might be prosecuted retroactively for helping their patients to die. When he told Max what had happened,

Max just shook his head. "You didn't do your homework, boy," he said. Then Max climbed into the Commodore taxi and drove the 3,000 kilometers back to Broken Hill, where he died a few weeks later: slowly, Philip said, in just the way he had hoped to avoid.

The only upside to the gruesome affair was the press coverage. Philip had introduced Max to a journalist at the Australian Broadcasting Corporation, and a few producers had made a film about his piteous ride home called *The Road to Nowhere*. In one scene, Max was filmed falling down at a gas station and being lifted up by a chance passerby. After the program aired, a local doctor called Philip to apologize for refusing to see Max and to say that he felt like shit about it. Philip told himself that he should never again underestimate the power of television in the battle for hearts and minds.

In the months after, Philip turned his attention to the question of what a "good death" was and what a good death might look like under the Northern Territory law. The law allowed him to administer lethal drugs intravenously, and Philip had at first assumed that he would offer this option to his patients. But the more he thought about it, the more he found it hard to imagine himself holding a syringe. More than that, Philip thought that patients should make the final gesture themselves. "I wanted to make it very clear that it was the individual making the decision," Philip said. "That it wasn't the case of some evil doctor pushing his will on a comatose or moribund patient. So I built a machine." Philip had read about Jack Kevorkian's Thanatron and had liked the idea of it, but he thought he could build something more sophisticated. His final product was a software program that ran off his silver Toshiba laptop and that he named Deliverance.

The second patient to find Philip, in March 1996, was Robert "Bob" Dent: a sixty-six-year-old with metastatic carcinoma of the prostate who said he was experiencing "a roller coaster of pain." By then, Philip had found a doctor who agreed to give a second opinion on the case, provided that his name was kept secret. He also found a psychiatrist—who flew in from Sydney to examine Bob—and who concluded that while Bob showed "elements of depression," he was not depressed, and as such was capable of making medical decisions. Philip approved Bob to die and told him to call when he was ready.

Bob called on September 22 and asked Philip to come for lunch at his home in a suburb called Tiwi. "Bring that machine around," Bob said. At lunch, Philip was so anxious that he sweated through his shirt and could eat only a bite or two of the ham sandwich that Bob's wife, Judy, made him. He thought he might lose his nerve. He could barely speak either. It was hard to talk without referencing the future. Conversation bound by the present tense felt turgid and strained. Even Bob noticed Philip's unease and tried to calm him down. The dying man told his trembling physician that things would be OK. After lunch, Bob and Philip watched TV for a while, which felt like forever, before Bob finally turned to the doctor. "You're here to do a job. Let's get on with it," he said. Then he stepped onto the veranda and lay down on a lounge chair.

As Judy watched, Philip knelt down beside Bob and pushed a needle into a vein on his arm. He was relieved when it slipped in without any trouble. The weight of the occasion made the air seem thick, and for some reason, Philip had expected to feel resistance against the glide of the syringe. Philip asked Bob once more if he was sure and Bob said he was, so Philip opened the Toshiba laptop and started running Deliverance. It was 2:30 p.m. Philip handed the laptop to Bob and then walked to the other side of the room, so that Bob could take Judy into his arms and start answering the questions on the screen.

> Are you aware that if you go ahead to the last screen and press the "Yes" button, you will be given a lethal dose of medications and die?
> YES.
> Are you certain you understand that if you proceed and press the "Yes" button on the next screen that you will die?

YES.

In fifteen seconds, you will be given a lethal injection . . . press "Yes" to proceed.

YES.

Exit.

The machine made a ticking sound as the barbiturates and muscle relaxants were released. Bob sighed and fell asleep and then, a few minutes later, stopped breathing. Across the room, Philip felt a staggering relief. And also pleasure. "It was a pleased feeling," he said. "It wasn't, 'Oh my God, I've broken some fundamental rule of killing.'" When he left Bob's house, Philip admitted later, he felt "this immense feeling of being alive . . . and almost immediately, this sexual urge. It was a way I could demonstrate to myself that I was alive. It wasn't me that was dead." It was primal and obvious. Carnality as proof of aliveness. Man spreads seed; lives forever. Reading his description years later, I shuddered. *He had liked it.*

Still, at the press conference announcing Bob's death, Philip was flustered and close to tears. "Nitschke, 49, looked terrible," reported the *Sydney Morning Herald.* "He had been told to wear a tie and trousers instead of his customary shorts, but his respectability could not hide his deep emotion." The writer noted that Philip had, of late, "been abused, labelled 'Dr. Death' and a murderer, and become an increasingly isolated figure within the medical hierarchy." Philip spoke of assisting Bob's death as "an act of love." He tried to stay calm.

Outside Australia, Philip found a more effusive reception. That October, the World Federation of Right to Die Societies met in Melbourne and feted him as a hero of the cause. Philip signed his name to a "Declaration on Physician Assisted Dying," alongside doctors from the United States, Canada, India, Japan, Switzerland, Britain, and the Netherlands. "We have the means to help those who may suffer severely from terminal illness," it read. "We know that, if we should find ourselves in such situations, we have the knowledge, and the access to drugs, to achieve self-deliverance, and we wish to extend this privilege to our patients."

Over the next months, Philip helped three patients to die with the Deliverance machine. But then, in March 1997, nine months after the Rights of the Terminally Ill Act came into effect, the Australian government repealed it, using a legal tool that allowed the federal government to overrule territory legislation. That day, Philip had to tell another patient—a fifty-six-year-old woman with a diffuse pelvic tumor and an antibiotic-resistant fistula that smelled so putrid it made her queasy—that he could no longer help her as he had promised to. He held another press conference: this one, on the steps of the Parliament building, where he burned copies of the Northern Territory constitution before a pack of reporters. A friend brought bottles of petrol in her handbag, which Philip used to douse the thick stacks of paper so that they would burn more spectacularly for the newspaper photographs.

Philip was despondent. He was tired and broke and sickened by the thought of returning to his former life, treating drifters and writing prescriptions for penicillin. So, in 1997, he founded the Voluntary Euthanasia Research Foundation (VERF), which he later renamed Exit International—after friends, who were alarmed by the doctor's obliviousness when it came to public relations and image crafting, urged him to avoid the historical taint of the "euthanasia" word. Nazis. Eugenicists. Kevorkian. Philip figured that while he wasn't able to inject patients with lethal drugs, there was nothing to stop him from educating very sick people who wanted to take their own lives. In 1997, he started running DIY Death workshops for sick and dying people, and his old colleagues started to distance themselves. Some told Philip that what he was doing was wrong. Others said that he was right, in theory, but that in reality he was holding back the assisted-death cause. A few admitted that they sometimes helped their own patients to hasten death—but said it wouldn't do anyone any good for Philip to be so public about it. Philip, in turn, said he hated the idea of doctors picking and choosing which patients to help, if any at all, according to their own personal criteria. Why should doctors be in charge of deciding who among them was sick enough, or sympathetic enough, or desperate enough? Or whose family was respectable and trustworthy enough?

It was around that time that a Mexican man named Samuelle wrote to Philip and said he wanted to help. A large, bearish man who lived in southeastern Mexico, Samuelle had read news articles about tourists coming to his region to buy Nembutal at veterinary supply stores. He thought he could make things more convenient for them, and make some money doing it. "Many people around the world are trying to die. And it's like . . . I have the key they need, so I can help them find the key," Samuelle explained in February 2017, after agreeing to be interviewed from his home on a flat street, off a tree-lined highway, in a valley that he did not want to name because he was afraid of being arrested.

In phone calls with Philip, Samuelle described himself as a hybrid hustler-philosophe. His own mother had died from cancer when he was a child, he said. She hadn't suffered much, but she had suffered some, and her death had left Samuelle sympathetic to the idea of assisted death. Later in life, Samuelle had read Daoist philosophy. Books by Lao-tzu. Through his reading, he had come to believe that Big Government and Big Society and Big Religion had a fear of free will and were trying to extinguish individual choice by colonizing the dying process. By wrapping it with institutional procedure. "I don't want to sound crazy about the New World Order," he said, "but . . . they want to control how we die. They don't want us to have that key that we can use at any moment." If people had the key, there could be chaos. Worse: nihilism. Soon Philip began referring people to Samuelle, who accepted payment by money transfer and, in return, mailed out bottles of Nembutal in unmarked brown envelopes. Philip designed a tiny Nembutal testing strip—a thin piece of plastic that looked like a pregnancy test—and started selling the tests through Exit International. He said they could confirm the purity of the drug, though a few of his detractors said they weren't very accurate, and most Exit members didn't bother. They trusted Philip's word.

Philip started getting recognized on the streets around Darwin. He was the subject of magazine profiles, just like the celebrity doctors of earlier eras: Dr. Spock, the child-rearing guru, and Dr. Ruth, the sex expert. He got fan mail and hate mail. Some people sent him photocopied pages of the Bible and Philip would feel glad that he lived in Australia instead of the United States, where he knew religious wackos were ready to murder a doctor for so much as an abortion. Now things were moving. He only needed to march forward—but to what? "It is interesting and important to ponder the type of world we are creating," he wrote in a 2005 book called *Killing Me Softly*. "Are we opening the floodgates for mass suicide, or are we setting a new agenda for aging? Will there be an avalanche of suicides, or will there be a wave of comfort that spreads rapidly through the swelling ranks of the elderly? Will society be better or worse off?"

FIONA STEWART, PHILIP'S new partner, helped to professionalize things. After she and Philip fell in love and she agreed to join his mission, she started to put Exit's affairs in order. Fiona helped Philip pay his taxes for the first time in three years. A lawyer by training, she instituted new rules about paperwork and record retention. In 2006, Fiona helped Philip to write a suicide manual, collecting all the information and advice that he normally shared in his seminars—and then set up a publishing house to print and distribute it. *The Peaceful Pill Handbook* had both of their names on the cover. Fiona wrote the sections on philosophy and Philip wrote the chapters about drugs. Afterward, when the handbook was banned across Australia, it was Fiona's idea to digitize it so that Exit could sell online subscriptions to its members. When Philip started giving seminars abroad, Fiona traveled with him and greeted attendees at the door. When journalists started calling their home with more frequency, she answered the phone and screened the calls. Once, when a BBC producer questioned Philip too pointedly, Fiona interrupted the interview to scream at him. It astonished her that her partner could be so unbothered by criticism and so indifferent to self-preservation. She wanted him to be careful.

With Fiona around to handle business matters, Philip had more time to interact with supporters. A top order of business was to find dying people—ideally, sympathetic ones—whose cases he could present to the media as proof of the Exit concept. In 2011, he got lucky. Philip met an elderly couple, Donald and Iris Flounders, who seemed like a perfect case in point. Don, who was seventy-eight, had mesothelioma and was in pain and wanted to die. Iris, his wife, wasn't very sick at all but told Philip that she had been married for almost sixty years and didn't want to live without Don. With Philip's guidance, Don and Iris acquired Nembutal and then gave an interview to Australia's ABC News about their plans to consume it. "We are quiet-living people and not excessively excitable," Don told the journalist. "I had no trouble whatsoever purchasing the poison. It will be completely painless."

In May, Don and Iris lay side by side and drank from their identical glass bottles. They died holding hands. Then, on cue, Philip went public. The extraordinary thing, he said later, was that most Australian newspapers reported on the double suicide with sympathy, and even a tacit approval. "After 60 Years of Life Together, Don and Iris Die Together," read a headline in the *Sydney Morning Herald*. "They listened to each other, finished each other's sentences and didn't ever want to be apart." The article, which included a photograph of Don and Iris cuddling in bed with their cat, mentioned Philip's role only in passing, and without the usual malice. It described Don as a suffering old man. It described Iris as someone struggling with the "ailments of old age"—not, as Philip might have feared, as a relatively healthy older woman driven to suicide

by preemptive grief and a fear of aloneness. It portrayed the couple's suicide pact as almost romantic. Something was changing.

Philip could feel the change in his audiences, too. By the time he met
Nigel Brayley, at a three-hundred-person Exit seminar in Perth, he was
used to seeing people who didn't look that old or that sick at his meetings, and he had relaxed his own rules about verifying age. Did it matter
that much if someone was a bit younger than fifty? Philip didn't think it
did. Still, he noticed Nigel because the man looked especially young, and
Philip pulled him aside for a moment to check him out. Nigel told Philip
that he was forty-five years old and that he had good reasons for wanting
to end his life. Basically, he said, his life was falling apart. Later, Philip
would insist that he asked Nigel what, specifically, was wrong, and that
Nigel had told him to mind his own business. A short while later, Nigel
emailed Philip to ask if he wanted a copy of his suicide note and Philip
replied to say that he would. It was only after Nigel's death, by Nembutal,
that Philip learned the whole story. At the time of the Exit seminar, Nigel
had been under criminal investigation in connection with the deaths of
a former girlfriend and his wife, who had mysteriously fallen from the
top of a quarry. He was also depressed. Before long, a journalist discovered that Philip and Nigel had exchanged emails and reported on Nigel's
connection to Exit. In response, the Medical Board of Australia held a
midnight meeting, where board members used their emergency powers
to suspend Philip's medical registration.

At first, Philip denied doing anything wrong. He argued that Nigel
had not been his patient and that, as such, he hadn't been under any
professional obligation to refer him for psychiatric help. He couldn't be
responsible for the medical fate of every man he crossed paths with, could
he? No physician was held to those standards. But soon, Philip started to
resent his own defensiveness. Why was he apologizing for Nigel? The
more Philip thought about it, the more it seemed to him that Nigel had
been smart to end his life. "What Nigel had done was simply balance

whether or not it was better to be dead or to be in prison for thirty years," he told me. "And Nigel came to the conclusion, as many of us might, in those situations . . . that death is the correct or preferred option. And that is a very good example of 'rational suicide.'" The important thing, Philip said, was that Nigel "died peacefully. Very effectively. And isn't now sitting, languishing in prison." Why argue with that?

Really, Philip thought, Nigel was a lot like the other people who contacted Exit for reasons that weren't, strictly speaking, medical. Sometimes, Philip got letters from prisoners who said they would rather die than spend the rest of their lives in jail cells. Sometimes, he heard from parents who did not want their children to watch them waste away. "People get cancers and they know what the final stages are going to be like, and they don't want their families to see them like that," he said. Once, Philip talked with an elderly woman who wanted to end things because her care was costing thousands of dollars a month and was eating through the savings that she had planned to leave her down-and-out daughter. "I'm going to die," the woman told Philip, "so my daughter can live." Philip didn't know if the woman's choice was right or wrong, but he decided that it didn't matter because it wasn't his choice anyway. He was pro-choice. That was enough. Yes, in an ideal world, maybe the woman wouldn't have to decide between healthcare and her daughter's well-being—but let's be real, this was not an ideal world. Why deny the woman a way out, in the meantime? Why expect her to suffer, heroically, in the service of—what? Some far-off social welfare revolution? Some wild dream that if thousands or millions of people suffered just like her, and people found out about it, the for-profit healthcare system would correct itself accordingly, or implode, or be burned down by the exasperated masses? Philip was a pragmatist. And soon he came to believe that man-made conditions like thirty-year prison sentences and poverty could be as awful and untreatable as any cancer. By extended logic, the people who suffered from those civilizational afflictions deserved his help as much as anyone else did.

With his medical license in suspension, Philip continued to give DIY Death seminars, but the seminars changed. Philip stopped speaking of Nembutal as a solution to material problems of the body—illness or infirmity or age—and instead described it in simpler terms: as a pharmacological tool that should be made available to the suffering. Philip's duty was to help people who suffered, but it was up to each sufferer to decide that she was suffering and to define her condition. For his part, Philip would take people at their word and he would not try to talk them out of it. He would even help, say, Stephen Hawking to die, if Stephen Hawking asked him to. "Of course! Of course. No one would blame me for that. Well, maybe they would. Every day he stays alive, the world benefits. I would imagine that people have said that to him. . . . Almost like you've got an obligation to live on and use your immense skill to benefit humankind. But the idea that you should stay alive to satisfy the rest of us is not the point." Philip came to think that efforts to suppress rational suicide were "a sign of an increasingly sick society." They were a sign that, maybe, society wasn't so confident in its reasons for insisting on life. "I don't know why people who commit suicide attract such anger and such resentment from the community," he said. "When I think about it, I think the most likely explanation is that what they are effectively saying to the rest of us is: 'We won't value the life that you live. We don't acknowledge the game that you're playing.'" The jig is up. There is no God. Life only matters if you think it does.

In October 2015, Australia's medical board announced that it would reinstate Philip's medical license, provided that he agreed to twenty-six conditions, one of which was that he stop sharing information about suicide with the public. The twenty-six conditions enraged Philip. In response, he called a press conference in Darwin to announce that he would burn his license and henceforth give up the practice of medicine. "It's a worthless document. It's a worthless document. And I'm giving evidence to suggest how worthless it is and showing my contempt for it," he said on the day of the burning. "It's effectively a document that impairs your ability to help people at the end of their lives." In the Darwin conference room, Philip stood solemnly beside a wooden podium, in a checkered dress shirt and patterned scarf, and raised both hands. In one, he held his medical license. In the other, he held a lighter. To the small crowd of reporters that was gathered, he seemed in high spirits, as if he took a certain joy in his persecution. As if the persecution itself were proof that he had been right all along. Someone asked Philip how he was feeling, and he shrugged. "Ah, a bit sad. A bit sad and a bit glad." Then he set the paper ablaze. He let it burn for a few undramatic seconds before dropping it into a metal garbage bin and watching the sparks die out. When it was over, Philip posed for press photographs. "Say when," he told the photographers, holding up the lighter.

After the press conference, Philip and Fiona decided to leave Australia for a while. Philip said he wanted to live somewhere more enlightened, in Europe, maybe. As a first stop, they rented a small house in London, where, one early morning in July, Fiona sat in the living room across from Philip with her phone pressed against her ear. "Yes, it is Exit. How can I help you? . . . Right. Right . . . Do you have a copy of *The Peaceful Pill Handbook*? . . . That explains your options and then you can come back to us if you have any questions. . . . Mm-hmm. Assisted suicide is illegal in the UK, so we can't help you. . . . Yes, you need to organize everything yourself. . . . Yeah, we agree." Fiona leaned forward and rested her elbows on the table. She looked dramatic, her hair cut short and spiky and red. Under the table, a tiny dog named Henny Penny wound herself around Fiona's legs. "It should give you peace of mind. . . . Well, if you get some options in place, I'm sure you'll feel even better and then you can get on with it. With living! . . . OK. Just get the book and I'm sure you'll be much better. . . . All right. Take care. Bye-bye!"

"Well, that was interesting," Fiona said, hanging up the phone and turning to Philip. The man on the line had said that he had non-Hodgkin's lymphoma and that he was dying, and that he wasn't interested in palliative care or hospice. He just wanted to die before he got very sick. The rub was that the man's wife was a palliative care physician and did not know what her husband was planning. On the phone, the man had told Fiona that he would keep his suicide plans a secret, "to protect her."

"That's interesting," Philip said.

Fiona frowned. "All right, what now?"

In recent weeks, the subject of Exit International's eligibility criteria had become a source of tension at home. Fiona was of the opinion that when a person applied to join Exit, or asked to buy *The Peaceful Pill Handbook*, it was her job to do at least a bit of verification. She usually asked the would-be buyer for proof of age, which she sometimes checked against a credit card, and an explanation of why he wanted the handbook in the first place. She asked what he was sick with. If a person's story didn't make sense or lacked detail, Fiona might ask the buyer for a copy of his medical records, or spend some time Googling his name, to see if anything weird came up, like a criminal record. Sometimes, if the tone of a person's request seemed off—if a person sounded unhinged or emailed her with frantic, lunatic prose—Fiona would refuse to sell him the handbook outright. "It's subjective," she said of her technique. The point was to protect Philip.

But Philip had come to believe that the background checks were wrong. They were also "a pain in the ass," he said, and sort of pointless because they didn't always work. Every so often, a young person with a mental illness would pretend to be old and sick, and Fiona would unwittingly sell him a copy of the book. Inevitably, the kid would end up killing himself. And inevitably, after he did, his family members would come forward to blame Philip for the suicide. Philip, in turn, would be impatient with their allegations. He would accuse the family members of being disgruntled people and of scapegoating him for their own failures. For their own inability to keep their loved one alive. "I might have once inappropriately, and perhaps inadvisably, used the phrase 'collateral damage,' referring to some of these unfortunate incidents," Philip said. "What I'm really trying to say is that you can't keep everybody safe."

ON NOVEMBER 2, 2016, I was sitting in my office in East London, reading the news, when I saw an article in the *Mirror* titled "Fears Grow for Man Who Disappeared After Reportedly Buying 'Euthanasia Drugs' Online." The article showed a picture of a twenty-seven-year-old named Joshua Smith: thin and pale and standing in a thicket of trees, smiling a little at the camera. It quoted Joshua's sister, Hannah, explaining that her brother had disappeared five days earlier. "We know from Josh's internet search history that he purchased a quick acting euthanasia drug, and we believe he took this with him on Tuesday morning," she said. "Josh is a loving, caring person who is very unwell." He was depressed and had become convinced that he would never be well again.

On Facebook, I found Hannah's profile and a group that she had started in her brother's name: "Joshua Smith: Missing—Stone, Staffordshire." In the days since the disappearance, Hannah wrote, she and police officers had studied grainy black-and-white security camera footage from a nearby scrap metal facility and, from it, concluded that Joshua had left his house at 8:35 on Tuesday morning. He had then walked down the road to the canal, where he either turned right or left or crossed over the bridge. On the Facebook page, people posted images of highlighted maps, with shading to represent the places where they had already searched for Joshua, on foot or by car. Someone named Alex said he had checked the local boatyard area: "every mooring, boat, building and outbuilding as well as the streams and any scrub or hedgerow or ditch."

That day, Philip emailed me with a link to the same article. "Too many teenagers telling us they've got lung cancer!" he wrote. "This is our newest!"

A few days later, I took an afternoon train to meet Hannah at her boyfriend's house, but when I got there, she told me that she was too tired and sad to talk, so I went back to London. A few days later, I traveled to meet her again, this time three hours northwest, at her mother's house in Stone, on a quiet street of boxy, rectangular houses and tidy lawns. Hannah and I sat on her bed, cross-legged and bent over her laptop. She wore pink socks.

Hannah had been the one to search through Joshua's emails after he went missing. There had been nothing odd in his inbox, but on a whim, she had checked his sent folder and found messages with clues. Joshua had apparently tried to buy *The Peaceful Pill* online handbook. Before he could, he was asked, by the seller, to identify his date of birth and his health diagnosis. Joshua had lied. He wrote back to say that his birthday was February 16, 1961, and that he was dying of lung cancer. He added that he suffered from rheumatoid arthritis. "My quality of life is decreasing rapidly. I would like to learn of alternative options to end my life with as little pain and as much dignity as possible."

After that, Joshua had exchanged emails with someone named Johnson. "Hello," he had written in one message. "I am looking to purchase Nembutal and I am informed that you are a reliable source."

"Thank you. Have a good week," he wrote in another email, after confirming that he had wired Johnson several hundred pounds and was awaiting his Nembutal shipment.

Hannah had never heard of Nembutal, but when she Googled it, she learned that it was a fast-acting drug, and also that American authorities sometimes used it to execute death-row prisoners. She went downstairs to tell her mother that it might be too late.

Joshua had been depressed for years. He had attempted to take his life once before, in 2012, but the pills had made his stomach burn and he had cried aloud. Hannah's boyfriend had found him in time to call an ambulance, and doctors had saved him. After that, Joshua's mother, Sara, tried to get him into a psychiatric program. She told doctors that she would agree to anything that might help. But Joshua was simply discharged from the hospital and told to come back in several weeks, for six cognitive behavioral therapy sessions that would be covered by the national healthcare system. On the day that Joshua was sent home, Sara sat in her car and cried because she was scared of what Joshua might do while he waited to see more doctors.

Joshua did his six therapy sessions, but he didn't feel better afterward. The sessions only lasted half an hour, and Joshua saw different experts each time. Each time, it was hard for him to express his feelings, and by the time he did, the session would be over and his feelings would be out there, exposed to the elements. Sara thought that Joshua's appointments "opened things up but then left him with nowhere to go." She asked the hospital again for more help, but nobody seemed to think that Joshua was in acute need. "Did they think I was some kind of hysterical mother?" Sara asked later. "They didn't take it seriously." In the meantime, Joshua kept a journal of all the ways he was attempting to be healthy again: exercising, eating a nutritious diet, meditating, not drinking, gardening. He loved gardening and was good at it. But still he admitted to searching online for ways to kill himself. In the end, Sara did get Joshua scheduled for another medical appointment, but then he was gone.

"I'm not angry with Josh for finding it too hard to carry on and wanting to end his life," Hannah told me, wiping her eyes. "No, I can't be angry at him because I would never want him to be in that amount of pain." She scrolled through pictures of her brother on her phone. "Why did you make it so hard to find you?" she said. "It's been thirteen days now. Where did you go?"

In the days following Joshua's disappearance, dozens of volunteers helped to search the neighborhood. It was late into fall and it was cold out, but bright. A detective from the police station gave instructions to a team of men in red puffy jackets who then fanned out into the forest, their walkie-talkies pressed against their lips and their boots pressed into the wet earth. Sara walked with them, slowly along the water, in her dark winter parka. She used a long wooden stick to push aside branches and poke at piles of leaves, maybe hoping and not hoping that she would strike something soft and doughy. Joshua's stepfather, Andy, brought along the dog. "Find him," he whispered into the animal's ear, coaxing him toward a tangled mound of shrubs. Twenty-five days after Joshua went missing, the search team found his body, lying under some trees.

After the memorial service, Sara sat on the sofa in the living room and rested her head on Andy's shoulder. Joshua had been having a few bad weeks, she said. His grandfather had died. He had gotten in a fight with his girlfriend. He had been crying a lot. And then he found *The Peaceful Pill*. "That encouraged him. They were suggesting *ways*," Sara said. "They are complicit." The drugs came on a Monday and Joshua took them on a Tuesday. "Without thinking, without pausing. Probably he took it so quickly, the day afterward, because if he had paused, his mind would have been changed. . . . I just hope it was quick and it was painless." Sara turned away and buried her face in Andy's chest.

"We do some checks," Philip said afterward. "But obviously . . . people will always slip in." He was in his new home: a large houseboat on a canal in the Netherlands, outside of Haarlem, where he and Fiona had decided to resettle. The houseboat had big windows and wooden floors and a large deck overlooking the water. It was cold, even inside the boat, and Philip wore a gray woolen hat. He said he had reviewed the emails sent by Joshua Smith and that the whole incident had got him thinking. The result of that thinking was a question: Who was to say that a twenty-seven-year-old like Joshua *shouldn't* have access to this information? Not him. Not Exit. Philip insisted that Joshua's emails had been carefully composed and well considered. "This is a person who may be lying, but he's not irrational . . . I think, well, I don't know. What do I feel about it? Joshua Smith got a peaceful death." In the months following, Philip would stick to this line, excusing his role in the suicide with a breezy abdication. It could not have been otherwise, he suggested. It could not have ended any other way.

Philip said he had been hearing more from people who wanted to die because they were young and mentally ill and lost in the world. Some were in their twenties, even. Fiona thought they should reject these people from Exit because they would only cause trouble, but Philip didn't think so. Already, he had turned away from Exit's founding rules: that a person be over fifty years old and that he be physically sick. Already, he was operating on a revised principle: that an Exit member need only have his own good reason for wanting to die. Now, even that watered-down condition seemed unfair. Why did a person need to have any reason at all, much less a good one, as judged by Philip?

"I don't feel comfortable saying 'no' to people," he said. "It's very arbitrary and I don't particularly feel comfortable with that. I feel that if we're going to go out there and teach people how to kill at eighteen, send them off to Afghanistan to kill people, which our society does. . . . Er, how can we seriously do that? And at the same time say, 'But oh no! You are not allowed to kill yourself!'" And so, Philip said, he was starting a new initiative: a subgroup called Exit Action, which could represent Exit's new "militant pro-euthanasia" position. With its launch, Philip would be ridding Exit International, once and for all, of its entry criteria. There would be no more age requirements. No more demands for proof of physical pathology. Anyone who wanted to die, was competent enough to understand the permanence of death, and was not in the throes of absolute madness—as revealed by crazy-sounding emails or phone calls—could buy the handbook and learn what Philip had to teach.

Fiona shifted loudly. "This has nothing to do with me," she said. She was sitting at the table in the kitchen, staring at her laptop. She was busy, she said, working on plans to translate *The Peaceful Pill* into Dutch, German, French, Italian, and Spanish. Fiona said that Philip had not asked for her opinion before announcing the new project on Twitter.

"I just did it," Philip agreed. "Because a part of the problem is that every time I talk about things like this, Fiona gets anxious. So it's better to just do it." They both laughed.

"I'm not into overt lawbreaking," said Fiona. "I see that civil disobedience only goes so far. But Philip is a child of the sixties." She smiled at him and cocked her head. "Maybe he's on to something. Don't put your foot down right away. Give him some rope and see if he hangs himself!"

Exit Action was important, Philip said, because it would signal the end of him playing nicely with other right-to-die activist groups. It would be the end of his respect for their slow, plodding ways. Good riddance. Philip said he'd had enough of the right-to-die mainstream, and even most of its fringe. All those people did was talk endlessly about eligibility criteria: proof of illness, proof of age, good reasons and bad ones. As a result, Philip said, Exit had already become "a pariah within the so-called progressive movement of people wanting to change legislation on end-of-life options. . . . They say, 'Oh, you've caused trouble and you've set back necessary changes.' That's an argument I'm quite dismissive of." He shrugged. "It's all very well to say I should shut up because it might allow things to happen a little quicker. But at the same time, I get annoyed by people who simply say that it's all about the ends, rather than the ideas. These ideas are important. Talking about those ideas will slow things down a bit, maybe, but ultimately will get us to a world that is a much better one."

Mostly, Philip said, he was tired of the old ways. "I'm sick to death of the traditional strategy of lobbying politicians: wheeling out sick people and sitting at the foot of the politicians, *begging*," he said. "No more of this, 'Please, can you help me, sir? Fill up my bowl of gruel some more.'" It wasn't good enough to manufacture pity. "That puts you on the back foot. Rather than saying: 'This is my right and I'm taking it. Try to stop me.'"

IN EARLY 2017, I flew to the Netherlands to see Philip. "Do your neighbors know what your business is?" I asked when I stepped inside the houseboat.

"Mm-hmm. Yeah. They've been very supportive."

"It's no big deal," Fiona interrupted, glaring up at me at me through new cat-eye glasses. "The guy next door, he has our competitor's book."

"Chabot." Philip shook his head. Dr. Boudewijn Chabot, a psychiatrist, had become famous in the Netherlands in the 1990s after he assisted in the death of a fifty-year-old patient who was grieving the death of her two young sons but was otherwise healthy. The woman had told Chabot that she could not accept the loss of her boys and wished only to lie forever in between their graves—and also that she had tried to end her life already. After the woman's suicide, Chabot was brought to trial and in 1994 was found guilty by the Dutch Supreme Court. Still, justices chose not to punish him, in a decision that was seen to validate the use of euthanasia for mental suffering. Chabot became famous. "The public seems to have an insatiable appetite for the details of his case," reported the *Independent*. In turn, Chabot used some of his fame to attack another rising Dr. Death, chiding Philip publicly for his technology-driven approach and questioning the accuracy of his Nembutal purity tests. "I was really annoyed," Philip said. "That annoyed me."

"I don't know," Fiona said. "I think he's fucked up. . . . But you can understand him being threatened. We've arrived on his turf!" Fiona had warned me, when she picked me up from the train station, that Western Europe's right-to-die community was an insular world unto itself: small and bitchy and racked by internecine clashes. "It's cutthroat. Fight to the death," she said. "All the sayings that are particularly good for euthanasia!" In Haarlem, Fiona had caused some drama of her own, accusing the country's largest pro-euthanasia activist group of profiting off Philip's research, while at the same time maintaining a certain public coolness toward Exit.

Still, they liked the Netherlands and thought it made sense for them to be there. The country had the most expansive assisted-dying laws in the world, and you could feel it on the ground. The idea of accessible euthanasia was tangible to the Dutch people. By 2016, it accounted for 4 percent of total deaths in the country, which meant that practically everyone knew someone who had been euthanized. To some, euthanasia was starting to feel like a national tradition, or at least a very ordinary way to die. Even the Dutch Reformed Church tolerated it. Church officials drew a distinction between the usual kind of suicide (*zelfmoord*, or "self-murder," which was a mortal sin) and this new kind of chosen death (*zelfdoding*, or "self-deathing").

For my part, I had come to the Netherlands see the machine. It lay outside, on the deck of the houseboat, exposed to the wind: a pyramid-shaped aluminum structure that was as long as a long human body and attached to a large gas tank. It was designed to kill a person using liquid nitrogen, which would be released into a holding tray at the bottom of the machine and then, upon contact with air, would turn into a gas and move through a vent into the main chamber, pushing out all the oxygen inside. If things went according to plan, Philip said, the user—who would be positioned lengthwise, inside, with the door closed—would breathe deeply and then feel "a sense of serene euphoria," and then lose consciousness. This was just a prototype, Philip told me as we walked around the exterior. The final appliance would be far more elegant: made of shiny recycled plastic, in customizable colors. It would also have a plate-glass window on top, so that a person could look up at the sky as he took his final breaths. Philip hoped to unveil the machine in Switzerland, which meant that the first user could die under the famous Swiss Alps, or even the northern lights. He had named his creation Sarco, because it looked like a sarcophagus.

"I mean, we've seen it portrayed in many fictional accounts," he said. "There's a classic scene out of *Soylent Green*. He goes into a very idealized environment with the right music, the right light. He lies back. Everything is beautiful. He watches graphic depictions of pleasant scenes and peacefully dies with the administration of the right drugs. . . . The sarcophagus machine is ideally going to provide that for people." More practically, the machine would reduce Exit's reliance on Nembutal dealers in Mexico and China. This was good news because the drugs were getting harder to access. The Mexican dealers were getting cagey. Online marketplaces were closing down. Scam sites were starting up.

The prototype was a bit bent out of shape, from Philip's first test of it. He had pumped in too much nitrogen too quickly and the thin metal siding had buckled under the pressure. Fiona had screamed and run to hide behind the houseboat, peeking out from around the corner every few minutes to gasp aloud and take a picture of Philip on her iPhone. It had looked like it was going to explode, but it hadn't exploded. "Look! Look at that!" Philip had called out when the test was over. His gas meter showed that oxygen levels inside the chamber had fallen to "0.5 percent!"

"Incompatible with life!" Fiona had cried, running forward to embrace him.

"From whence you came!"

Philip thought the Sarco would appeal to Exit members who didn't want to order illegal things on the Internet or lie to their doctors to get pills, and who were freaked out by the idea of plastic bags and asphyxiation. It might also draw the kind of person who wanted to make his death a bit of a show. "I can see it appealing to the romantic," Philip said. "People who care about the aesthetic, who want to die beautifully." The Sarco didn't look like a coffin; it looked like a vessel, ready to take off and fly. Maybe death by Sarco would feel ritualistic, modern but also somehow practiced and ancient. Maybe a person's whole community would come out to watch. At an early presentation of the device, one Exit volunteer said she thought the machine was "a little Auschwitzy," but Philip thought it wasn't, because it had an escape hatch.

I ran my hand along the cool aluminum siding. Philip said the prototype had cost hundreds of thousands of dollars to build but that his plan was for future Sarcos to be 3-D printed in people's homes or communities, using a digital design that Exit would make free and open-source. The technology was already there. According to Philip's vision, each printed Sarco would also require a four-digit code, which Exit would send the would-be user after he passed a simple online test that measured his mental capacity and ability to make end-of-life decisions. Philip was still hazy on the details of the capacity test and its feasibility. It would make use of artificial intelligence, he said. He was still figuring it out. But already, some news outlets had written cheery articles about the machine. *Newsweek*, in its piece, had compared Philip to the billionaire founder of Tesla: "the Elon Musk of Assisted Suicide."

"Would it be legal to sell?" I asked.

"It seems to me that there shouldn't be any real issues," Philip said. It was like selling someone a rope. When a man hangs himself, nobody blames the owner of the hardware store.

Philip believed that once the Sarco was unleashed into the world, there would be no point in even arguing about physician-assisted death anymore. What would be the point? Critics could debate first principles all they liked, but their talk would literally be irrelevant because they could not prevent anyone from printing his own Sarco, in his own basement, and using the machine to die with. Quickly. Painlessly. As I listened to Philip talk, I thought about San Francisco and its fabled start-up scene: all its odd-man engineer-founders, preaching the virtues of their special designs alongside a larger politics of gadget-mediated progress. In California, too, optimism and techno-libertarianism could blend together into something that looked like spiritual rebirth. Philip understood this. In a promotional video he made for the Sarco, he featured breathy testimony from a white-haired Exit member who declared that the Sarco was "utopia. It's *Brave New World* stuff."

Back inside the houseboat, Philip and Fiona were fighting. "Fiona? Shut up, Fiona."

"You've *got* to let Katie have a photo with the tulips!"

Philip sighed and gestured toward the door and then handed me a plastic motorcycle helmet. He had bought the motorcycle as a gift to himself, on his seventieth birthday. It had a little sidecar on it, where Fiona usually sat with her knees pulled into her chest, and Philip said I should sit there, too. For a while, we drove in silence, past fields of the country's renowned tulips. Some stood in full and perfect bloom. Others had already wilted on their stems. Why, Philip wondered aloud, had nobody picked them before they died? We stopped and walked around in a patch of yellow and red flowers, and Philip took a picture of me with my phone. We spoke very little. It occurred to me that I had never seen Philip in the wild before, alone and off duty. He was quiet and a little shy—as if, stripped of a chance to be outraged, or to pantomime outrage, or to deflect the outrage of others, his instinct was not to say much at all.

Because he was away from Fiona, who always brushed off questions about sales of *The Peaceful Pill Handbook*, I asked Philip how the business was doing. He said that the book was bringing in around half a million dollars a year and that, after more than ten years in circulation, its profits were "as regular as clockwork." For the sake of appearances, he and Fiona had organized things so that their work was split in two; he ran Exit International as a nonprofit, with an annual salary of $0, and Fiona ran the for-profit publishing wing. It was all the same to him, because anything she earned was shared between the two of them. As we walked back, through the tulips and toward the motorcycle, Philip told me that when it came to Exit and its eligibility criteria, Fiona seemed to be coming around to his view of things. Just the other day, she had sold a copy of the handbook to a thirty-something woman in Canada who said she was unable to sleep because she was afraid of nuclear war. The woman wanted to have Nembutal in her cupboard, in case of apocalypse. "That makes perfect sense to me," Philip said.

Philip thought the right-to-die movement was speeding toward a historic shift that it would not and could not and definitely should not turn back from: a pivot from a medical model of assisted dying to a rights-based model. "I'll explain the difference," he said. "The 'medical model' is where we see this as a service that you provide the sick. If a person gets sick enough, and all the doctors agree, the person who is very sick and keen to die gets lawful help to die. The laws are quite complex because they have to decide whether you're sick enough. . . . Now, the rights model, which I'm strongly in favor of, says that this has got *nothing* to do with sickness. The idea is: having a peaceful death is a human right. And as a right, it's not something that you have to ask permission for. In other words, it's something you have simply because you're a person of this planet. The rights model, of course, means that doctors don't necessarily have to be involved."

The more Philip thought about it, the more he believed that the medical profession was in way over its head. Doctors had made themselves judge and jury in a process that had more to do with the human spirit than the human body. More to do with meaning, and the search for it, than physical pain. And what did doctors know about the meaning of life anyway? "Doctors love it. They can't help themselves," Philip said. "And I find that insufferable paternalism of the medical profession difficult to deal with." Lawmakers had played their part, too. They had let it happen. Now, Philip thought, doctors and legislators were running a mutually beneficial racket: each delegating decision-making and gatekeeping powers to the other, so that together they could maintain control over death and dying. Because they were afraid of the alternative. Only a doctrine of rational suicide—a philosophy that accepted peaceful death as a human right—would correct the injustice. Embraced by the masses, rational suicide would be a slap in the face to doctors who claimed to advocate for patient autonomy but still clung to its ill-defined limits. It would expose old, religious ways of thinking and exorcise them from hospitals. Not even Kevorkian had thought so boldly, Philip said. Until the end, Kevorkian had insisted that doctors be involved. That doctors be in charge! That doctors know best.

After leaving Philip's houseboat, I took the train across the Netherlands and spoke with Dutch doctors and lawyers and legislators. I wanted to understand what it meant for this tiny European country to be at the euthanasia vanguard. By the time of my visit, some people outside the Netherlands were already looking at the country with alarm. International newspapers like the *Daily Mail* ran headlines about Dutch doctors who granted euthanasia requests from patients with anorexia, personality disorders, severe tinnitus, feelings of being "meaningless," and trauma resulting from sexual abuse. They quoted experts who pointed out, correctly, that the percentage of approved euthanasia requests was rising, and that some doctors granted approvals to patients they didn't know very well— and that more than 99 percent of assisted deaths were judged by authorities, after the fact, to have been carried out correctly. In the Netherlands, wrote the psychiatrist and philosopher Scott Kim, "the doctor is virtually always right when it comes to euthanasia."

In his 2014 book, *Being Mortal*, the physician and writer Atul Gawande noted that, historically, the Netherlands was quick to embrace euthanasia but relatively slow to provide high-quality palliative care. As such, Gawande wrote, the Dutch "may have reinforced beliefs that reducing suffering and improving lives through other means is not feasible when one becomes debilitated or seriously ill"—and, in doing so, led sick patients to assume that they could find relief from pain only in death. Gawande referred to the country's high euthanasia rate as "a measure of failure" and said that he was "less worried about the abuse of these powers than I am about dependence on them." What if euthanasia became the new Dutch normal?

In reviewing Gawande's book in the *New York Review of Books*, Dr. Marcia Angell, a former editor at the *New England Journal of Medicine*, criticized the author for failing to clarify just what about euthanasia he found so morally wanting. Why, she asked, "does Gawande simply assert that the one in thirty-five assisted deaths in the Netherlands are too many? Given the prevalence of terrible deaths from cancer, as Gawande describes so well in his book, why is it not the right number?"

While I was in Amsterdam, some doctors mentioned an ethics professor named Theo Boer, at the Protestant Theological University, who had served for ten years on the country's euthanasia oversight committee before resigning in protest. I wrote to Boer and asked if we could speak. "My concern is that euthanasia is increasingly becoming *the* way to die for cancer patients," he told me later, in stilted English. "So gradually there has taken place a paradigm shift from 'euthanasia as the last resort' to 'euthanasia as the preferred option.'" Many patients were asking for death without even considering palliative care, which he said had improved significantly in Dutch hospitals since the 1990s.

"So what?" I asked.

"I think there is nothing wrong with a good taboo," Boer said carefully. Without it, "we will end up in a society where elderly people are killed. You may say, 'Is there anything wrong with that?' Well then, in that case, your question already includes or illustrates the paradigm shift."

"Is your concern that the value of human life will be degraded in a way that cannot be reversed?" I asked. "Or is it something more extreme? Like, some sort of nihilistic crisis of civilization because we've lost human worth. I don't mean to sound hyperbolic . . ."

"Interesting. Life is miserable. It is often completely miserable. It is challenging. And what I see is an increasing atmosphere in which death is considered to be the solution to all major and serious suffering. Kant was the champion of autonomy. He is the one we have to thank for the idea of autonomy in our society. . . . But he said, don't kill yourself. That would be putting all your autonomy to an end." Boer was silent for a moment. "I don't know that it can be proven, but what I do see is that the supply of euthanasia creates a certain demand."

I NEXT SAW PHILIP IN December, in Toronto, at a death technology conference that he was hosting in a rented conference room, in a nondescript strip mall, on a quiet street in the semi-suburban north of the city. Philip asked me to keep the location a secret. I arrived early and found a seat next to an older man in red suspenders. He held out his hand. "Hello! Neal Nicol."

"Ah." I knew the name. Jack Kevorkian's former assistant. I placed my outstretched hand in his. "What are you presenting on today?" I asked.

"My original presentation was titled 'Erotic Asphyxiation.' But really it's just jugular strangulation." With one hand, Neal grabbed my lower arm. With the other, he pretended to strangle himself. Then he offered me a cinnamon mint from a silver tin in his shirt pocket.

The rented space had hard yellow lighting and bookshelves lined with self-help literature. On the counter, by the drip coffee, someone had left a plastic container of assorted Danish pastries. This was the New Technologies in Self-Deliverance (NuTech) conference, held every other year since 1999, by "a loose assembly of individuals interested in, and working on, the development of practical solutions for stakeholders (rational adults) who are interested in access to a peaceful, reliable (and non-medical) death." In the 1990s, NuTech members had perfected the helium-gas-tank-and-plastic-bag-hood method and shared the informa-tion with activist groups around the world. This year, NuTech would be featuring a handful of DIY death inventors. "Know a better way to die?" Philip had tweeted in his announcement of the event.

Philip took the stage and the room grew still. Around me were about two dozen people: many, grandees of the fringiest right-to-die fringe. "In the twenty-year history of this organization, I would have expected more action," Philip said gravely. "You look at any field and you think, 'Well, *that* wasn't there ten years ago.'" Everything was being mecha-nized. Technology was advancing apace. But euthanasia was still hung up on plastic bags and illegally imported veterinary medicines. Philip said they needed new solutions. If they were going to "demedicalize death," they were going to have to technify it.

The mood in the room was fizzy when the presentations began. A man named Richard unveiled "the Rebreather": a plastic mask attached to a container filled with tiny black-and-white CO_2-absorbent pellets, which Richard said could cause death by nitrogen gas asphyxiation. An Aus-tralian named Davy discussed his design for a "Life Quality Monitor," which involved reverse engineering a standard pacemaker to initiate a forced ventricle fibrillation (lethal) whenever certain preset physiological criteria were reached. Neal Nicol presented, to a grimacing audience, his cruder contraption. It was made of a tennis sweatband, a tensor bandage, and two tablespoons, designed to fit around the neck and cut off blood flow through the carotid arteries. The design, Neal admitted, was clumsy, but it was meant to help people who couldn't afford anything fancier and didn't want to break the law: "a little old lady," he suggested. "An eighty-one- or eighty-two-year-old widow who is in an assisted-living facility and is on Social Security." Philip presented last, with a shoebox-size prototype of the Sarco, looking purple and shiny and extraterrestrial. "Wildly impractical," Neal hissed in my ear.

The next day, Philip ran one of his standard DIY Death seminars on the second floor of a quiet Unitarian Universalist church in downtown Toronto. He often used Unitarian churches as meeting venues. In 1988, the small Unitarian Universalist Association had broken with the broader religious fold to endorse physician-assisted death as a means of preventing "unnecessary suffering and/or loss of dignity." Now the liberal Unitarians were relaxed about renting out church properties to Exit and other right-to-die groups. Philip liked the spaces because they tended to have lots of available seating.

When I arrived, there were already several dozen people sitting in straight-backed chairs with faded green upholstery. Fiona was standing by the door, selling copies of *The Peaceful Pill Handbook*. Philip was setting up his now familiar PowerPoint presentation. "Can everybody read this?"

A peaceful death is everyone's right
Philip Nitschke, MD, PhD

He began. "The right of a rational adult to a peaceful death, at the time of one's choosing, is fundamental." As such, he explained, it could not be taken away. And it was not dependent on how sick a person was. In fact, because it was a human right, it had no eligibility criteria at all. Philip smiled. "Eligible to die? Now, that's a quaint notion."

The End

I could have filled this book with confessions. With all the tiny disclo-
sures I've received over the last several years, often from near strangers. About people who died terribly, in ways they did not want and that
confused them. Violent deaths. Ugly deaths. Long deaths. Or about people who ended their own lives, to avoid all that. And the people who
helped them. Many people told me about promises they made to parents
and grandparents, to help them die if they develop Alzheimer's or otherwise lose their minds. Whether and how they will keep their word is
another matter. I'm left to wonder if the promises are even sincere, or just
another way to announce, "I am also scared." If they are sincere, what then?
Will everyone be OK afterward, certain in the feeling that what they did
was merciful? Or will they come to think that what they did was illegal
and wrong and strange? Who can say? What I know is this: It would be
hard to exaggerate how many people told me that they wish simply for
the same rights as their cherished dogs—to be put out of their misery
when the time is right.

Only a small minority of people will choose and qualify for physician-
assisted death, in the states and countries where it is legal. Elsewhere,

another small faction will opt for what they call rational suicide. More people, I think, will consider hastened death, or wish for it, or plead for it. According to a 2017 survey by the Kaiser Family Foundation, about half of Americans think that patients do not have enough control over end-of-life medical decisions. Endings, of course, are not always controllable. Still, it is worth asking whether this is an acceptable and philosophically coherent status quo.

In the United States, the law inches forward. Every few months, another state legislature considers passing a death with dignity law of its own, and once in a while one does. It seems likely that the Oregon model will expand outward, and eastward. Already, right-to-die lobbyists in DC and Portland are beginning to speak with a bit more confidence. In turn, religious institutions are digging their heels in. In October 2019, leading representatives of the major Abrahamic monotheistic religions met with Pope Francis at the Vatican to sign a joint declaration condemning assisted death and euthanasia as against "the dignity of the dying patient." Some Catholic bishops—diminishing in local relevance but reanimated by a "politics of life"—have formally banned priests from being at a person's bedside to offer comfort and counsel during an assisted death.

National medical groups are reacting in much the same way. At a June 2019 meeting, the American Medical Association's House of Delegates voted 392–162 to reaffirm the group's opposition to physician-assisted death. "The wheels are coming off the bus on assisted suicide," warned one doctor-delegate. "We do not have the luxury of time to continue to fail to act. . . . Unless we're willing to embrace widespread euthanasia." Also in 2019, the National Hospice and Palliative Care Organization began a reexamination of its long-standing opposition to the practice. "The fact that we were even *looking* at this policy caused such outrage," Edo Banach, the group's CEO, told me. "I was getting calls from Catholic bishops!" Banach was new in the job, a lawyer and a liberal who supported the death with dignity cause. Nevertheless, in the course of his deliberation, he was persuaded to leave things as they were. The choice, he said, was more practical than anything else. Hospice care in the United States wasn't what it should be; many hospice agencies were underresourced and underperforming. "I want to make sure that if anyone provides hospice care, it's the best kind of care that we can provide," Banach said. "Only then can I have the bandwidth to actually have a debate over whether we should endorse or not endorse assisted death." Banach also worries about money. What if the NHPCO endorsed aid in dying, and then conservative politicians used that as an excuse to cut hospice Medicare funding? "That's really something you need to weigh. I hate to say it." Banach said that when it comes to questions about assisted death, he usually changes the subject. "I dodge a lot. I actually don't want to talk about this."

Inside the states where aid in dying is legal, physicians like Dr. Lonny Shavelson are still trying to streamline the process. In February 2020, Lonny hosted the country's first National Clinicians Conference on Medical Aid in Dying in Berkeley, California. I watched from the balcony as three hundred people, many of them white-haired clinicians, filed into a wood-paneled auditorium with green velvet curtains. Lonny gave an introductory address from a podium on a large stage. "This is history making," he said. Still, he warned the crowd that "we who practice aid-in-dying have no monopoly on a good death. We have no corner on death with dignity." Seated to my right, Dr. Timothy Quill—the palliative care physician who in 1991 admitted to prescribing lethal drugs to his patient Diane, and then wrote about it in a medical journal, and then was celebrated and castigated across the country—nodded and clapped.

Over the course of two days, the conference attendees heard lectures on "The Pharmacology and Physiology of Aid in Dying," "Family Conflicts and Social Complexity in Aid in Dying Requests," and "Practice Pragmatics: Creating an Efficient and Effective Work Flow for Aid in Dying." Some attended a working dinner on "Billing Considerations for Aid-in-Dying Care." And though Lonny had initially threatened to ban all philosophers from the meeting—because, he said, they had been philosophizing for years and years, and now it was time for ordinary doctors to step in and get their hands dirty—he eventually admitted a few, to discuss "Ethical Challenges in Aid-in-Dying Care." At the end of the gathering, Lonny took the stage again to announce the formation of a new national body, the American Clinicians Academy on Medical Aid in Dying, which would bring together practitioners to share knowledge and develop best practices. "This is not a fiction," Lonny said, beaming before the crowd. "I got the website!"

Within days, of course, several cases of COVID-19 had been confirmed in California, and the coronavirus started spreading. Within weeks, the state and country had closed down. Back at his Berkeley home office, Lonny wasn't sure what to expect. Amid all the virus deaths, would other patients still want his help to die? He found that they did. "We're seeing roughly the same number of requests as before coronavirus," he told me in April. The main difference was that he and Thalia were now doing assisted deaths via telemedicine.

Away from the public eye, new questions about the practice of physician-assisted death continue to emerge. Should doctors actively present the option of assisted death to their dying patients—because, of course, doctors are meant to present us with all of our options? Or should they wait until their patients ask about it, lest the simple act of providing information be interpreted as an endorsement or a sign that the doctor has lost hope? Can assisted death ever be something that hospitals advertise? If a doctor refuses to assist in death, should he have to refer an inquiring patient to a doctor who will? Is physician-assisted death better carried out by a small number of specialized physicians or by family doctors? The specialists would quickly become skillful, but the family doctors are more accessible. Also, specialization might ghettoize assisted death—and make it seem like something separate from normal end-of-life medicine.

We can go on: Down the line, should aid-in-dying patients be allowed to donate organs? Of course, that would require that the patients die in a hospital, via injection, to preserve the health of the vital parts—so we would need to change the death with dignity rules. While we're at it, why not go one step further to really maximize the chances of successful transplant: allowing organs to be removed from patients who are under anesthesia but still living, in such a way that the surgery itself would kill them? No doubt, some charitable patients would want the option of "death by donation," as researchers call it. The question is whether the state should allow it: whether death by donation would amount to an odious ethical breach or would just be an efficient way to make the best of a bad situation. For the good of us all.

As they are, existing Oregon-style death with dignity laws are defective. They grant rights to some patients but not to others, in ways that can seem arbitrary and unwise. A breast cancer patient who can swallow lethal medication might have the right to end her life with a doctor's help, but not a brain cancer patient whose tumor has robbed him of his ability to move and to swallow. A person with six months left to live might be declared eligible for assistance, but not a chronically ill person in ten times more pain. Why should someone who is approved to die be made to wait for fifteen days, suffering the whole way through? And what do we do about all the people who would rather be dead than have dementia? Right-to-die opponents see these deficiencies as a sign that we must rescind the laws, to prevent an inevitable slippery-slope expansion. Proponents see the same evidence as proof that we should expand the laws—and redraw the line in the sand, between eligible and ineligible, at a place that is more flexible to the different ways that people hurt.

Even then, the center might not hold. As this book went to print, the Canadian Parliament was working to extend its already liberal Bill C-14 legislation, after a provincial court ruled that it was unconstitutional to require that a patient's death be "reasonably foreseeable." The government was also debating an amendment of the law's eligibility criteria, to include "mature minors" under eighteen years old and patients with mental illnesses. "It could not be otherwise," warned the columnist Andrew Coyne in the *Globe and Mail*. "Once you have accepted the logic of legalization—that death is no longer to be viewed as a terrible tragedy, something we should wish if possible to prevent, but as a blessing, a release from suffering we should wish to assist—all else follows."

The end point to all this might be something that looks like Belgium or the Netherlands. In those countries, euthanasia rates hold steady—but the practice is now accompanied by a whiff of collective unease. In January 2020, three Belgian doctors were put on trial for "manslaughter by poisoning" after assisting in the death of a thirty-eight-year-old woman who prosecutors said did not meet the law's requirements. The patient, Tine Nys, reportedly suffered from a handful of psychiatric disorders and a heroin addiction and had tried to end her life on several occasions. Her longtime psychiatrist had rejected her request to die, presumably because he did not believe that she was incurable. In the end, though, it didn't matter, because Nys searched the country and found three willing physicians, including Dr. Lieve Thienpont, the psychiatrist whom I met at the Vonkel house in Ghent. When Nys asked again to die, Thienpont said yes.

The case was described in the Belgian media as a kind of ultimatum on euthanasia in the country. It marked the first time that health professionals were charged for violating Belgium's euthanasia law. But just a month after the trial began, the three doctors were acquitted. According to an Associated Press report, when the jury announced its decision, around a hundred courtroom spectators "broke out in wild applause."

Around that time, I wrote to all the women whom I had met through Dr. Thienpont at the Vonkel patient support group. On the phone with Ann, I learned that Emily—who was the same age as me, who had dreamed of living in Scotland, who had tried to love her dog Spike so much that she would want to live again—had died by euthanasia a few months earlier. Emily had been approved on the basis of her mental suffering. "She tried so hard, so hard, so hard. And she didn't succeed," Ann said. "She tried very hard to find another meaning in life. . . . She got her dog, Spike, but she always had the feeling that she couldn't love the dog enough." By the time she died, Emily had stopped coming to group meetings at Vonkel because she didn't want to make the others sad.

After speaking to Ann, I started a correspondence with Emily's mother, Veerle. I asked her whether she had supported her daughter's euthanasia request. "I remember I tried to convince her to wait for one more year," Veerle wrote. "She would try alternative therapies. . . . I was willing to go to the end of the world with her if that could help her." But Emily did not want to wait a year. "She had already contacted Lieve Thienpont. She made it quite clear that she would feel alienated from me if I kept on trying to change her mind. I knew that she needed me to respect her autonomy. . . . She did not want to be kept alive, living like a zombie, because of all the drugs she would need to take to not kill herself." When Emily finally scheduled a day to die, Veerle said, "she came home with a bottle of champagne in her hands" and was "joyful."

Elsewhere, impatience with the law is growing. In Britain, a former Supreme Court justice, Lord Jonathan Sumption, made national news by declaring that there was "no moral obligation to obey the law" when it came to assisted suicide. Sumption was not advocating for the legalization of physician-assisted death per se—in fact, he said the existing ban was good and necessary, to prevent abuse—but he argued that "courageous friends and families" would and should continue to help loved ones, on the sly. "I think the law should be broken from time to time," the former justice said. He acknowledged that his position amounted to an "untidy compromise."

I can imagine Philip Nitschke laughing in the face of it. I'm sure he'd call the compromise a cop-out. When we last spoke, Philip seemed in good spirits. He was still at work on the Sarco. *The Peaceful Pill eHandbook* had been translated into French, German, Dutch, Italian, and Spanish. And, at long last, Exit International had been granted admission into the World Federation of Right to Die Societies, an international consortium of several dozen advocacy groups that had previously rebuffed Philip's petitions. At the federation's annual meeting in Cape Town, Philip gave a speech titled "The Death of the Medical Model." "A right is a right," he told the crowd of movement dignitaries. "You don't have to go and beg a doctor for that." The speech, Philip said, did not go down well. "I was damn near chucked out."

The only thing still troubling him were signs of renewed police interest in Exit International. In the summer of 2019, Australian officers visited the homes of several elderly Exit members, demanding that they turn over their imported suicide drugs. Then, a few months later, French media reported that 130 bottles of Nembutal had been seized from private homes in a series of "nationwide raids" carried out by hundreds of police officers. Major outlets claimed that "American authorities" had tipped off their French counterparts after discovering shipments of Nembutal en route to France, disguised as cosmetics.

A NUMBER OF COUNTRIES and states are currently considering death with dignity laws of their own. These debates have all the makings of good moral melodrama: life and death, a contest of first principles, competing appeals to mercy. Also, a sense of urgency. Elsewhere, laws are passing now; people are dying under them. What happens in the United States will reveal something about where this whole thing is headed. Historically, physician-assisted death has been the domain of small Western European countries with national public healthcare systems, bountiful social safety nets, and relatively low levels of cultural diversity. That's not many places and it's not America. Here, big and messy politics get in the way. This is philosophy as practiced on the streets, and at scale.

But the United States is a uniquely imperfect laboratory to be experimenting with these moral principles. Unlike other countries where physician-assisted death is legal, the United States offers no universal healthcare access. In states like Oregon, there is a right to die but not a corresponding right to medical care. Already, stories have appeared in local newspapers about people who were denied exotic and expensive treatments by their health insurance companies but who qualified for a state-subsidized assisted death. "In this profit-driven economic climate, is it realistic to expect that insurers are going to do the right thing, or the cheap thing?" asked Helena Berger, president of the American Association of People with Disabilities, in a 2017 article.

Dr. Wim Distelmans, the well-known Belgian oncologist and supporter of euthanasia, phrased things more starkly. When I asked him about physician-assisted dying in America, he physically recoiled. "It's a developing country," he said. "You shouldn't try to implement a law of euthanasia in countries where there is no basic healthcare." This echoes much of the liberal, secular opposition to assisted death, from skeptics who are less fearful of old perils—Nazis, midcentury eugenic passions, Malthusian panic on the hospital ward—and instead worried about poverty and its perversions.

Within the United States, a new surge of interest in physician-assisted death has landed at a precarious moment, when the country's population is aging. In 2010, the number of people in America over sixty-five years old was around 40 million, but by 2030 that number will have doubled to almost one in five people. The sclerotic healthcare system cannot bear the strain. Already, in 2017, Americans spent more than $3.5 trillion on healthcare: more than 17 percent of the entire country's gross domestic product, and about double, per capita, what the average OECD country pays. Up to a quarter of all Medicare spending goes to patients in just *the last year* of their lives. Given this context, even some supporters worry that well-meaning death with dignity laws will be warped by a debased logic of financial utilitarianism. They imagine that a right to die will become a duty to die cheaply. For the greater good. For the children.

Because clinging to life, at enormous communal expense, may come to look like a terrible kind of vanity.

At the same time, it seems that Americans fight harder than anyone to evade and ignore death. According to the 2017 Kaiser Family Foundation study, about 70 percent of Americans report that they "generally avoid" talking about death. Just 22 percent of people aged sixty-five and older have ever discussed end-of-life wishes with a healthcare provider. National death phobia is so institutionalized that, in 2009, a rather technical policy debate about how American physicians should be reimbursed by Medicare for counseling their patients on living wills and end-of-life care options (the proposed fee was $86 for an initial thirty-minute appointment) was hijacked by conservative lawmakers and vice presidential candidate Sarah Palin, who argued that such counseling sessions amounted to government-run "death panels," deciding who could live and who must die. In response, the Obama administration withdrew the provision and deleted references to end-of-life planning from its healthcare law. And still, the mythical death panels endured. In 2013, three years after the passage of the Affordable Care Act, 40 percent of Americans still falsely believed that the law gave Washington the authority to make end-of-life decisions on behalf of seniors, and 21 percent weren't sure. "Rallying a party base against death makes for a creepy sort of populism," wrote the historian Jill Lepore. "But if harnessing the fear of death for political gain is a grotesque tactic, it may also be a savvy one."

In Oregon, at least, aid-in-dying proponents are buoyed by evidence that the worst slippery-slope predictions of the 1990s have not played out. The law has restrained itself. A study in the *Journal of Medical Ethics* revealed that the rates of physician-assisted death in the state "showed no evidence of heightened risk for the elderly, women, the uninsured . . . people with low educational status, the poor, the physically disabled or chronically ill, minors, people with psychiatric illness, including depression, or racial or ethnic minorities." Assisted death has also not replaced palliative care and hospice care. In fact, the opposite seems true. In

Oregon, referrals for hospice increased after the Death with Dignity law passed, and hospice utilization in the state is now among the highest in the country.

Broadly, in the states where physician-assisted death is legal, it has remained rare and has mostly been used by patients who are very close—weeks or days—to the end. The bioethicist Dr. Arthur Caplan, once one of the country's most ardent critics of assisted dying, was so persuaded by this evidence that he now supports the passage of additional death with dignity laws. "Money was the source of my concern," he told me. "But Oregon and Washington didn't have those abuses. Killing poor people—it didn't happen. There was no 'Mom was trundled off to save money . . .' None of that. So I flipped."

EARLY IN 2020, I called Maia Calloway to wish her a happy New Year. She and Tevye had spent New Year's Eve at her dad's house in Colorado. They watched the Times Square ball drop on TV and then went to bed. On the phone, Maia told me that she would never see the ball drop again, because this would definitely be her last year of life. She was, at that very moment, putting together final arrangements for her death in Switzerland, at a new clinic called Pegasos, which offers "peaceful, dignified and caring assisted death" for 10,000 ($11,000), tax included. Months earlier, she had started another crowdsourcing campaign, this time on GoFundMe, titled "Good Life-Good Death," and had managed to raise more than $7,000: some of it through small donations from strangers: $25, $5. "Your funds will help me to pay for all the fees associated with getting me to Switzerland," she wrote on the campaign page. "Due to daily spinal degeneration, I will not be able to make the 15-hour international flight for much longer."

In the photo that she posted above the text, Maia is seen in her wheelchair. The chair is facing away from the camera, but Maia has turned her head back over her shoulder, toward it. Her lips are parted and her expression is a little startled, as if she was surprised to see a camera there. She looks like the girl in the famous Vermeer painting *Girl with a Pearl Earring*. She looks beautiful. I recognized the image right away. It was a photo that I had taken in New Mexico. Moments before, Maia had moved her wheelchair to the edge of the Rio Grande gorge and looked down into it. There she was, as she had promised she would be—the dying woman, literally staring into the abyss.

"We can't save other people," Maia told me. "We can't rescue other people. We can't prevent other people's suffering because that suffering is inevitable. So what is the difference in preventing your own suffering?" She paused. "I don't want to live in assisted living. Being turned over on a bed. With a catheter. Give me freedom!" Sometimes, Maia said, she still had dreams of outrunning her body and becoming a bird and taking flight. Was the impulse so different from others that I wrote about in this book? Everyone was running from something. Avril from her age, Debra from her disease, Adam from his mind. But toward what?

Almost everyone I met while researching this book told me that they were looking for dignity in dying. Almost always, they used that very word: "dignity." What did it mean? The word, and its appeal for definition, have been at the heart of this work. In the end, of course, "dignity" does not mean any one thing—but in the stories I collected here, I can see a unifying thread. It is that people find dignity in authenticity. They find it in consistency and equilibrium and a kind of narrative coherence. It mattered to the people I met that they lived as themselves, as they defined themselves, until the very final moment, even if that meant sacrificing days or weeks or years of life. It mattered how their lives wrapped up. In this way, a chosen death became a kind of authorial act. It let a person play herself out, until the end.

And so it would be for Maia. This was the penultimate stage of her hero's journey. The only way forward was to conclusion. "I know I've been saying that for a long time," she told me softly. "But I mean it."

Before I sent this book to print, I also wrote again to Derek Humphry, the activist and Hemlock Society founder. In a way, Derek's publication of *Final Exit: The Practicalities of Self-Deliverance and Assisted Suicide for the Dying*, the surprise 1991 bestseller, had set things in motion for my entire project. When we spoke, Derek told me that he still sells several copies of the book every day. By mid-2019, he had sold around 2 million, in twelve languages. In an era of Internet scams, he said, lots of people were still looking for old-fashioned advice: about gas canisters and plastic bags and prescription drug combinations.

I have a secondhand, dog-eared copy of *Final Exit* and had noticed that, in it, Derek listed his personal phone number. I asked him if he'd ever gotten a call from a reader.

He told me that, almost thirty years after the book's first publication, he still receives a phone call or two almost every day, usually from people who are terminally ill and want to know what they can do if staying alive becomes too hard. Derek takes the calls from his two-bedroom home near Eugene, Oregon, by the Willamette River. On a clear day, he can look out the window at the Cascade Mountains and wonder if this—an elderly man answering phone calls from strangers—is the best we can do.

ACKNOWLEDGMENTS

This project took on a crazed life of its own, but it began many years ago with an assignment from an editor in London. I am forever indebted to my former documentary film team at VICE—and especially to directors Yonni Usiskin and Matt Shea—for bringing me along on a wild journalistic ride into the "euthanasia underground."

This book would likely not exist had Simon Sebag Montefiore not encouraged me to write it, at a bar in West London. Thank you. It would certainly not exist if Georgina Capel, my agent, had not urged me to put pen to paper—even though, as she acknowledged at our first meeting, the whole subject matter was "a bit fucked up." Thank you also to William Callahan, at InkWell, who joined as an agent when I moved to New York City.

Anna deVries, at St. Martin's Press, edited this book with enormous thoughtfulness. Thank you to her and the rest of the SMP team, including Sally Richardson, Jennifer Weis, Jennifer Fernandez, and Alex Brown. Equal thanks to Mike Harpley and the team at Atlantic Books, in the UK. Tom Colligan fact-checked every sentence with extraordinary rigor.

A version of Chapter 4 was published in *California Sunday* in March

2019 under the title "Her Time." Kit Rachlis, my wonderful and generous editor, helped me turn a pile of notes into a story. Doug McGray gave it a home at his magazine.

Over the course of five years, my research involved many trips across the United States and abroad. I was supported, financially and otherwise, by a fellowship at New America—and by guidance from Anne-Marie Slaughter, Peter Bergen, Awista Ayub, and Azmat Khan.

Several of my brilliant friends and family members read drafts of this book along the way. I owe infinite thanks to Kathryn Olivarius (who read *many* drafts), as well as Deborah Basckin, Jeff Howard, Linda Kinstler, Emily Miner, and Nabiha Syed—and also Dr. Sally Engelhart, Dr. Brad Segal, and Dr. Jennifer Shaw.

Many others helped me through the process with their conversation and counsel and spare bedrooms. Among them were Dr. Atul Gawande, Ian Cobain, Rebecca Davis, Carlos Beltran, Becky Bratu, Ed Ou, Haimy Assefa, Sutton Raphael, Bob Bikel, Owain Rich, Ali Withers, Ali Velshi, Seyward Darby, Alissa de Carbonnel, Ben Judah, Josie Delap, Mark MacKinnon, Robert Steiner, Timothy Garton Ash, Adam Ellick, Mark Allen, Laura Corwin, Jeeshan Chowdhury, Simon Ostrovsky, Danny Gold, Phoebe Barghouty, Alice Robb, Daniel Medina, Emily Goligoski, Kate Godfrey, Claire Ward, Julia Belluz, Lauren Wagner, Claire Schneiderman, Julia Webster, Aviva Levy, Katie Reisner, Haley Cohen, Nana Ayensu, and Jen Percy.

When I was a little girl, my parents, Susan Paul and Ken Engelhart, read to me every night. They have supported me always, and in everything. Thank you to my siblings, Luke Engelhart and Sally Engelhart. And to my partner, Layth Ashoo, for his incredible, almost unimaginable, patience.

While writing this book, I had the privilege of meeting many people in many countries who shared their homes and minds and lives with me. Not all of the stories they told made their way into print—but all had a deep impression on me and helped to shape this book. If you are reading this, you know who you are. I am grateful to you.

A TIMELINE

January 1942: Switzerland begins permitting assisted death, provided that the assistance is not inspired by "selfish motives."

August 1980: Derek Humphry founds the Hemlock Society in California.

1981: Following a court ruling, the Netherlands effectively stops prosecuting doctors for assisting in patient deaths.

September 1982: In the United States, Medicare begins funding hospice care.

January 1988: An anonymous gynecology resident publishes "It's Over, Debbie" in *JAMA: Journal of the American Medical Association*.

June 1990: A Michigan doctor named Jack Kevorkian helps his first patient, Janet Adkins, to die in the back of his Volkswagen van.

March 1991: Derek Humphry publishes *Final Exit: The Practicalities of Self-Deliverance and Assisted Suicide for the Dying*.

March 1991: In an essay in the *New England Journal of Medicine*, Rochester, New York, doctor Timothy Quill admits to prescribing lethal medication to a cancer patient who wanted to end her life.

November 1994: Oregon voters pass Measure 16 (Oregon Death with Dignity), making the state the first place in the world to legalize, by vote, what was then called "assisted suicide."

March 1995: Pope John Paul II issues his "Evangelium vitae," calling assisted death a "violation of the divine law."

July 1996: In Australia, the Rights of the Terminally Ill Act comes into effect in the Northern Territory.

September 1996: In Australia, Dr. Philip Nitschke becomes the first doctor in the world to legally assist in a patient's death.

March 1997: In Australia, the government repeals the Rights of the Terminally Ill Act. Dr. Philip Nitschke founds the Voluntary Euthanasia Research Foundation and runs his first Exit workshop, in Melbourne.

May 1997: Colombia's Supreme Court decriminalizes assisted death involving terminally ill patients.

June 1997: The US Supreme Court rules on two assisted-death cases, from Washington and New York. The justices decide not to overrule state-level bans on physician-assisted death.

May 1998: The Dignitas assisted-death clinic is founded in Switzerland. It accepts foreign, nonresident patients.

April 2002: Legalized euthanasia and physician-assisted death come into effect in the Netherlands.

May 2002: Belgium legalizes euthanasia and physician-assisted death.

2004: The Final Exit Network is founded.

2005: End-of-Life Choices (previously known as the Hemlock Society) merges with Compassion in Dying to become Compassion & Choices.

July 2006: Dr. Philip Nitschke and Fiona Stewart publish *The Peaceful Pill Handbook*.

November 2008: Washington State legalizes physician-assisted death.

March 2009: In Luxembourg, legal euthanasia and physician-assisted death come into effect.

December 2009: In the United Kingdom, Dr. Michael Irwin founds the Society for Old Age Rational Suicide (SOARS).

December 2009: In *Baxter v. Montana*, the Montana Supreme Court rules that state law protects doctors who help terminally ill patients to die.

May 2013: Vermont's Death with Dignity Act comes into effect.

February 2014: Belgium extends legalized euthanasia to terminally ill children.

February 2015: In *Carter v. Canada*, Canada's Supreme Court overturns the country's ban on physician-assisted death.

September 2015: In the United Kingdom, MPs rejected a physician-assisted-dying bill.

June 2016: The California End of Life Option Act comes into effect.

June 2016: Doctors in Seattle meet to develop the lethal medication cocktail known as DDMP.

June 2016: In Canada, the Parliament passes Bill C-14, legalizing physician-assisted death.

October 2016: Dutch health minister Edith Schippers says she supports the legalization of assisted death for elderly citizens who feel they have "completed life."

December 2016: The Colorado End of Life Options Act comes into effect.

February 2017: The Washington, DC, Death with Dignity Act comes into effect.

April 2018: Hawaii's Our Care, Our Choice Act comes into effect.

June 2019: The American Medical Association reaffirms its opposition to physician-assisted death.

June 2019: Maine's Death with Dignity Act comes into effect.

August 2019: New Jersey's Aid in Dying for the Terminally Ill Act comes into effect.

September 2019: A provincial court in Quebec, Canada, strikes down a restriction that limits physician-assisted death to terminally ill patients.

NOTES

INTRODUCTION

3 **Betty had learned about the Mexican drug**: Philip Nitschke and Fiona Stewart, *The Peaceful Pill eHandbook* (n.p.: Exit International US, 2008). The online handbook is updated up to six times a year, "ensuring," the authors write, "that readers have access to the most up-to-date important information on euthanasia and assisted suicide developments globally," accessed December 2019, http://www.peacefulpillhandbook.com.

3 **Environmental regulations on the automobile industry**: Neil B. Hampson, "United States Mortality Due to Carbon Monoxide Poisoning, 1999–2014. Accidental and Intentional Deaths," *Annals of the American Thoracic Society* 13, no. 10 (October 2016): 1768–1774; Joshua A. Mott et al., "National Vehicle Emissions Policies and Practices and Declining US Carbon Monoxide–Related Mortality," *JAMA: Journal of the American Medical Association* 288, no. 8 (August 2002): 988–995; David M. Studdert et al., "Relationship Between Vehicle Emissions Laws and Incidence of Suicide by Motor Vehicle Exhaust Gas in Australia 2001–06: An Ecological Analysis," *PLOS Medicine* 7, no. 1 (January 2010), http://www.ncbi.nlm.nih.gov/pubmed/20052278.

3 **Coal gas ovens had been replaced**: "The Coal Gas Story: United Kingdom Suicide Rates, 1960–81," *British Journal of Preventative Social Medicine* 30, no. 2 (June 1976): 86–93; Matthew Miller, "Preventing Suicide by Preventing Lethal Injury: The Need to Act on What We Already Know," *American Journal of Public Health* 102, no. 1 (March 2012): e1–e3. The author notes that the same phenomenon is observed in relation to pesticides. In Sri Lanka, for instance, suicide by pesticide declined after the most lethal pesticides were banned.

4 **First-generation sleeping pills**: Wallace B. Mendelson, "A Short History of Sleeping Pills," *Sleep Review*, August 16, 2018, http://sleeppreviewmag.com2018/08/history-sleeping-pills/.

4 **Betty warned her friends**: Robert Rivas, "Survey of State Laws Against Assisting in a

Suicide," Final Exit Network, 2007, www.finalexitnetwork.org/Survey_of_State_Laws_Against_Assisting_in_a_Suicide_2017_update.pdf.

5 **a larger political crusade for "patient autonomy"**: The patient autonomy debate in America, as it pertains to euthanasia, is sometimes dated to 1870, when a man named Samuel Williams (not a doctor) gave a speech in favor of legalizing euthanasia at the Birmingham Speculative Club. The address may have gone unnoticed were it not reprinted as a book (reviewed favorably and widely circulated) in 1972. Dr. Ezekiel J. Emanuel writes that "Williams's articles were praised by the most prominent British literary and political journals of the day as 'remarkable.'" Ezekiel J. Emanuel, "The History of Euthanasia Debates in the United States and Britain," *Annals of Internal Medicine* 121, no. 10 (1994): 793–802.

5 **this modern history begins in 1975**: For more on the Quinlan case and the patient autonomy movement, see *In re Quinlan: In the Matter of Karen Quinlan, an Alleged Incompetent*, 70 NJ 10, 355 A.2d 647 (NJ 1976), argued January 26, 1976, decided March 31, 1976; Jill Lepore, *The Mansion of Happiness: A History of Life and Death* (New York: Knopf, 2012); Jill Lepore, "The Politics of Death," *New Yorker*, November 22, 2009; Robert D. McFadden, "Karen Ann Quinlan, 31, Dies; Focus of '76 Right to Die Case," *New York Times*, June 12, 1985; M. L. Tina Stevens, "The Quinlan Case Revisited: A History of Culture Politics of Medicine and the Law," *HEC Forum* 21, no. 2 (1996): 347–366; Tom L. Beauchamp, "The Autonomy Turn in Physician-Assisted Suicide," *Annals of the New York Academy of Sciences* 913, no. 1 (September 2000): 111–126; Haider Warraich, *Modern Death: How Medicine Changed the End of Life* (New York: St. Martin's Press, 2017); Gregory E. Pence, "Comas," chap. 2 in *Classical Cases in Medical Ethics: Accounts of the Cases and Issues That Define Medical Ethics* (New York: McGraw-Hill, 2008).

5 **On the other side, lawyers representing the hospital doctors**: Lepore, "Politics of Death."

6 **Supreme Court, which reversed the lower-court decision**: *In re Quinlan*.

6 **though others would call it "passive euthanasia"**: For instance, see William F. Smith, "In re Quinlan, Defining the Basis for Terminating Life Support Under the Right of Privacy," *Tulsa Law Review* 12, no. 1 (1976): 150–167.

6 **He said he prayed that the young woman's**: Robert Hanley, "Quinlan Funeral Is a Quiet Farewell," *New York Times*, June 15, 1985; Karin Laub, "Karen Ann Quinlan Buried After 10 Years in Coma," Associated Press, June 15, 1985.

6 **In 1983, twenty-five-year-old Nancy Cruzan**: For more on the Nancy Cruzan case and its legacy, see *Cruzan v. Director, Missouri Department of Health*, 497 US 261 (1990); George J. Annas, "Nancy Cruzan and the Right to Die," *New England Journal of Medicine* 323 (September 1990): 670–673; Ronald Dworkin, "The Right to Death," *New York Review of Books*, January 31, 1991; Jacqueline J. Glover, "The Case of Ms. Nancy Cruzan and the Care of the Elderly," *Journal of the American Geriatric Society* 38, no. 5 (May 1990): 588–593.

6 **This time, the patient's fate was**: *Cruzan v. Director, Missouri Department of Health*. For more on the legacy of the case, see Alexander Morgan Capron, "Looking Back at Withdrawal of Life-Support Law and Policy to See What Lies Ahead for Medical Aid-in-Dying," *Yale Journal of Biology and Medicine* 94, no. 4 (December 1990): 781–791; Tamar Lewin, "Nancy Cruzan Dies, Outlived by a Debate over the Right to Die," *New York Times*, December 27, 1990.

7 **Her tongue swelled and her eyelids**: James M. Hoefler, *Deathright: Culture, Medicine, Politics and the Right to Die* (New York: Routledge, 2018); *The Death of Nancy Cruzan*, produced by *Frontline*, PBS (PBS Video, 1992), VHS.

7 **"Even a dog in Missouri"**: Lewin, "Nancy Cruzan Dies."

7 **That same year, a twenty-six-year-old named Terri Schiavo:** For more on Terri Schiavo's case, see Joan Didion, "The Case of Theresa Schiavo," *New York Review of Books*, June 9, 2005; Rebecca Dresser, "Schiavo's Legacy: The Need for an Objective Standard," *Hastings Center Report* 35, no. 3 (May–June 2005): 20–22.

7 **Terri's feeding tube would be inserted:** "Judge Rules Man May Let Wife Die," Reuters, August 9, 2001; "Brain-Damaged Florida Woman Receiving Fluids," CNN, October 22, 2003; "Brain-Damaged Woman Receives Feeding Tube," Associated Press, October 23, 2003; "Florida Court Strikes Down Terri's Law," CNN, September 23, 2004; Abby Goodnough, "Florida Steps Back into Fight over Feeding Tube for Woman," *New York Times*, February 24, 2005; "Bush Signs Schiavo Legislation," Associated Press, March 21, 2005; "Florida Judge Rejects State Custody Bid in Schiavo Case," CNN, March 24, 2005; Abby Goodnough, "Supreme Court Refuses to Hear Schiavo Case," *New York Times*, March 25, 2005.

7 **the patient autonomy movement even further:** Also relevant is the 1990 Patient Self-Determination Act, which required most hospitals and nursing homes to educate patients about their end-of-life options and their right to make healthcare decisions, and to provide them with advance directive paperwork. US Congress, House, Patient Self-Determination Act of 1990, HR 4449, 101st Cong. (1990), https://www.congress.gov/bill/101st-congress/house-bill/4449.

7 **in the vocabulary of political lobbyists and patients:** Kathryn Tucker and David Leven, "Aid in Dying Language Matters," End of Life Choices New York and Disability Rights Legal Center, May 2016, accessed January 2, 2019, https://www.albanylaw.edu/event/End-of-Life-Care/Documents/Materials%20Death%20w%20dignity.pdf.

7 **After a string of legal challenges:** "Oregon Death with Dignity Act: A History," Death with Dignity National Center, accessed March 2020, https://www.deathwithdignity.org/oregon-death-with-dignity-act-history/; Eli D. Stutsman, "Oregon Death with Dignity Act: Four Challenges That Ensured the Law's Success," Death with Dignity National Center, May 6, 2015, https://www.deathwithdignity.org/news/2015/05/oregon-death-with-dignity-act-challenges/; Ben A. Rich, "Oregon Versus Ashcroft: Pain Relief, Physician-Assisted Suicide, and the Controlled Substances Act," *Pain Medicine* 3, no. 4 (2002): 353–360.

7 **and a repeal campaign backed by nearly $2 million:** Timothy Egan, "Assisted Suicide Comes Full Circle, to Oregon," *New York Times*, October 26, 1997; Timothy Egan, "The 1997 Elections: Right to Die; in Oregon, Opening a New Front in the World of Medicine," *New York Times*, November 6, 1997.

8 **A year later, in 1998, an eighty-four-year-old:** Dr. Peter Reagan published a description of the case in 1999. Peter Reagan, "Helen," *Lancet* 353 (1999): 1265–1267; see also Myrna C. Goldstein and Mark A. Goldstein, *Controversies in the Practice of Medicine* (Westport, CT: Greenwood Press, 2001), 321–323; Timothy Egan, "First Death Under an Assisted-Suicide Law," *New York Times*, March 26, 1998.

8 **A quarter of patients who made those requests:** Anthony L. Back et al., "Physician-Assisted Suicide and Euthanasia in Washington State. Patient Requests and Physician Responses," *JAMA: Journal of the American Medical Association* 275, no. 12 (March 27, 1996): 919–925. Of the 1,453 physicians who were sent questionnaires, 828 responded, for a response rate of 57 percent.

8 **In a separate 1995 study of Michigan oncologists:** David J. Doukas et al., "Attitudes and Behaviors on Physician-Assisted Death: A Study of Michigan Oncologists," *Journal of Clinical Oncology* 13, no. 5 (1995): 1055–1061. Another study, of Oregon physicians in 1995, found that 21 percent had "previously received requests for assisted suicide" and that 7 percent had complied with them. Melinda A. Lee et al., "Legalizing Assisted Suicide:

Views of Physicians in Oregon," *New England Journal of Medicine* 334 (February 1, 1996): 310–315.

In 2000, researchers conducted an expanded study, surveying 3,299 oncologists on their attitudes to physician-assisted death and euthanasia. The survey found that an overwhelming 62.9 percent of oncologists "had received requests for euthanasia or physician-assisted suicide during their career." Over that time, "3.7% of surveyed oncologists had performed euthanasia and 10.8% had performed physician-assisted suicide." Of the oncologists who had performed euthanasia, 57 percent had done so only once and 12 percent had done so five or more times. Of note: Oncologists "who believed that they had received adequate training in end-of-life care" were less likely to have performed euthanasia or physician-assisted death, compared to colleagues "who reported not being able to obtain all the care that a dying patient needed." Study authors hypothesized that "physicians with better training in end-of-life care may feel more capable of providing optimal palliative care and less need to resort to euthanasia or physician-assisted suicide." A limitation of the study is its low response rate of 39.8 percent. Ezekiel J. Emanuel et al., "Attitudes and Practices of U.S. Oncologists Regarding Euthanasia and Physician-Assisted Suicide," *Annals of Internal Medicine* 133, no. 7 (October 3, 2000): 527–532.

9 **"While doctors, religious leaders and politicians"**: Egan, "First Death Under an Assisted-Suicide Law."

9 **"There was a lot of fear that the elderly"**: Katie Hafner, "In Ill Doctor, a Surprise Reflection of Who Picks Assisted Suicide," *New York Times*, August 11, 2012.

9 **Under the Oregon Death with Dignity Act**: "Oregon's Death with Dignity Act (DWDA)," Oregon Health Authority, accessed January 2020, http://oregon.gov/oha/PH/PROVIDER PARTNERRESOURCES/EVALUATIONRESEARCH/DEATHWITHDIGNI TYACT/PAGES/faqs.aspx; see also Kathryn Tucker, "Aid in Dying: Guidance for an Emerging End-of-Life Practice," *Medical Ethics* 142, no. 1 (July 2012): 218–224.

9 **Prognostication is a fuzzy science**: For instance, see Nicola White et al., "A Systematic Review of Predictions of Survival in Palliative Care: How Accurate Are Clinicians and Who Are the Experts?" *PLOS One* 11, no. 8 (2016). Authors reviewed existing English-language studies of prognostic accuracy in palliative settings. They found wide variation in estimates and concluded that "clinicians' predictions are frequently inaccurate. No sub-group of clinicians was consistently shown to be more accurate than any other."

In 2000, Nicholas Christakis and Elizabeth Lamont surveyed 343 physicians who were responsible for providing survival estimates to 468 patients. They found that "of 468 predictions, only 92 (20%) were accurate (within 33% of actual survival); 295 (63%) were overoptimistic, and 81 (17%) were overpessimistic. Overall, physicians overestimated survival by a factor of 5.3." Nicholas A. Christakis and Elizabeth B. Lamont, "Extent and Determinants of Error in Physicians' Prognoses in Terminally Ill Patients," *Western Journal of Medicine* 172, no. 5 (May 2000): 310–313.

9 **If her doctor suspects that her judgment is impaired**: Hawaii is the only state that requires a mental health evaluation for all applicants.

10 **In 1995, the Vatican called assisted death**: Pope John Paul II, "Evangelium vitae," *Encyclicals*, March 25, 1995.

10 **The American Medical Association also declared**: "Physician-Assisted Suicide," American Medical Association, accessed January 2020, http://www.ama-assn.org/delivering -care/ethics/physician-assisted-suicide.

10 **Doctors in Portland came to assume**: National Academies of Sciences, Engineering, and

Medicine 2008, *Physician-Assisted Death: Scanning the Landscape: Proceedings of a Workshop* (Washington, DC: National Academies Press, 2018), 46.

10 **the US Supreme Court ruled on two assisted-death cases:** *Vacco v. Quill*, 521 US 793 (June 26, 1997); *Washington v. Glucksberg*, 521 US 702 (June 26, 1997). For context, see Kathryn Tucker, "In the Laboratory of the States: The Progress of Glucksberg's Invitation to States to Address End-of-Life Choice," *Michigan Law Review* 106, no. 8 (June 2008): 1593–1611.

11 **Instead, the Supreme Court sent the issue back:** In *Washington v. Glucksberg*, Chief Justice William Rehnquist, delivering the opinion of the court, wrote, "Finally, the State may fear that permitting assisted suicide will start it down the path to voluntary and perhaps even involuntary euthanasia." Summarizing an earlier ruling by the court of appeals, he wrote, "Thus, it turns out that what is couched as a limited right to 'physician assisted suicide' is likely, in effect, a much broader license, which could prove extremely difficult to police and contain. Washington's ban on assisting suicide prevents such erosion." Justice David Souter added, "The case for the slippery slope is fairly made out here, not because recognizing one due process right would leave a court with no principled basis to avoid recognizing another, but because there is a plausible case that the right claimed would not be readily containable by reference to facts about the mind that are matters of difficult judgment, or by gatekeepers who are subject to temptation, noble or not." *Washington et al., Petitioners v. Harold Glucksberg et al.*, Supreme Court of the United States, June 26, 1997, https://www.law.cornell.edu/supct/html/96-110.ZO.html.

11 **Any given principle, US Supreme Court:** Benjamin N. Cardozo, *The Nature of the Judicial Process* (New Haven, CT: Yale University Press, 1921), 51.

11 **"The law has taken my rights away":** "Diane Pretty loses right to die case," *Guardian*, April 29, 2002, https://www.theguardian.com/society/2002/apr/29/health.medicineandhealth.

11 **"in the way she always feared":** Sandra Laville, "Diane Pretty dies in the way she always feared," *Telegraph*, May 13, 2002, https://www.telegraph.co.uk/news/uknews/1394038/Diane-Pretty-dies-in-the-way-she-always-feared.html.

11 **it wasn't until 2008 that a second state:** There is some variation between state laws. For instance, Hawaii's Our Care, Our Choice Act requires a mental health assessment and a twenty-day waiting period (as opposed to Oregon's fifteen-day waiting period).

12 **According to a 2017 Gallup survey:** Jade Wood and Justin McCarthy, "Majority of Americans Remain Supportive of Euthanasia," Gallup, June 12, 2017, https://news.gallup.com/poll/211928/majority-americans-remain-supportive-euthanasia.aspx.

12 **the numbers have remained small:** Public Health Division, Center for Health Statistics, "Oregon Death with Dignity Act: 2019 Summary," Oregon Health Authority, February 25, 2020, https://www.oregon.gov/oha/PH/PROVIDERPARTNERRESOURCES/EVALUATIONRESEARCH/DEATHWITHDIGNITYACT/Documents/year22.pdf.

12 **Almost all have health insurance:** Hospice is a philosophy of end-of-life care that is generally focused on alleviating the symptoms of a dying patient (comfort care), rather than curative treatment. Hospice care is often provided in a patient's home, by an interdisciplinary team of doctors, nurses, social workers, chaplains, and volunteers—though it can also be provided in hospitals, nursing homes, and assisted-living facilities. In the United States, Medicare covers hospice for patients with a life expectancy of six months or less. In most states, Medicaid (for low-income patients) also covers hospice benefits.

12 **They note that African Americans are generally less likely:** African Americans experience disparities in both quality of and access to end-of-life care, including palliative and

hospice care. In 2009, for instance, just 33 percent of African American decedents used hospice service prior to their deaths—compared with 44 percent of white decedents. Cheryl Arenella, "Hospice and Palliative Care for African Americans: Overcoming Disparities," *Journal of Palliative Medicine* 19, no. 2 (February 1, 2016): 126. For more on racial disparities in hospice care, see K. T. Washington et al., "Barriers to Hospice Use Among African Americans: A Systematic Review," *Health and Social Work* 33, no. 4 (November 2008); Stephen J. Ramey and Steve H. Chin, "Disparity in Hospice Utilization by African American Patients with Cancer," *American Journal of Hospice and Palliative Medicine* 29, no. 5 (October 2011): 346–354; Jessica Rizzuto and Melissa Aldridge, "Racial Disparities in Hospice Outcomes: A Race or Hospice-Level Effect?" *Journal of the American Geriatrics Society* 66, no. 2 (February 2018): 407–413.

13 **The vast majority cite**: Public Health Division, Center for Health Statistics, "Oregon Death with Dignity Act: 2018 Summary," Oregon Health Authority, February 15, 2019, www.healthoregon.org/dwd. Annual reports are published each year and available online. Ganzini and colleagues have surveyed reasons for choosing physician-assisted suicide among Oregon patients: Linda Ganzini et al., "Oregonians' Reasons for Requesting Physician Aid in Dying," *Archives of Internal Medicine* 169, no. 5 (2009): 489–492.

13 **I did some reporting on the subject**: I worked with two colleagues, the directors Yonni Usiskin and Matt Shea, on a feature-length documentary film called *Time to Die*, which won Best Feature at London's Fragments film festival. I am endlessly grateful to Yonni and Matt for their genius and collaboration and for allowing me to use some of our reporting in this book. *Time to Die*, directed by Yonni Usiskin and Matt Shea (London: VICE, 2019), documentary film.

14 **I was surprised to find**: Others defend the status quo on data collection by pointing out that states do not demand physician reports and patient statements for many other end-of-life decisions, for example, the decision to withhold or withdraw life-sustaining treatment.

15 **"despair suicide," which is most suicides**: See, for instance, Silke Bachmann, "Epidemiology of Suicide and the Psychiatric Perspective," *International Journal of Environmental Research and Public Health* 15, no. 7 (July 6, 2018): 1425; World Health Organization Department of Mental Health, *Preventing Suicide: A Resource for Primary Health Care Workers* (Geneva: World Health Organization, 2000), http://www.who.int/mental_health /media/en/59.pdf.

18 **their catchphrase euphemism "death with dignity"**: I found several texts especially useful when thinking about "dignity" in this context. For historical and philosophical overviews, see Michael Rosen, *Dignity: Its History and Meaning* (Cambridge, MA: Harvard University Press, 2018); Paul Formosa and Catriona Mackenzie, "Nussbaum, Kant and the Capabilities Approach to Dignity," *Ethical Theory and Moral Practice* 17, no. 5 (November 2014): 875–892; Sebastian Muders, "Natural Good Theories and the Value of Human Dignity," *Cambridge Quarterly of Healthcare Ethics* 25 (2016): 239–249; and, of course, Albert Camus, *The Myth of Sisyphus and Other Essays* (New York: Vintage, 1991).

For more discussion of dignity as it applies to dying and physician assistance in death, see Scott Cutler Shershow, *A Critique of the Right-to-Die Debate* (Chicago: University of Chicago Press, 2014); Margaret P. Battin, *The Least Worst Death: Essays in Bioethics on the End of Life* (Oxford: Oxford University Press, 1994); Margaret P. Battin, *Ending Life: Ethics and the Way We Die* (Oxford: Oxford University Press, 2005); Sheldon Solomon et al., *The Worm at the Core: On the Role of Death in Life* (New York: Random House, 2015); Ernst Becker, *The Denial of Death* (New York: Free Press, 1973); Elisabeth Kübler-Ross,

On Death and Dying: What the Dying Have to Teach Doctors, Nurses, Clergy and Their Own Families (New York: Scribner, 1969); Clair Morrissey, "The Value of Dignity in and for Bioethics: Rethinking the Terms of the Debate," *Theoretical Medicine and Bioethics* 37, no. 3 (June 2016): 173–192; Susan M. Behuniak, "Death with 'Dignity': The Wedge That Divides the Disability Rights Movement from the Right to Die Movement," *Politics and the Life Sciences* 30, no. 1 (Spring 2011): 17–32; Mara Buchbinder, "Access to Aid-in-Dying in the United States: Shifting the Debate from Rights to Justice," *American Journal of Public Health* 108, no. 6 (June 2018): 754–759; Ronald Dworkin et al., "Assisted Suicide: The Philosopher's Brief," *New York Review of Books*, March 27, 1997; Yale Kamisar, "Assisted Suicide and Euthanasia: An Exchange," *New York Review of Books*, November 6, 1997; Yale Kamisar, "Are the Distinctions Drawn in the Debate About End-of-Life Decision Making 'Principled'? If Not, How Much Does It Matter?" *Journal of Law, Medicine and Ethics* 40, no. 1 (Spring 2012); Yale Kamisar, "Some Non-religious Views Against Proposed 'Mercy Killing' Legislation Part 1," *Human Life Review* 1, no. 2 (1976): 71–114; Peter Allmark, "Death with Dignity," *Journal of Medical Ethics* 28, no. 4 (August 1, 2002); J. David Vellemen, "A Right of Self-Determination," *Ethics* 109, no. 3 (April 1999): 606–628; Peter Singer, "Voluntary Euthanasia: A Utilitarian Perspective," *Bioethics* 17, no. 5 (2003); Gorsuch, *Future of Assisted Suicide*; Ezekiel Emanuel, "Whose Right to Die?" *The Atlantic*, March 1997.

Researchers have studied the effects of terminal illness on perceptions of personal dignity: Harvey M. Chochinov et al., "Dignity in the Terminally Ill: A Developing Empirical Model," *Social Science and Medicine* 54 (2002): 433–443; Harvey M. Chochinov et al., "Dignity in the Terminally Ill: A Cross-Sectional, Cohort Study," *Lancet* 360 (2002): 2026–2030. The authors found, in a sample of 213 patients with terminal cancer, that patients who reported feeling a loss of dignity due to their illness were more likely to acknowledge having lost the "will to live." They write, "Preservation of dignity should be an overall aim of treatment and care in patients who are nearing death."

18 **"We oppose euthanasia and assisted suicide":** Chris Good, "GOP Approves Abortion Amendment, Keeps Silent on Cases of Rape," ABC News, August 21, 2012.

19 **in the country that spends more per capita on healthcare:** "U.S. Health Care Spending Highest Among Developed Countries," Johns Hopkins Bloomberg School of Public Health, January 7, 2019, http://www.jhsph.edu/news/news-releases/2019/us-health-care-spending-highest-among-developed-countries.html. "The paper finds that the U.S. remains an outlier in terms of per capita health care spending which was $9,892 in 2016. That amount was about 25 percent higher than second-place Switzerland's $7,919. It was also 108 percent higher than Canada's $4,753, and 145 percent higher than the Organization for Economic Cooperation and Development (OECD) median of $4,033. And it was more than double the $4,559 the U.S. spent per capita on health care in 2000—the year whose data the researchers analyzed for a 2003 study."

I. MODERN MEDICINE

22 **He would say that this had less to do:** According to a survey of California's 270 hospitals, eighteen months after the implementation of the End of Life Option Act, more than 60 percent banned physicians from participating. Cindy L. Cain et al., "Hospital Responses to the End of Life Option Act: Implementation of Aid in Dying in California," *JAMA Internal Medicine* 179, no. 7 (April 2019): 985–987; JoNel Aleccia, "Legalizing Aid in Dying

Doesn't Mean Patients Have Access to It," NPR, January 25, 2017, https://www.npr.org /sections/health-shots/2017/01/25/511456109/legalizing-aid-in-dying-doesnt-mean-patients -have-access-to-it; Stephanie O'Neill, "Aid-in-Dying Requires More Than Just a Law, Californians Find," NPR, June 8, 2017, https://www.npr.org/sections/health-shots/2017/06 /08/530944807/aid-in-dying-requires-more-than-just-a-law-californians-find; Jessica Nutik Zitter, "Should I Help My Patients Die?" *New York Times*, August 5, 2017; Lindsey Holden, "When SLO Woman Could No Longer Fight for Her Life, She Chose to Fight for Her Death," *San Luis Obispo Tribune*, October 3, 2018, https://www.sanluisobispo.com /news/health-and-medicine/article218638260.html; Laura A. Petrillo et al., "How California Prepared for Implementation of Physician-Assisted Death: A Primer," *American Journal of Public Health* 107, no. 6 (June 2017): 883–888; Paula Span, "Aid in Dying Soon Will Be Available to More Americans. Few Will Choose It," *New York Times*, July 8, 2019, https:// www.nytimes.com/2019/07/08/health/aid-in-dying-states.html.

Access issues exist in a number of states. For instance, in Vermont, few doctors outside of Burlington are willing to provide physician-assisted death and few pharmacies have agreed to obtain or compound the drugs. Nearly a year after Washington, DC, legalized aid in dying, just 2 out of 11,000 licensed physicians in the district had formally registered to assist patients. JoNel Aleccia, "Terminally Ill, He Wanted Aid-in-Dying. His Catholic Hospital Said No," Kaiser Health News, January 29, 2020, https://khn.org/news /when-aid-in-dying-is-legal-but-the-medicine-is-out-of-reach/; Fenit Nirappil, "A Year After D.C. Passed Its Controversial Assisted Suicide Law, Not a Single Patient Has Used It," *Washington Post*, April 10, 2018, https://www.washingtonpost.com/local/dc-politics/a -year-after-dc-passed-its-assisted-suicide-law-only-two-doctors-have-signed-up/2018/04 /10/823cf7e2-39ca-11e8-9c0a-85d477d9a226_story.html.

24 **VITAS's chief medical officer told me:** VITAS's chief medical officer confirmed that while hospice doctors could not "prescribe, manage, prepare, dispense, deliver, administer, or assist in ingestion of aid-in-dying medications" or act as consulting physicians in aid-in-dying cases, staff members could, if requested, be present at a patient's bedside during and after ingestion. A VITAS spokesperson declined to comment on the case of Bradshaw Perkins Jr., citing patient privacy laws. Rules vary from hospice to hospice. At some institutions, staff members are not permitted to be present during ingestion of the drugs but may enter the room after ingestion. Other hospices forbid staff from being present at all.

24 **Some criticized Lonny for running a boutique death clinic:** For example, Wesley J. Smith, "Death Doctor to Charge $2000 for Suicide Prescription," *National Review*, June 6, 2016, https://www.nationalreview.com/corner/death-doctor-charge-2000-suicide -prescription/.

24 **Marc did some research and found that:** US Congress, House, Assisted Suicide Funding Restriction Act of 1997, HR 1003, 105th Cong. (1997), https://www.congress.gov /bill/105th-congress/house-bill/1003; JoNel Aleccia, "At Some Veterans Homes, Aid-in-Dying Is Not an Option," NPR, February 13, 2018, https://khn.org/news/california-joins -states-that-would-evict-veterans-who-seek-aid-in-dying-option/.

24 **a move supported by then president Bill Clinton:** Assisted Suicide Funding Restriction Act of 1997, HR 1003, 105th Cong., 1st sess., *Congressional Record* 143, no. 45, S3255.

26 **About a third of people didn't make it through:** Lonny's estimates are roughly consistent with a study conducted by Kaiser Permanente Southern California. Huong Q. Nguyen et al., "Characterizing Kaiser Permanente Southern California's Experience with the California End of Life Option Act in the First Year of Implementation," *JAMA Internal Medicine* 178, no. 3 (March 2018): 417–421. In July 2019, Oregon amended its death with dignity leg-

islation to remove the fifteen-day waiting period for gravely ill patients. "This improvement will result in fewer Oregonians suffering needlessly at the end of their lives," said Democratic senator Floyd Prozanski, who sponsored the legislation. Sarah Zimmerman, "Oregon Removes Assisted Suicide Wait for Certain Patients," Associated Press, July 24, 2019, https://abcnews.go.com/Health/wireStory/oregon-removes-assisted-suicide-wait-patients-64548415.

27 **"We have a bit of paperwork":** "End of Life Option Act," California Department of Public Health, modified July 9, 2019, https://www.cdph.ca.gov/Programs/CHSI/Pages/End-of-Life-Option-Act-.aspx; see Laura Petrillo et al., "How California Prepared for Implementation of Physician-Assisted Death: A Primer," *American Journal of Public Health* 107, no. 6 (June 2017): 883–888.

29 **Cory Taylor observed:** Cory Taylor, *Dying: A Memoir* (New York: Tin House Books, 2017).

30 **"The road to death":** Nigel Barley, *Dancing on the Grave: Encounters with Death* (London: John Murray, 1995). I first saw reference to Barley's work in Sallie Tisdale, *Advice for Future Corpses: A Practical Perspective on Death and Dying* (New York: Gallery Books, 2018).

32 **"pain" and "suffering" were two different things:** See Charlotte Mary Duffee, "Pain Versus Suffering: A Distinction Currently Without a Difference," *Journal of Medical Ethics* (December 24, 2019).

33 **the American philosopher Margaret Pabst Battin:** Margaret Pabst Battin, *Ending Life: Ethics and the Way We Die* (Oxford: Oxford University Press, 2005), 90, 92; Margaret Pabst Battin, "The Least Worst Death," *Journal of Medical Ethics* 22, no. 3 (July 1996): 183–187; Margaret Pabst Battin, *The Least Worst Death: Essays in Bioethics on the End of Life* (Oxford: Oxford University Press, 1994). See also Margaret Pabst Battin et al., eds., *Physician Assisted Suicide: Expanding the Debate* (London: Routledge, 1998); Margaret Pabst Battin and Timothy Quill, eds., *The Case for Physician-Assisted Dying: The Right to Excellent End-of-Life Care and Patient Choice* (Baltimore: Johns Hopkins University Press, 2004); Margaret Pabst Battin, *The Ethics of Suicide: Historical Sources* (Oxford: Oxford University Press, 2015).

34 **Lonny grew up in the wake:** Lonny Shavelson, *A Chosen Death: The Dying Confront Assisted Suicide* (New York: Simon and Schuster, 1995).

35 **In 1992, a suicide manual:** Derek Humphry, *Final Exit: The Practicalities of Self-Deliverance and Assisted Suicide for the Dying* (New York: Dell, 1992).

35 **He liked *The Enigma of Suicide*:** George Howe Colt, *The Enigma of Suicide: A Timely Investigation into the Causes, the Possibilities for Prevention and the Paths to Healing* (New York: Touchstone, 1991), 383.

35 **a doctor in Michigan named Jack Kevorkian:** Jack Kevorkian, *Prescription Medicine: The Goodness of Planned Death* (New York: Prometheus Books, 1991); Detroit Free Press Staff, *The Suicide Machine* (Detroit: Detroit Free Press, 1997); Neal Nicol and Harry Wylie, *Between the Dying and the Dead: Dr. Jack Kevorkian, the Assisted Suicide Machine and the Battle to Legalize Euthanasia* (Madison: University of Wisconsin Press, 2006).

36 **"I realized," Lonny would later write:** Shavelson, *A Chosen Death*, 12.

37 **in the words of the reporter Randy Shilts:** Randy Shilts, "Talking AIDS to Death," in *The Best American Essays 1990*, ed. Justin Kaplan (New York: Ticknor and Fields, 1990), 243. See also Randy Shilts, *And the Band Played On: Politics, People and the AIDS Epidemic* (New York: St. Martin's Griffin, 2007).

37 **Governor Jerry Brown, a former Jesuit seminary student:** Patrick McGreevy, "After Struggling, Jerry Brown Makes Assisted Suicide Legal in California," *Los Angeles Times*,

October 5, 2015, https://www.latimes.com/local/political/la-me-pc-gov-brown-end-of-life
-bill-20151005-story.html; Ian Lovett and Richard Perez-Pena, "California Governor Signs
Assisted Suicide Bill into Law," *New York Times*, October 5, 2015, https://www.nytimes
.com/2015/10/06/us/california-governor-signs-assisted-suicide-bill-into-law.html.

37 **the writings of South African archbishop and Nobel peace laureate Desmond Tutu:** Harriet Sherwood, "Desmond Tutu: I Want Right to End My Life Through Assisted Dying,"
Guardian, October 7, 2016, https://www.theguardian.com/society/2016/oct/07/desmond-tutu
-assisted-dying-world-leaders-should-take-action; Peter Granitz, "Desmond Tutu Joins
Advocates to Call for Right to Assisted Death," NPR, January 4, 2017.

37 **In 2016, 191 Californians:** "California End of Life Option Act 2016 Data Report," "California End of Life Option Act 2017 Data Report," and "California End of Life Option
Act 2018 Data Report," California Department of Public Health, modified July 9, 2019,
https://www.cdph.ca.gov/Programs/CHSI/Pages/End-of-Life-Option-Act-.aspx.

38 **but there were problems with the drugs:** Details come from interviews with a number of prescribing physicians in California, Oregon, and Washington, in addition to
state-published annual reports. For more on the history of aid-in-dying drug development,
see Jennie Dear, "The Doctors Who Invented a New Way to Help People Die," *The Atlantic*, January 22, 2019, https://www.theatlantic.com/health/archive/2019/01/medical-aid
-in-dying-medications/580591/; Catherine Offord, "Accessing Drugs for Medical Aid-
in-Dying," *The Scientist*, August 17, 2017, https://www.the-scientist.com/bio-business
/accessing-drugs-for-medical-aid-in-dying-31067; JoNel Aleccia, "Northwest Doctors
Rethink Aid-in-Dying Drugs to Avoid Prolonged Deaths," Kaiser Health News, March
5, 2017, https://www.seattletimes.com/seattle-news/health/northwest-doctors-rethink
-aid-in-dying-drugs-to-avoid-prolonged-deaths/; JoNel Aleccia, "Dying Drugs to Prevent Prolonged Deaths," Kaiser Health News, February 21, 2017, https://khn.org/news
/docs-in-northwest-tweak-aid-in-dying-drugs-to-prevent-prolonged-deaths/; JoNel Aleccia,
"In Colorado, a Low-Price Drug Cocktail Will Tamp Down Cost of Death with Dignity,"
Kaiser Health News, December 19, 2016, https://khn.org/news/in-colorado-a-low-price
-drug-cocktail-will-tamp-down-cost-of-death-with-dignity/.

38 **once, in Oregon, 104 hours:** "Oregon Death with Dignity: Data Summary 2016," Oregon
Health Authority, February 2017, https://www.oregon.gov/oha/PH/PROVIDERPART
NERRESOURCES/EVALUATIONRESEARCH/DEATHWITHDIGNITYACT
/Documents/year19.pdf.

38 **By 2011, however, pharmacists were struggling:** In an interview, Lundbeck spokesperson
Anders Schroll told me that the company acquired the rights to an intravenous formulation of pentobarbital in 2009 and that it was designed to treat severe cases of epilepsy.
In 2011, the company "became aware that pentobarbital, or Nembutal, the brand name,
was being misused for capital punishment" and "started to look into ways to prevent
the misuse." He said that Lundbeck viewed capital punishment as being "against our
values" and hypothesized that prison doctors had allowed for its use in death-penalty
cases. Around the same time, Lundbeck officials learned that pentobarbital was being
used for physician-assisted death, which Schroll also described as a "misuse." In response,
Lundbeck established a new delivery model, so that only approved customers could purchase it, for epileptic treatment, from specialty pharmacies. See also "Lundbeck Over-
hauls Pentobarbital Distribution Program to Restrict Misuse," Lundbeck, media release,
July 1, 2017, https://investor.lundbeck.com/news-releases/news-release-details/lundbeck
-overhauls-pentobarbital-distribution-program-restrict. See also Sean Riley, "Navigating
the New Era of Assisted Suicide and Execution Drugs," *Journal of Law and the Biosciences*

4, no. 2 (August 2017): 424–434; Roxanne Nelson, "When Dying Becomes Unaffordable," Medscape, November 9, 2017, https://www.medscape.com/viewarticle/888271; Kimberly Leonard, "Drug Used in 'Death with Dignity' Is Same Used in Executions," *US News and World Report*, October 16, 2015, https://www.usnews.com/news/articles/2015 /10/16/drug-shortage-creates-hurdle-for-death-with-dignity-movement; David Nicholl, "Lundbeck and Pentobarbital: Pharma Takes a Stand," *Guardian*, July 1, 2011, https:// www.theguardian.com/commentisfree/cifamerica/2011/jul/01/pentobarbital-lundbeck -execution-drug; Offord, "Accessing Drugs for Medical Aid-in-Dying."

39 **That same year, the European Union placed an export ban on the drug**: European Commission, "Commission Extends Control over Goods Which Could Be Used for Capital Punishment or Torture," media release IP/11/1578, December 20, 2011, https://ec .europa.eu/commission/presscorner/detail/en/IP_11_1578; David Brunnstrom, "EU Puts Squeeze on Drug Supplies for U.S. Executions," Reuters, December 20, 2011, https:// www.reuters.com/article/eu-executions-drugs/eu-puts-squeeze-on-drug-supplies-for-u-s -executions-idUSL6E7NK30820111220.

39 **Then Akorn Pharmaceuticals**: April Dembosky, "Pharmaceutical Companies Hiked Price on Aid in Dying Drug," KQED, March 22, 2016, https://www.kqed.org/stateofhealth /163375/pharmaceutical-companies-hiked-price-on-aid-in-dying-drug.

39 **A lethal dose of Seconal that**: Bausch Health companies declined to be interviewed for this book. A spokesperson wrote, in response to my interview request, that "since the topic of your book is in regard to an off-label use of the product, we are unable to participate or comment."

39 **A *JAMA Oncology* article called**: Veena Shankaran et al., "Drug Price Inflation and the Cost of Assisted Death for Terminally Ill Patients: Death with Indignity," *JAMA Oncology* 3, no. 1 (January 2017): 15–16; David Grube and Ashley Cardenas, "Insurance Coverage and Aid-in-Dying Medication Costs: Reply," *JAMA Oncology* 3, no. 8 (August 2017): 1138.

40 **So-called compound drugs had**: US Department of Health and Human Services, Food and Drug Administration, "Compounded Drug Products That Are Essentially Copies of a Commercially Available Drug Product Under Section 503A of the Federal Food, Drug and Cosmetic Act: Guidance for Industry," January 2018, https://www.fda.gov/media /98973/download.

41 **At the end of their meeting, the Seattle doctors**: Carol Parrot and Lonny Shavelson, "The Pharmacology and Physiology of Aid in Dying" (presentation, National Clinicians Conference on Medical Aid in Dying, February 14, 2020).

41 **They found compound pharmacists**: At the time of my visit to Berkeley, a single compound pharmacist in the Bay Area was supplying most of Northern California. The pharmacist met me on the condition that I not name him or the pharmacy. "Most pharmacists are scared," he told me. Some don't understand the law. Others are worried about compounding medication that hasn't been subject to more rigorous testing. Still others worry that, because the End of Life Option Act is controversial, they will lose business if they start filling lethal prescriptions and other clients find out.

The pharmacist told me that he filled about three aid-in-dying prescriptions each week and that he found the process more stressful than his normal work. "I was scared at the start. I'm actually dispensing something that will be used to end their lives." On a few occasions, he said, he found himself tangled up in family dramas. Angry daughters or wives would call him and shout down the line—"No, we don't want it!"—only to have the patient call five minutes later to ask for the drugs. Often, patients called with tons of questions about how the death would work. "You have to talk to your doctor," the pharmacist would say. But sometimes, the patients persisted. They said that doctors weren't returning their calls. The pharmacist said that Lonny was his favorite doctor to work with because he communicated things clearly to his patients—so they didn't ask very much of him.

When I asked the pharmacist if the work was lucrative, he said that it was. "People don't want to talk about this. . . . It's tough to quantify, but our costs are probably $100, give or take. We sell for about $500 to $700."

41 In Oregon, between 1998 and 2015: Charles Blanke et al., "Characterizing 18 Years of the Death with Dignity Act in Oregon," *JAMA Oncology* 3, no. 10 (October 2017): 1403–1406; Luai Al Rabadi et al., "Trends in Medical Aid in Dying in Oregon and Washington," *JAMA Network Open* 2, no. 8 (August 2019), https://jamanetwork.com/journals/jamanetworkopen/fullarticle/2747692.

41 One awoken person reportedly: Leonard, "Drug Used in 'Death with Dignity.'"

42 In Canada and Belgium, patients almost always: Government of Canada, "Fourth Interim Report on Medical Assistance in Dying in Canada," April 2019, https://www.canada.ca/en/health-canada/services/publications/health-system-services/medical-assistance-dying-interim-report-april-2019.html; Jennifer Gibson, "The Canadian Experience," in *Physician-Assisted Death: Scanning the Landscape. Proceedings of a Workshop* (Washington, DC: National Academies Press, 2018); Christopher Harty et al., "Oral Medical Assistance in Dying (MAiD): Informing Practice to Enhance Utilization in Canada," *Canadian Journal of Anesthesia* 66 (2019): 1106–1112; C. Harty et al., "The Oral MAiD Option in Canada," Canadian Association of MAiD Assessors and Providers, April 2018, https://camapcanada.ca/wp-content/uploads/2019/01/OralMAiD-Med.pdf; Sigrid Dierickx, "Euthanasia Practice in Belgium: A Population-Based Evaluation of Trends and Currently Debated Issues" (PhD diss., Faculty of Medicine and Pharmacy, Vrije Universiteit Brussel, 2018), https://www.worldrtd.net/sites/default/files/newsfiles/Sigrid_Dierickx.pdf; R. Cohen-Almagor, "Belgian Euthanasia Law: A Critical Analysis," *Journal of Medical Ethics* 35, no. 7 (2009): 436–439.

42 In the 1990s, Oregon legislators added a "self-administration" requirement: Kathryn Tucker, who was legal director of Compassion & Choices in 1997—and who argued *Washington v. Glucksberg* before the Supreme Court—writes, "Thus, efforts to enact statutory permission for AID over the past twenty-five years have succeeded in only a handful of states and only when written with a 'kitchen sink' approach to regulation of the practice, in order to survive opponents' claims that the measures lack sufficient safeguards. The history of Oregon's Death with Dignity Act exemplifies this reality. Oregon's effort followed failed attempts to pass somewhat similar measures in Washington (1991) and California (1992). Having seen those efforts fail in campaigns where opponents claimed there were insufficient safeguards, the drafters of the Oregon measure included an array of procedural hurdles, including multiple written and oral requests, mandatory second opinions, and a lengthy waiting period, among others. . . . Unfortunately, it appears that the continued introduction of Oregon-style bills has resulted in even more restrictions being added to such measures, as seen in the 2018 Hawaii measure, the Our Care, Our Choice Act, which adds a mandatory counseling requirement and extends the mandatory waiting period from fifteen to twenty days." Kathryn L. Tucker, "Aid in Dying in North Carolina," *North Carolina Law Review* 97 (2019).

In an interview, Tucker told me that, as an advocate, she understands the need for pragmatism. "I see and appreciate that the broad public support for aid in dying is dependent on these bright lines. . . . The three bright lines that I think are important are mental competency, terminal illness, and patient self-administration." Tucker believes that the self-administration requirement, beyond being politically useful, ensures that the patient's personal autonomy is protected. "Ensuring that it is the patient's wish, the patient's volition, is fundamentally essential. And so when the patient is the last actor, that is certain."

"But," I added, "everything else in medicine is done by consent." You don't, for instance, require a surgery patient to make an initial incision on her chest as proof of her consent.

"I hear you," Tucker said. "Everyone would prefer that the physician would be empowered to administer. I get that. It may be that as time goes by and we know more and more about this practice, and people become more familiar and comfortable, this will be the first bright line to shift."

42 **In fact, in other countries, if an aid-in-dying patient**: In the Netherlands, for instance, patients who choose the oral protocol must have an IV cannula inserted prior to taking the medication. If death has not resulted within two hours of ingestion, the physician may switch to the IV protocol. Between 2013 and 2015, the intravenous backup was used in 9 percent of cases. In Canada, physicians have referred to this process as "backup IV rescue." C. Harty et al., "The Oral MAiD Option in Canada: Part 1, Medication Protocols," Canadian Association of MAiD Assessors and Providers, April 18, 2018, https://camapcanada .ca/wp-content/uploads/2019/01/OralMAiD-Med.pdf.

43 **What if he got things wrong?**: "I'm really leery," a physician named Stephanie Marquet told me, of Lonny's research methods, in 2019. "If your sample size is too small, please don't draw conclusions. Just say: 'Anecdotally . . .'" Marquet argued that large aid-in-dying organizations like Compassion & Choices should be funding high-quality research into lethal drug protocols.

44 **As he took on more patients, he started meeting**: Mara Buchbinder writes, "The requirement that patients self-administer and ingest the lethal medication, a safeguard designed to ensure that participation in AID is voluntary, was a major barrier for some patients who hoped to pursue AID. Such obstacles were most pronounced for patients with neurologic conditions such as amyotrophic lateral sclerosis (ALS), which results in progressively declining mobility and often entails swallowing difficulties in later stages." She quotes another physician as reflecting, "That doesn't make sense to me. It seems like it puts undue stress on my patients and it also prevents a patient who really needs this program from being able to access it. I feel like it was designed with the cancer patients in mind." Mara Buchbinder, "Access to Aid-in-Dying in the United States: Shifting the Debate from Rights to Justice," *American Journal of Public Health* 108, no. 6 (June 2018): 754–759. See also National Academies of Sciences, Engineering, and Medicine, *Physician-Assisted Death: Scanning the Landscape: Proceedings of a Workshop* (Washington, DC: National Academies Press, 2018); Amanda M. Thyden, "Death with Dignity and Assistance: A Critique of the Self-Administration Requirement of California's End of Life Option Act," *Chapman Law Review* 20, no. 2 (2017).

44 **"affirmative, conscious, and physical act"**: The state of California's Health and Safety Code states the following, with respect to medical aid in dying: "'Self-administer' means a qualified individual's affirmative, conscious, and physical act of administering and ingesting the aid-in-dying drug to bring about his or her own death." California Department of Consumer Affairs, Physician Assistant Board, "Division 1, Section 1: Part 1.85: End of Life Option Act," Health and Safety Code, https://www.pab.ca.gov/forms_pubs/end_of_life.pdf.

44 **In other states, patients were required**: Thaddeus Pope, "Medical Aid in Dying: Six Variations Among U.S. State Laws" (presentation, Berkeley, California, January 2020), http://

thaddeuspope.com/maid/popearticles.html. Indeed, some have argued that intravenous self-administration would technically be legal in states that do not explicitly require "ingestion" of lethal drugs. See also James Gerhart et al., "An Examination of State-Level Personality Variation and Physician Aid in Dying Legislation," *Journal of Pain and Symptom Management* 56, no. 3 (September 2018).

45 **A few days later, the board's executive director**: A spokesperson from the California Medical Board told me, in an email, "that ingestion includes the patient self-administering the medication by mouth, feeding tube, or rectally. This has been determined through reviewing definitions of 'ingest' and through consultations with physicians." He confirmed that "intravenous administration is not considered ingestion" but that rectal administration can be.

47 **an academic paper I had come across**: Emily B. Rubin et al., "States Worse Than Death Among Hospitalized Patients with Serious Illnesses," *JAMA Internal Medicine* 176, no. 19 (2016): 1557–1559.

48 **Lonny tried to be sensitive to**: For more on race and medical aid in dying, see Cindy L. Cain and Sara McCleskey, "Expanded Definitions of the 'Good Death'? Race, Ethnicity and Medical Aid in Dying," *Sociology of Health and Illness* 41, no. 6 (2019): 1175–1191; Terri Laws, "How Race Matters in Physician-Assisted Suicide Debate," Religion and Politics, September 3, 2019, https://religionandpolitics.org/2019/09/03/how-race-matters -in-the-physician-assisted-suicide-debate/; Vyjeyanthi S. Periyakoil et al., "Multi-Ethnic Attitudes Toward Physician-Assisted Death in California and Hawaii," *Journal of Palliative Medicine* 19, no. 10 (October 2016): 1060–1065; Fenit Nirappil, "Right-to-Die Law Faces Skepticism in Nation's Capital: 'It's Really Aimed at Old Black People,'" *Washington Post*, October 17, 2016, https://www.washingtonpost.com/local/dc-politics/right -to-die-law-faces-skepticism-in-us-capital-its-really-aimed-at-old-black-people/2016/10 /17/8abf6334-8ff6-11e6-a6a3-d50061aa9fae_story.html?utm_term=.bbc0abbe01ad.

50 **"I felt like this is definitely not right with the circle of life"**: For more on the hospice movement's historic opposition to aid in dying, see Timothy E. Quill and Margaret P. Battin eds., *Physician-Assisted Dying: The Case for Palliative Care and Patient Choice* (Baltimore: Johns Hopkins University Press, 2004). See also Peter Hudson et al., "Legalizing Physician-Assisted Suicide and/or Euthanasia: Pragmatic Implications," *Palliative and Supportive Care* 13 (2015): 1399–1409.

51 **"What are we asking of our medical profession?"**: Daniel P. Sulmasy, "Ethics and the Psychiatric Dimensions of Physician-Assisted Suicide: A View from the United States," chap. 3 in *Euthanasia and Assisted Suicide: Lessons from Belgium*, ed. David Albert Jones et al. (Cambridge: Cambridge University Press, 2017).

51 **Since the 1970s, the goal of hospice**: For more on this history, see Ann Neumann, *The Good Death: An Exploration of Dying in America* (Boston: Beacon Press, 2017); Haider Warraich, *Modern Death: How Medicine Changed the End of Life* (New York: St. Martin's Press, 2017).

52 **By the time assisted dying was**: US Department of Health and Human Services, Centers for Disease Control and Prevention, "Long-Term Care Providers and Services Users in the United States," *Vital and Health Statistics* 3, no. 43 (February 2019): 73; National Hospice and Palliative Care Organization, "NHPCO Facts and Figures," 2018, https:// 39k5cm1a9u1968hg74aj3x51-wpengine.netdna-ssl.com/wp-content/uploads/2019/07 /2018_NHPCO_Facts_Figures.pdf.

52 **The National Hospice and Palliative Care Organization**: "Statement on Legally Accelerated Death," National Hospice and Palliative Care Organization, November 4, 2018,

https://www.nhpco.org/wp-content/uploads/2019/07/Legally_Accelerated_Death_Position
_Statement.pdf.

52 In 1993, the palliative care physician Dr. Timothy Quill: Timothy Quill, *Death and Dignity: Making Choices and Taking Charge* (New York: W. W. Norton, 1993).

54 "Centuries from now," wrote Dr. Ira Byock: Ira Byock, "Physician-Assisted Suicide Won't Atone for Medicine's 'Original Sin,'" *Stat*, January 31, 2018, https://www.statnews .com/2018/01/31/physician-assisted-suicide-medicine/. See also Ira Byock, "Words Matter: It Is Still Physician-Assisted Suicide and Still Wrong," *Maryland Medicine* 17 (January 4, 2017), http://irabyock.org/wp-content/uploads/2014/06/Byock-Maryland-Medicine-vol -17-4-January-2017.pdf; Ira Byock, "Physician-Assisted Suicide Is Not Progressive," *The Atlantic*, October 25, 2012, https://www.theatlantic.com/health/archive/2012/10/physician -assisted-suicide-is-not-progressive/264091/.

55 Back in 1997, the US Supreme Court ruled: *Washington v. Glucksberg*, 521 US 702 (June 26, 1997). See also Kathryn L. Tucker, "In the Laboratory of the States: The Progress of Glucksberg's Invitation to States to Address End-of-Life Choice," *Michigan Law Review* 106, no. 8 (June 2008): 1593–1611; Robert A. Burt, "The Supreme Court Speaks—Not Assisted Suicide but a Constitutional Right to Palliative Care," *New England Journal of Medicine* 337 (October 1997): 1234–1236.

55 From then on, "palliative sedation," which had always occurred: In 1935, the founders of the Voluntary Euthanasia Society in Britain thought legalization of physician-assisted death was unnecessary because "all good doctors do it anyway." The following year, the royal physician Lord Dawson euthanized King George V in the presence of Queen Mary. Colin Brewer, "Assisted Dying: 'All Good Doctors Do It Anyway,'" *BMJ* 345 (2012).

55 became a mainstream medical intervention: For more on palliative sedation, see Sam Rys et al., "Continuous Sedation Until Death: Moral Justification of Physicians and Nurses—A Content Analysis of Opinion Pieces," *Medicine, Health Care and Philosophy* 16 (2013): 533–542; Judith A. C. Rietjens et al., "Terminal Sedation and Euthanasia: A Comparison of Clinical Practices," *Archives of Internal Medicine* 166 (April 2006); Timothy Quill, "Myths and Misconceptions About Palliative Sedation," *American Medical Association Journal of Ethics* 8, no. 9 (September 2006): 577–581; Molly L. Olsen et al., "Ethical Decision Making with End-of-Life Care: Palliative Sedation and Withholding or Withdrawing Life-Sustaining Treatments," *Mayo Clinic Proceedings* 85, no. 10 (October 2010): 949–954; Henk ten Have and Jos V. M. Welie, "Palliative Sedation Versus Euthanasia: An Ethical Assessment," *Journal of Pain and Symptom Management* 47, no. 1 (January 2014); Timothy Quill et al., "Last-Resort Options for Palliative Sedation," *Annals of Internal Medicine* 151 (2009): 421–424; Sophie M. Bruinsma et al., "The Experiences of Relatives with the Practice of Palliative Sedation: A Systematic Review," *Journal of Pain and Symptom Management* 44, no. 3 (September 2012); James Rachels, "Active and Passive Euthanasia," *New England Journal of Medicine* 292 (1975): 78–80; Donna L. Dickenson, "Practitioner Attitudes in the United States and United Kingdom Toward Decisions at the End of Life: Are Medical Ethicists out of Touch?" *Western Journal of Medicine* 174, no. 2 (2001): 103–109. Some researchers argue that palliative sedation does not, in fact, hasten death. For example, see M. Maltoni et al., "Palliative Sedation Therapy Does Not Hasten Death: Results from a Prospective Multicenter Study," *Annals of Oncology* 20 (2009): 1163–1169.

55 It was formally endorsed by: Timothy W. Kirk and Margaret M. Mahon, "National Hospice and Palliative Care Organization (NHPCO) Position Statement and Commentary on the Use of Palliative Sedation in Imminently Dying Terminally Ill Patients," *Journal of Pain and Symptom Management* 39, no. 5 (May 2010): 914–923; "Statement on Palliative

Sedation," American Academy of Hospice and Palliative Medicine, December 5, 2014, http://aahpm.org/positions/palliative-sedation.

55 **"between 1% and 52%"**: Kirk and Mahon, "National Hospice and Palliative Care Organization (NHPCO) Position Statement."

56 **But bioethicists have long insisted**: For more on the double effect and moral justifications for palliative and terminal sedation, see Glanville Williams, "Euthanasia," *Medico-Legal Journal* 41, no. 1 (1973): 14–34; Yale Kamisar, "Active v. Passive Euthanasia: Why Keep the Distinction?" *Trial* 29, no. 3 (1993): 32–38; Margaret P. Battin, "Terminal Sedation: Pulling the Sheet over Our Eyes," *Hastings Center Report* 38, no. 5 (2008): 27–30; Timothy Quill et al., "The Rule of Double-Effect: A Critique of Its Role in End-of-Life Decision Making," *New England Journal of Medicine* 337, no. 24 (December 1997): 1768–1771; Charles E. Douglas et al., "Narratives of 'Terminal Sedation,' and the Importance of the Intention-Foresight Distinction in Palliative Care Practice," *Bioethics* 27, no. 1 (2013): 1–11; Paul Rosseau, "The Ethical Validity and Clinical Experience of Palliative Sedation," *Mayo Clinic Proceedings* 75 (2000): 1064–1069; Joseph Boyle, "Medical Ethics and Double Effect: The Case of Terminal Sedation," *Theoretical Medicine* 25 (2004): 51–60; Susan Anderson Fohr, "The Double Effect of Pain Medication: Separating Myth from Reality," *Journal of Palliative Medicine* 1, no. 4 (1998); Rita L. Marker, "End-of-Life Decisions and Double Effect: How Can This Be Wrong When It Feels So Right?" *National Catholic Bioethics Quarterly* 11, no. 1 (2011): 99–119; Franklin G. Miller et al., "Assisted Suicide Compared with Refusal of Treatment: A Valid Distinction?" *Annals of Internal Medicine* 132, no. 6 (2000): 470–475.

2. AGE

65 **what William Osler, in his classic**: William Osler, *The Principles and Practice of Medicine* (New York: McGraw-Hill, 1996).

67 **that, according to national polls**: "Assisted Suicide: Public Attitudes at Odds with UK Law," NatCen: Social Research That Works Today, May 19, 2011, http://www.natcen.ac.uk/blog/assisted-suicide-public-attitudes-at-odds-with-uk-law.

67 **Dr. Sherwin Nuland observed**: Sherwin Nuland, *How We Die: Reflections on Life's Final Chapter* (New York: Knopf, 1994).

68 **Dr. Atul Gawande has written**: Atul Gawande, *Being Mortal: Medicine and What Matters in the End* (New York: Metropolitan Books, 2014).

68 **In 1909, the word "geriatrics" entered the medical lexicon**: I. L. Nascher, *Geriatrics: The Diseases of Old Age and Their Treatment* (Philadelphia: P. Blakiston's Son, 1914); John E. Morley, "A Brief History of Geriatrics," *Journals of Gerontology* 59, no. 11 (November 2014); John C. Beck and Susan Vivell, "Development of Geriatrics in the United States," chap. 5 in *Geriatric Medicine*, ed. C. K. Cassel and J. R. Walsh (New York: Springer, 1984).

68 **The unusual word appeared alongside**: Carole Haber, "Anti-Aging Medicine: The History," *Journals of Gerontology* 59, no. 6 (June 2014); Eric Grundhauser, "The True Story of Dr. Voronoff's Plan to Use Monkey Testicles to Make Us Immortal," Atlas Obscura, October 13, 2015, https://www.atlasobscura.com/articles/the-true-story-of-dr-voronoffs-plan-to-use-monkey-testicles-to-make-us-immortal; Adam Leith Gollner, *The Book of Immortality: The Science, Belief, and Magic Behind Living Forever* (New York: Scribner, 2013).

68 **Most researchers no longer spoke of curing**: The "compression of morbidity" theory was first proposed by Dr. James Fries in 1980. James F. Fries, "Aging, Natural Death, and the

Compression of Morbidity," *New England Journal of Medicine* 303, no. 3 (August 1980): 130–135; also explained in Anthony J. Vita et al., "Aging, Health Risks and Cumulative Disability," *New England Journal of Medicine* 338 (April 1998): 1035–1041; V. Mor, "The Compression of Morbidity Hypothesis: A Review of Research and Prospects for the Future," *Journal of the American Geriatric Society* 53, no. 9 (2005): S308–S309; James F. Fries et al., "Compression of Morbidity 1980–2011: A Focused Review of Paradigms and Progress," *Journal of Aging Research* (August 2011). For criticism of the theory, see Eileen M. Crimmins and Hiram Beltran-Sanchez, "Mortality and Morbidity Trends: Is There Compression of Morbidity?" *Journals of Gerontology, Series* B, 66, no. 1 (December 2010): 75–86; Colin Steensma et al., "Evaluating Compression or Expansion of Morbidity in Canada," *Health Promotion and Chronic Disease Prevention in Canada* 37, no. 3 (2017): 68–76; Carol Jagger, "Compression or Expansion of Morbidity—What Does the Future Hold?" *Age and Ageing* 29 (2000): 93–94; Kenneth Howse, "Increasing Life Expectancy and the Compression of Morbidity: A Critical Review of the Debate" (Oxford Institute of Ageing Working Paper, July 2006), https://www.ageing.ox.ac.uk/files/workingpaper _206.pdf; Stefan Walter et al., "No Evidence of Morbidity Compression in Spain: A Time Series Study Based on National Hospitalization Records," *International Journal of Public Health* 61, no. 1 (September 2016).

69 **There was, Nuland wrote, "a nice Victorian reticence"**: Nuland, *How We Die*.

69 **"Compression of morbidity is a quintessentially American idea"**: Ezekiel Emanuel, "Why I Hope to Die at 75," *The Atlantic*, October 2014.

69 **Today, around a fifth of elderly Americans**: Alvin C. Kwok et al., "The Intensity and Variation of Surgical Care at the End of Life: A Retrospective Cohort Study," *Lancet* 378, no. 9800 (October 2011): P1408–P1413.

71 **Once, she published an examination**: Avril Henry, "Chaucer's 'A B C': Line 39 and the Irregular Stanza Again," *Chaucer Review* 18, no. 2 (1983): 95–99.

73 **Philip Roth called old age**: Philip Roth, *Everyman* (New York: Vintage International, 2006).

73 **Jean Améry, the journalist and Holocaust survivor**: I came across the reference in Vivian Gornick, *The Situation and the Story: The Act of Personal Narrative* (New York: Farrar, Straus and Giroux, 2001); Jean Améry, *On Aging: Revolt and Resignation* (Bloomington: Indiana University Press, 1994).

73 **As Avril waited, a line from a T. S. Eliot**: T. S. Eliot, "The Love Song of J. Alfred Prufrock," in *The Waste Land and Other Poems* (New York: Signet Classic, 1998).

74 **"I may still not suffer from one serious specific illness"**: Michael Irwin, "Approaching Old Age," SOARS, 2014, https://www.mydeath-mydecision.org.uk/wp-content/uploads /2016/07/Approaching-Old-Old-booklet.pdf, 78. The original site is no longer active but can be accessed via the Wayback Machine. Michael Irwin, "European Support for Rational Suicide in Old Age," Society for Old Age Rational Suicide, accessed March 3, 2020, https://web.archive.org/web/20190204001345/http://soars.org.uk/index.php/about.

74 **"rational and positive act"**: Irwin, "European Support for Rational Suicide in Old Age." Some scholars have considered the idea of "rational" death, for elderly adults, in a context of scarce resources and medical rationing—and have argued that, in the face of scarcity, care for older adults should be scaled back. This modern academic discussion dates back to the 1980s. For context, see, for instance, Margaret P. Battin, "Age Rationing and the Just Distribution of Health Care: Is There a Duty to Die?" *Ethics* 97, no. 2 (1987): 317–340; Norman Daniels, "Justice Between Age Groups: Am I My Parents' Keeper?" *Milbank Memorial Fund Quarterly* 61, no. 3 (1983): 489–522; Dennis McKerlie, "Justice Between Age-Groups: A Comment on Norman Daniels," *Journal of Applied Philosophy* 6, no. 2

(1989): 227–234; Henry J. Aaron et al., *Painful Prescription: Rationing Hospital Care*, Studies in Social Economics (Washington, DC: Brookings Institution Press, 1984).

75 **1516 book *Utopia*:** Thomas More, *Utopia* (New York: Penguin Books, 1965). See also Friedrich Nietzsche, who wrote that a physician should administer "a fresh dose of disgust" to a sick man who "continues to vegetate in a state of cowardly dependency on doctors" and who allows himself to become a "parasite" on society. "In certain cases it is indecent to go on living." Friedrich Nietzsche, *Complete Works*, vol. 16 (New York: Russell, 1964).

75 **Irwin held small meetings across south England:** Martin Beckford, "'Dr Death' Calls for Assisted Suicide for Those Who Are Not Terminally Ill," *Telegraph*, August 16, 2010, https://www.telegraph.co.uk/news/uknews/law-and-order/7944884/Dr-Death-calls-for-assisted-suicide-for-those-who-are-not-terminally-ill.html; "Retired GP Admits to Helping People to Die in the Past," BBC, April 4, 2011, https://www.bbc.co.uk/news/uk-12960984; "Right-to-Die Activist Nan Maitland 'Died with Dignity,'" BBC, April 4, 2011, https://www.bbc.com/news/uk-12959664.

75 **In 2010, the British novelist Martin Amis:** Maurice Chittenden, "Martin Amis Calls for Euthanasia Booths on Street Corners," *Times*, January 24, 2010, https://www.thetimes.co.uk/article/martin-amis-calls-for-euthanasia-booths-on-street-corners-mct9qdm0ft9.

75 **Amis said that he had meant to be "satirical":** Caroline Davies, "Martin Amis in New Row over 'Euthanasia Booths,'" *Guardian*, January 24, 2010, https://www.theguardian.com/books/2010/jan/24/martin-amis-euthanasia-booths-alzheimers.

76 **In a conference center in New Orleans:** Deborah Brauser, "'Rational Suicide' Talk Increasing Among 'Healthy' Elderly," Medscape, April 8, 2015, https://www.medscape.com/viewarticle/842819. See also Robert McCue et al., "Rational Suicide in the Elderly: Mental Illness or Choice?" *American Journal of Geriatric Psychiatry* 23, no. 3 (March 2015): S41–S42.

77 **When suicide was mentioned in the *Diagnostic and Statistical Manual*:** *Diagnostic and Statistical Manual of Mental Disorders: DSM-5* (Arlington, VA: American Psychiatric Association, 2013).

78 **After the conference, Dr. McCue and Dr. Meera Balasubramaniam:** Robert E. McCue and Meera Balasubramaniam, eds., *Rational Suicide in the Elderly* (Basel: Springer International, 2017). See also Meera Balasubramaniam, "Rational Suicide in Elderly Adults: A Clinician's Perspective," *Journal of the American Geriatrics Society* 66, no. 5 (March 2018). For a critique of McCue and Balasubramaniam's works, see Elizabeth Dzeng and Steven Z. Pantilat, "What Are the Social Causes of Rational Suicide in Older Adults?" *Journal of the American Geriatrics Society* 66, no. 5 (May 2018): 853–855. For more on the subject, see Naomi Richards, "Old Age Rational Suicide," *Sociology Compass* 11, no. 2 (2017); Paula Span, "A Debate over 'Rational Suicide,'" *New York Times*, August 31, 2018, https://www.nytimes.com/2018/08/31/health/suicide-elderly.html?login=email&auth=login-email&login=email&auth=login-email.

78 **In a 2018 paper:** J. Yager et al., "Working with Decisionally Capable Patients Who Are Determined to End Their Own Lives," *Journal of Clinical Psychiatry* 79, no. 4 (May 2018).

79 **As it was, there were big, epistemological gaps:** Heather Uncapher et al., "Hopelessness and Suicidal Ideation in Older Adults," *Gerontological Society of America* 38, no. 1 (1998).

80 **Already, global suicide rates for elderly:** Ismael Conejero et al., "Suicide in Older Adults: Current Perspectives," *Clinical Interventions in Ageing* 13 (2018): 691–699.

80 **Nearly 10 percent of Americans aged sixty-five and over:** Library of Congress, Congressional Research Service, *Poverty Among Americans Aged 65 and Older*, by Zhe Li and Joseph Dalaker, R45791, July 1, 2019. The briefing notes, "The poverty rate among Americans aged 65 and older has declined by almost 70% in the past five decades. In 2017, approxi-

mately 9.2% of Americans aged 65 and older had income below the poverty thresholds. However, the number of aged poor has increased since the mid-1970s as the total number of elderly has grown. In 2017, 4.7 million people aged 65 and older lived in poverty."

80 **Medicare does not cover assisted-living facilities:** "Medicare vs. Medicaid," A Place for Mom, modified June 2018, https://www.aplaceformom.com/planning-and-advice/articles/senior -care-costs; "Does Medicare Pay for Assisted Living?" AARP, accessed March 2020, https:// www.aarp.org/health/medicare-qa-tool/does-medicare-cover-assisted-living/; Jennifer J. Salopek, "Medicare Home Health Benefits: What Caregiving Costs Are Covered," AARP, October 11, 2019, https://www.aarp.org/caregiving/financial-legal/info-2019/medicare-home -health-care-benefits.html.

80 **about a quarter of Medicare spending:** Gerald F. Riley and James D. Lubitz, "Long-Term Trends in Medicare Payments in the Last Year of Life," *Health Services Research* 45, no. 2 (April 2010): 565–576. In 2018, researchers published an article in *Science* offering context for this "one quarter" figure, noting that "less than 5% of spending is accounted for by individuals with predicted mortality above 50%." Liran Einav et al., "Predictive Modeling of U.S. Health Care Spending in Late Life," *Science* 360, no. 6396 (June 2018): 1462–1465.

80 **what the philosopher Paul Menzel called:** Paul T. Menzel, *Strong Medicine: The Ethical Rationing of Health Care* (Oxford: Oxford University Press, 1990).

81 **In early 2019, Dr. Michael Irwin started a new organization:** Michael Irwin, Ninety Plus, modified 2020, https://ninetyplus.org.uk/.

81 **Currently, three countries in Europe have assisted-dying laws:** Polypathology is also referred to as "multimorbidity" in scientific reports. According to Belgium's Federal Commission for the Control and Evaluation of Euthanasia, patients with polypathology accounted for 13.2 percent of total euthanasia cases in 2016–2017, making it the second-most frequently cited diagnosis after cancer. Commission Fédérale de Contrôle et d'Évaluation de l'Euthanasie, "Huitième rapport aux chambres législatives années 2016–2017," October 2018, https://organesdeconcertation.sante.belgique.be/sites/default /files/documents/8_rapport-euthanasie_2016-2017-fr.pdf.

In the Netherlands, the Dutch regional review committees have separate categories for patients who suffer from multiple disorders related to age and those who suffer from a combination of disorders. In 2018, the commission received notification of 6,126 euthanasias; 205 involved patients with "multiple geriatric disorders" and 738 involved patients with a "combination of disorders." Regional Euthanasia Review Committee, "Annual Report 2018," April 2019, https://www.euthanasiecommissie.nl/binaries/euthanasiecommissie /documenten/jaarverslagen/2018/april/11/jaarverslag-2018/RTE_jv2018_English.pdf. See also Woulter Beekman, *The Self-Chosen Death of the Elderly* (United Kingdom: Society for Old Age Rational Suicide, 2011); Els van Wijngaarden et al., "Assisted Dying for Healthy Older People: A Step Too Far?" *BMJ* 357 (May 19, 2017).

Luxembourg's law is based largely on the Belgian law, though euthanasia cases in the country have been limited. Some Swiss clinics and physicians also accept patients with polypathology related to advanced age. See Sigrid Dierickx, "Euthanasia Practice in Belgium: A Population-Based Evaluation of Trends and Currently Debated Issues" (PhD diss., Faculty of Medicine and Pharmacy, Vrije Universiteit Brussel, 2018), https://www.worldrtd .net/sites/default/files/newsfiles/Sigrid_Dierickx.pdf.

82 **Edith Schippers, proposed a measure:** Dan Bilefsky and Christopher F. Schuetz, "Dutch Law Would Allow Assisted Suicide for Healthy Older People," *New York Times*, October

13, 2016; "Netherlands May Extend Assisted Dying to Those Who Feel 'Life Is Complete," Reuters, October 12, 2016.

82 **Wilders told the Dutch newspaper:** Quoted in Paul Ratner, "Dutch May Allow Assisted Suicide for Terminally Ill Patients," Big Think, October 14, 2016, http://bigthink.com/paul-ratner/dutch-may-allow-assisted-suicide-for-people-who-have-completed-life.

82 **Pia Dijkstra announced that:** Janene Pieters, "D66 Working on a Bill for Assisted Suicide at End of a 'Completed Life,'" *NL Times*, September 2, 2019, https://nltimes.nl/2019/09/02/d66-working-bill-assisted-suicide-end-completed-life.

82 **In 2016, a number of Dutch academics published a study:** Els van Wijngaarden et al., "Caught Between Intending and Doing: Older People Ideating on a Self-Chosen Death," *BMJ Open* 6, no. 1 (2016).

83 **which Prince Charles once coolly compared:** "Prince of Wales Always Outspoken on Modern Architecture," *Telegraph*, May 12, 2009, https://www.telegraph.co.uk/news/uknews/theroyalfamily/5311155/Prince-of-Wales-always-outspoken-on-modern-architecture.html.

85 **Avril found the right-to-die group Exit International:** Exit International, "About Exit," modified 2020, https://exitinternational.net/about-exit/history/.

86 **She also read that for $185:** Philip Nitschke and Fiona Stewart, *The Peaceful Pill eHandbook* (n.p.: Exit International US, 2008).

89 **At 8: 49 p.m., on Friday:** I have reconstructed these details through multiple interviews: with Avril, police officers, Avril's former caregivers, and local healthcare workers. I have also reviewed police and medical records. I was helped enormously by a digital recording of an inquest later carried out by Exeter's senior coroner, which the coroner later shared with me; it included extensive testimony from involved law enforcement officials and healthcare workers.

91 **Interpol "had intercepted some information":** Later, nobody at the Devon and Cornwall Police Department would speak to me about the encounter, though a spokesperson did confirm the main events of the evening at Avril's home. My freedom of information request about departmental correspondence with Interpol was also rejected. A media officer would "neither confirm nor deny that it holds the information."

Interpol is headquartered in Lyon, France, and does not maintain national bureaus of its own. Britain's National Crime Agency (NCA), which works with Interpol on matters of "serious and organized crime," does house the country's Interpol National Central Bureau. Nobody at Interpol or the NCA would speak to me. Through a freedom of information request to the UK Home Office, I discovered that British Border Force agents had seized three shipments of pentobarbital at UK ports of entry in April 2016, the month of the police visit to Avril's home.

91 **In notes that the doctor typed up that evening:** I received a copy of the "Devon Doctors Group OOH Call Incident Report," dated April 15, 2016, 4:36 a.m., which includes the physician's record of the evening's events.

95 **He said they did the visit on behalf of** *either* **Homeland Security:** Around the same time, a spokeswoman for the Department of Homeland Security Immigration and Customs Enforcement told me, in an email, that DHS was not involved, either with the specific visit to Sarah's home or with a broader investigation into Nembutal sales. A DEA spokeswoman explained, by email, that "due to ongoing litigation, we're unable to comment on this issue."

95 **Driving home afterward, a number of them hit a police roadblock:** Eleanor Ainge Roy, "New Zealand Police Set Up Roadblocks to Question Euthanasia Group," *Guardian*, October 25, 2016, https://www.theguardian.com/world/2016/oct/25/new-zealand

-police-set-up-roadblocks-to-question-euthanasia-group-members-say; "Woman Who Sparked Controversial Police Investigation into Euthanasia Supporters Identified as Annemarie Treadwell," *New Zealand Herald*, October 28, 2016, https://www.nzherald .co.nz/nz/news/article.cfm?c_id=1&objectid=11737581; Tom Hunt, "Police Admit Using Checkpoint to Target Euthanasia Meeting Attendees," Stuff, October 27, 2016, https://www.stuff.co.nz/national/crime/85752421/police-admit-using-checkpoint-to -target-euthanasia-meeting-attendees; Matt Stewart, "Wellington Euthanasia Lobbyist, Accused of Aiding Suicide, Seeks Global Backing," Stuff, April 24, 2017, https://www .stuff.co.nz/national/health/91852436/wellington-euthanasia-lobbyist-accused-of-aiding -suicide-seeks-global-backing; Matt Stewart and Tom Hunt, "Checkpoint 'Targets' Advised to Take Class Action Against Police After IPCA Ruling," Stuff, March 15, 2018, https://www.stuff.co.nz/national/health/euthanasia-debate/102280034/ipca-police -not-justified-in-using-illegal-checkpoint-to-target-euthanasia-group-members; "Operation Painter: Findings in Privacy Investigation," Scoop, March 15, 2018, https:// www.scoop.co.nz/stories/PO1803/S00228/operation-painter-findings-in-privacy -investigation.htm?from-mobile=bottom-link-01.

96 **In October 2016, Suzy:** "A Trial Is to Be Held for Lower Hutt Woman Susan Austen, Charged with Aiding a Suicide," May 12, 2017, Stuff, https://www.stuff.co.nz/national /crime/92501870/a-trial-is-to-be-held-for-a-woman-charged-with-aiding-a-suicide; "Susan Austen Trial: Police Bugs Recorded Exit Meeting at Suspect's Home," Stuff, February 16, 2018, https://www.stuff.co.nz/national/crime/101479354/suzy-austen-had-email-translated -after-customs-intercepted-parcel; "Austen Trial: Dead Woman Believed in Personal Choice over Living and Dying," Stuff, February 20, 2018, https://www.stuff.co.nz/national/crime /101581275/austen-trial-dead-woman-believed-in-personal-choice-over-living-and-dying; Tom Hunt, "The Susan Austen Interview—from Teacher to Campaigner to Unlikely Criminal," Stuff, May 13, 2018, https://www.stuff.co.nz/dominion-post/news/103857083/the -susan-austen-interview—from-teacher-to-campaigner-to-unlikely-criminal.

96 **After a two-week criminal hearing, she was acquitted on charges:** "Susan Austen Not Guilty of Assisting Suicide," *New Zealand Herald*, February 23, 2018, https://www.nzherald .co.nz/nz/news/article.cfm?c_id=1&objectid=12000695; Melissa Nightingale, "Convicted Euthanasia Advocate: 'I Was Made a Scapegoat,'" *New Zealand Herald*, January 10, 2019, https://www.nzherald.co.nz/nz/news/article.cfm?c_id=1&objectid=12166426&ref=rss.

97 **In the 1990s, scholars who studied them observed:** Alec Wilkinson, "Notes Left Behind," *New Yorker*, February 8, 1999.

3. BODY

100 **the work of Joseph Campbell:** Joseph Campbell, *The Hero with a Thousand Faces* (New York: Pantheon Books, 1949).

100 **at Lifecircle, one of Switzerland's:** At the time of publication, operations at Lifecircle were paused, following the criminal trial of its founder and head physician, Dr. Erika Preisig. Preisig was prosecuted for her assistance in the 2016 suicide of a sixty-year-old woman suffering from psychiatric disorders. In July 2019, the public prosecutor's office in Basel found Preisig not guilty of homicide but warned that she had "narrowly" escaped conviction. The president of the court chastised Preisig for her failure to consult with a psychiatrist about the patient. (Preisig said she had tried to refer the patient for psychiatric assessment but could not find a willing physician.) Preisig was given a fifteen-month suspended prison sentence for several legal breaches related to her handling of therapeutic products. Céline Zünd, "Erika Preisig échappe à une condamnation pour homicide," *Le Temps*, July 9, 2019, https://www.letemps.ch/suisse/erika-preisig-echappe-une -condamnation-homicide.

101 In January 2016, a lawmaker in Colorado: "Colorado," Death with Dignity National Center, accessed March 2020, https://www.deathwithdignity.org/states/colorado/.

101 Maia started researching online, and soon: *Choosing to Die*, directed by Charlie Russell (London: BBC, 2011), television broadcast.

101 Maia learned that assisted death has been legal in Switzerland: Samia A. Hurst and Alex Mauron, "Assisted Suicide and Euthanasia in Switzerland: Allowing a Role for Non-Physicians," *BMJ* 326, no. 7383 (2003): 271–273; George Mills, "What You Need to Know About Assisted Suicide in Switzerland," *Local*, May 3, 2018, https://www.thelocal.ch /20180503/what-you-need-to-know-about-assisted-death-in-switzerland.

102 Article 115 of the Swiss Federal Code: The code reads, "Any person who for selfish motives incites or assists another to commit or attempt to commit suicide is, if that other person thereafter commits or attempts to commit suicide, liable to a custodial sentence not exceeding five years or to a monetary penalty." "Swiss Criminal Code," Federal Assembly, Swiss Confederation, accessed March 2020, https://www.admin.ch/opc/en/classified -compilation/19370083/202003030000/311.0.pdf.

102 Swiss authorities have since interpreted the law: The euthanasia clinic Dignitas, for instance, defines selfish motives as, "for example, if through assisting in suicide someone could inherit assets earlier or would get rid of a financial obligation of support." Dignitas guidelines argue that "normal financial compensation for assistance with suicide" would also be exempt from the "selfish motive" criteria. "Legal Basis," Dignitas, accessed March 2020, http://www.dignitas.ch/index.php?option=com_content&view=article&id =12&Itemid=53&lang=en.

102 The clinics require that their patients: For instance, see Lifecircle's guidance: "Guide to Eternal Spirit," Lifecircle, December 2019, https://www.lifecircle.ch/fileadmin/eternal _spirit/docs/en/Guide_en.pdf.

102 This means that foreigners can fly into Zurich: "Swiss Parliament Rejects Tighter Controls on Assisted Suicide," Reuters, September 26, 2012, https://www.reuters.com/article /us-swiss-politics-suicide/swiss-parliament-rejects-tighter-controls-on-assisted-suicide -idUSBRE88P15320120926.

102 By 2016, people from around the world: DeMond Shondell Miller and Christopher Gonzalez, "When Death Is the Destination: The Business of Death Tourism—Despite Legal and Social Implications," *International Journal of Culture, Tourism and Hospitality Research* 7, no. 3 (2013): 293–306; Saskia Gauthier et al., "Suicide Tourism: A Pilot Study of the Swiss Phenomenon," *Journal of Medical Ethics* 41, no. 8 (2015): 611–617; Samuel Blouin, "'Suicide Tourism' and Understanding the Swiss Model of the Right to Die," Conversation, May 23, 2018, http://theconversation.com/suicide-tourism-and-understanding-the-swiss-model-of -the-right-to-die-96698.

102 According to one study from the University of Zurich: Gauthier et al., "Suicide Tourism."

102 by 1.6 million people: Tim Glanfield, "TV Ratings: Terry Pratchett: Choosing to Die Watched by 1.64m Viewers," RadioTimes, June 14, 2011, https://www.radiotimes .com/news/2011-06-14/tv-ratings-terry-pratchett-choosing-to-die-watched-by-1-64m -viewers/.

103 "Grandfather goes to Dignitas": See, for instance, *Tod nach plan* (A planned death), directed by Hanspeter Bäni (Switzerland, 2010), documentary film; *Manon: The Last Right?*

by Marie-Josée Lévesque et al. (Quebec: Télé-Québec, 2004); *EXIT: Le droit de mourir* (Exit: The right to die), directed by Fernand Melgar (First Run / Icarus Films, 2006), documentary; *The Suicide Tourist*, directed by John Zaritsky (Boston: PBS, 2010), television broadcast; *How to Die: Simon's Choice*, directed by Rowan Deacon (London: BBC, 2016), television broadcast; *Right to Die*, produced by Vikram Gandhi et al. (New York: VICE on HBO, 2017); *Scientist David Goodall Chooses Euthanasia at 104 Years Old*, produced by Lisa McGregor (Australia: ABC Australia, 2018); *End Game*, directed by Rob Epstein and Jeffrey Friedman (Netflix, 2018), documentary film.

Footage of assisted deaths carried out in Switzerland is also popular on YouTube. For instance, the 2010 death of Michèle Causse has been watched more than 2.3 million times. "Assisted Suicide of Michèle Causse," YouTube, uploaded May 30, 2014, https://www.youtube.com/watch?v=JfyxUO4ZsDo.

103 **Ludwig Minelli, referred to assisted dying as "the last human right"**: Imogen Foulkes, "Dignitas Boss: Healthy Should Have Right to Die," BBC News, July 2, 2010, https://www.bbc.com/news/10481309.

103 **after locals complained of human ashes washing up**: Foulkes, "Switzerland Plans New Controls"; BBC News, July 2, 2010, https://www.bbc.com/news/10461894; Roger Boys, "Ashes Dumped in Lake Zurich Put Dignitas Back in the Spotlight," London *Times*, May 1, 2010, https://www.thetimes.co.uk/article/ashes-dumped-in-lake-zurich-put-dignitas-back-in-the-spotlight-wftlfdc06fk.

103 **"Lifecircle is committed to the dignity of mankind"**: "Support and Promote Quality of Life," Lifecircle, accessed March 2020, https://www.lifecircle.ch/en/.

109 **The spinal tap looked normal**: A spinal tap (also called a lumbar puncture) is used to obtain and test cerebrospinal fluid (CSF), a colorless liquid that surrounds the spinal cord and brain. Elevated levels of certain proteins in a CSF sample may be suggestive of MS. However, the National Multiple Sclerosis Society notes that "in people with a confirmed diagnosis of MS, 5–10% do not show abnormalities in the CSF. Therefore, CSF analysis by itself cannot confirm or exclude a diagnosis of MS." "Cerebrospinal Fluid (CSF)," National Multiple Sclerosis Society, accessed March 2020, https://www.nationalmssociety.org/Symptoms-Diagnosis/Diagnosing-Tools/Cerebrospinal-Fluid-(CSF).

110 **a relapsing and remitting form of the disease**: The National Multiple Sclerosis Society notes, "RRMS—the most common disease course—is characterized by clearly defined attacks of new or increasing neurologic symptoms. These attacks—also called relapses or exacerbations—are followed by periods of partial or complete recovery (remissions). During remissions, all symptoms may disappear, or some symptoms may continue and become permanent. However, there is no apparent progression of the disease during the periods of remission." "Relapsing-Remitting MS (RRMS)," National Multiple Sclerosis Society, accessed March 2020, https://www.nationalmssociety.org/What-is-MS/Types-of-MS/Relapsing-remitting-MS.

113 **Maia applied for Social Security disability and was rejected**: Between 2004 and 2013, just 36 percent of Social Security Disability Insurance applicants were approved. Around a quarter were approved on their initial claim. Another 13 percent were approved after a hearing or appeal. Social Security Administration, "Annual Statistical Report on the Social Security Disability Insurance Program, 2014," November 2015, https://www.ssa.gov/policy/docs/statcomps/di_asr/2014/di_asr14.pdf.

113 **According to US Census data, MS patients were about 50 percent more likely to be poor**: Jonathan D. Campbell et al., "Burden of Multiple Sclerosis on Direct, Indirect Costs and

Quality of Life: National US Estimates," *Multiple Sclerosis and Related Disorders* 3, no. 2 (2014): 227–236.

113 **"Insurance is a *huge* problem"**: See also Dennis N. Bourdett et al., "Practices of US Health Insurance Companies Concerning MS Therapies Interfere with Shared Decision-Making and Harm Patients," *Neurology Clinical Practice* 6, no. 2 (2016): 177–182. The authors write, "Increasingly, we find ourselves altering the care we provide our patients because of rules regarding coverage of MS DMTs [Disease Modifying Treatments] and spending hours dealing with insurance companies that refuse to cover treatments that we have pre-scribed." They describe surveying seventeen physicians treating MS patients in a handful of states. "They estimated that their staff spent 20–30 hours per month addressing prob-lems related to insurance coverage for MS drugs. The neurologists indicated that they usually spent 1–1.5 hours per week on insurance denials."

114 **She preferred to read articles**: Gary R. Cutter et al., "Causes of Death Among Persons with Multiple Sclerosis," *Multiple Sclerosis and Related Disorders* 4 (2015): 484–490.

115 **Another was a *New York Times* profile**: N. R. Kleinfield, "The Lonely Death of George Bell," *New York Times*, October 17, 2015, https://www.nytimes.com/2015/10/18/nyregion/dying-alone-in-new-york-city.html.

116 **When Maia looked for information**: For instance, see the websites for Not Dead Yet (not-deadyet.org), Care Not Killing (carenotkilling.org.uk), and Euthanasia Prevention Coalition (epcc.ca).

116 **the early histories of the American right-to-die movement**: For instance, see Ian Dow-biggen, *A Merciful End: The Euthanasia Movement in Modern America* (Oxford: Oxford University Press, 2003); Kevin Yuill, *Assisted Suicide: The Liberal, Humanist Case Against Legalization* (Houndmills, Basingstoke, UK: Palgrave Macmillan, 2013), 60–82.

117 **A 2019 report by the National Council on Disability**: National Council on Disability, "The Danger of Assisted Suicide Laws," October 9, 2019, https://ncd.gov/sites/default/files/NCD_Assisted_Suicide_Report_508.pdf.

117 **In recent years, aid-in-dying supporters**: For more on the subject of disability and aid-in-dying legislation, see Andrew Batavia, "The New Paternalism: Portraying People with Disabilities as an Oppressed Minority," *Journal of Disability Policy Studies* 12, no. 2 (2001): 107–113; Susan M. Behuniak, "Death with 'Dignity': The Wedge That Divides the Dis-ability Rights Movement from the Right to Die Movement," *Politics and the Life Sciences* 30, no. 1 (2011): 17–32; Diane Coleman, "Assisted Suicide Laws Create Discriminatory Double Standard for Who Gets Suicide Prevention and Who Gets Suicide Assistance: Not Dead Yet Responds to Autonomy, Inc.," *Disability and Health Journal* 3 (2010): 39–50; Ann Neumann, *The Good Death: An Exploration of Dying in America* (Boston: Bea-con Press, 2017); Alicia Ouellette, "Barriers to Physician Aid in Dying for People with Disabilities," *Laws* 6, no. 23 (2017); Anita Silvers, "Protecting the Innocents: People with Disabilities and Physician-Assisted Dying," *Western Journal of Medicine* 166, no. 6 (1997): 407–409.

117 **have tried to assuage these fears**: For instance, Compassion & Choices has published "nine facts you need to know" about disability and medical aid in dying. The webpage notes that "two out of three people living with a disability support medical aid in dy-ing according to surveys in Connecticut, New Jersey and Massachusetts." Compassion & Choices, "Medical Aid in Dying and People with Disabilities," accessed March 2020, https://compassionandchoices.org/resource/medical-aid-dying-people-disabilities/.

117 **In a 2007 peer-reviewed study**: Margaret Battin et al., "Legal Physician-Assisted Dying in

Oregon and the Netherlands: Evidence Concerning the Impact on Patients in 'Vulnerable' Groups," *Journal of Medical Ethics* 33, no. 10 (2007): 591–597.

118 **In 2016, Disability Rights Oregon**: Compassion & Choices, "Death with Dignity and People with Disabilities," accessed March 2020, https://www.deathwithdignity.org/death-dignity-people-disabilities/.

119 **an essay that the bioethicist Ezekiel Emanuel**: Ezekiel Emanuel, "Whose Right to Die?" *The Atlantic*, March 1997.

119 **In November 2016, Colorado voters passed**: Colorado Department of Public Health and Environment, "Medical Aid in Dying," accessed March 2020, https://www.colorado.gov/pacific/cdphe/medical-aid-dying.

120 **Under Canada's Bill C-14**: Julia Nicol and Marlisa Tiedemann, "Bill C-14: An Act to Amend the Criminal Code and to Make Related Amendments to Other Acts (Medical Assistance in Dying)," Library of Parliament, No. 42-1-C14-E, April 2016, https://lop.parl.ca/staticfiles/PublicWebsite/Home/ResearchPublications/LegislativeSummaries/PDF/42-1/c14-e.pdf.

120 **A patient was considered to be suffering grievously**: Canadian Association of MAID Assessors and Providers, "The Clinical Interpretation of 'Reasonably Foreseeable,'" June 2017, https://camapcanada.ca/wp-content/uploads/2019/01/cpg1-1.pdf.

120 **Later, in 2019, a Canadian provincial court ruled**: Tu Thanh Ha and Kelly Grant, "Quebec Court Strikes Down Restriction to Medically Assisted Dying Law, Calls It Unconstitutional," *Globe and Mail*, September 11, 2019, https://www.theglobeandmail.com/life/health-and-fitness/article-quebec-court-strikes-down-parts-of-laws-on-medically-assisted-death/; *Truchon c. Procureur général du Canada*, QCCS 3792 (Quebec 2019), https://d3n8a8pro7vhmx.cloudfront.net/dwdcanada/pages/4439/attachments/original/1568236478/500-17-099119-177.pdf?1568236478.

120 **In America, however, MS patients can**: For more on multiple sclerosis and aid in dying, see Deborah Brauser, "More Than 50% of Patients with MS Surveyed Would Consider Physician-Assisted Death," Medscape, October 12, 2016, https://www.medscape.com/viewarticle/870154; Ruth Ann Marrie et al., "High Hypothetical Interest in Physician-Assisted Death in Multiple Sclerosis," *Neurology* 88, no. 16 (2017); Neil Scolding, "Physician-Assisted Death Should Be Available to People with MS—NO," *Multiple Sclerosis Journal* 23, no. 13 (2017): 1679–1680; Kim Louise Wiebe, "Physician-Assisted Death Should Be Available to People with MS—YES," *Multiple Sclerosis Journal* 23, no. 13 (2017): 1677–1678.

120 **Oregon data shows that in 2019**: Oregon Health Authority, "Oregon Death with Dignity Act: 2019 Data Summary," February 25, 2020, https://www.oregon.gov/oha/PH/PROVIDERPARTNERRESOURCES/EVALUATIONRESEARCH/DEATHWITHDIGNITYACT/Documents/year22.pdf.

For more on ALS and aid in dying, see Leo H. Wang et al., "Death with Dignity in Washington Patients with Amyotrophic Lateral Sclerosis," *Neurology* 87, no. 20 (2016): 2117–2122; James A. Russell and Mario F. Dulay, "Hastened Death in ALS: Damaged Brains and Bad Decisions?" *Neurology* 87, no. 13 (2016): 1312–1313; Jonathan Katz and Hiroshi Mitsumono, "ALS and Physician-Assisted Suicide," *Neurology* 87, no. 11 (2016): 1072–1073. See also James A. Russell, "Physician-Hastened Death in Patients with Progressive Neurodegenerative or Neuromuscular Disorders," *Seminars in Neurology* 38, no. 5 (2018): 522–532.

120 **That same year in Colorado**: Center for Health and Environmental Data, "Colorado End-of-Life Options Act, Year Three," 2020, https://www.colorado.gov/pacific/cdphe/medical-aid-dying.

120 One told me that, given the increased risk: For instance, see H. Hoang et al., "Psychiatric Co-morbidity in Multiple Sclerosis: The Risk of Depression and Anxiety Before and After MS Diagnosis," *Multiple Sclerosis Journal* 22, no. 3 (2016): 347–353; Anthony Feinstein and Bennis Pavisian, "Multiple Sclerosis and Suicide," *Multiple Sclerosis Journal* 23, no. 7 (2017): 923–927; Ruth Ann Marrie, "What Is the Risk of Suicide in Multiple Sclerosis?" *Multiple Sclerosis Journal* 23, no. 6 (2017): 755–756.

125 On the National MS Society website: National Multiple Sclerosis Society, "Cognitive Changes," accessed March 2020, https://www.nationalmssociety.org/Symptoms-Diagnosis/MS-Symptoms/Cognitive-Changes.

126 and into a secondary progressive phase: Gabrielle Macaron and Daniel Ontaneda, "Diagnosis and Management of Progressive Multiple Sclerosis," *Biomedicines* 7, no. 3 (2019).

126 It was like the C. S. Lewis quote: C. S. Lewis, *A Grief Observed* (New York: HarperOne, 2001).

127 That year, she finally qualified for Medicare: Social Security Administration, "Will a Beneficiary Get Medicare Coverage?" accessed March 2020, https://www.ssa.gov/disabilityresearch/wi/medicare.htm.

127 One study from 2007 showed that: L. Iezzoni and L. Ngo, "Health, Disability, and Life Insurance Experiences of Working-Age Persons with Multiple Sclerosis," *Multiple Sclerosis Journal* 13, no. 4 (2007): 534–546.

128 I spoke with Bari Talente: "Making Health Care More Affordable: Lowering Drug Prices and Increasing Transparency," written statement of Bari Talente, JD, Executive Vice President of Advocacy, National Multiple Sclerosis Society, to United States House of Representatives, Committee on Education and Labor, September 26, 2019, https://edlabor.house.gov/imo/media/doc/TalenteTestimony092619.pdf; Daniel M. Hartung et al., "The Cost of Multiple Sclerosis Drugs in the US and the Pharmaceutical Industry," *Neurology* 84, no. 21 (2015): 2185–2192; Lisa Rapaport, "U.S. Prices for Multiple Sclerosis Drugs Are on the Rise," Reuters, August 27, 2019, https://www.reuters.com/article/us-health-ms/u-s-prices-for-multiple-sclerosis-drugs-are-on-the-rise-idUSKCN1VH2I5.

128 because the medications are so expensive: "2019 Employer Health Benefits Survey," Kaiser Family Foundation, September 25, 2019, https://www.kff.org/report-section/ehbs-2019-section-9-prescription-drug-benefits/.

128 Even elderly people on Medicare: Mark Miller, "Medicare Part D No Match for Runaway Specialty Drug Costs: Study," Reuters, February 7, 2019, https://www.reuters.com/article/us-health-ms/u-s-prices-for-multiple-sclerosis-drugs-are-on-the-rise-idUSKCN1VH2I5; Juliette Cubanski et al., "The Out-of-Pocket Cost Burden for Specialty Drugs in Medicare Part D in 2019," Kaiser Family Foundation, February 1, 2019, https://www.kff.org/medicare/issue-brief/the-out-of-pocket-cost-burden-for-specialty-drugs-in-medicare-part-d-in-2019/.

129 voluntarily stopping eating and drinking: Timothy Quill, "Voluntary Stopping of Eating and Drinking (VSED), Physician-Assisted Death (PAD), or Neither in the Last Stage of Life? Both Should Be Available as a Last Resort," *Annals of Family Medicine* 13, no. 5 (2015): 208–209; Timothy Quill et al., "Voluntarily Stopping Eating and Drinking Among Patients with Serious Advanced Illness—Clinical, Ethical, and Legal Aspects," *JAMA Internal Medicine* 178, no. 1 (2018): 123–127.

129 In 2016, the lobby group: Compassion & Choices, "The Facts: Medical Aid-in-Dying in the United States," December 2016, https://www.lwvbn.org/notices/DeathDyingConcurrence/G-Fact%20Sheet%20Aid%20in%20Dying%20in%20US%20Compassion%20and%20Choices%20Support.pdf.

130 **According to 2019 Oregon Death with Dignity:** Oregon Health Authority, "Oregon Death with Dignity Act: 2019 Data Summary."

132 **a line from the writer Julian Barnes:** Julian Barnes, *Nothing to Be Frightened Of* (New York: Vintage, 2009).

133 **In July 2018, Maia sent me a link:** Rob Kuznia, "In Oregon, Pushing to Give Patients with Degenerative Diseases the Right to Die," *Washington Post*, March 11, 2018, https://www.washingtonpost.com/national/in-oregon-pushing-to-give-patients-with-degenerative-diseases-the-right-to-die/2018/03/11/3b6a2362-230e-11e8-94da-ebf9d112159c_story.html.

136 **In 2008, Debbie had become a celebrity:** "Debbie Purdy," BBC Radio 4, February 26, 2019, https://www.bbc.co.uk/programmes/m0002r4f; Martin Beckford, "Debbie Purdy Demands Director of Public Prosecutions Spell Out Law on Assisted Suicide," *Telegraph*, October 2, 2008, https://www.telegraph.co.uk/news/uknews/3123290/Debbie-Purdy-demands-Director-of-Public-Prosecutions-spell-out-law-on-assisted-suicide.html; Afua Hirsch, "Prison Fear for Relatives Who Assist Suicide," *Guardian*, October 29, 2008, https://www.theguardian.com/society/2008/oct/29/assisted-suicide-right-to-die.

137 **However, if she had to travel alone:** Martin Beckford and Rosa Prince, "Debbie Purdy Wins House of Lords Victory to Have Assisted Suicide Law Clarified," *Telegraph*, July 31, 2009, https://www.telegraph.co.uk/news/uknews/law-and-order/5942603/Debbie-Purdy-wins-House-of-Lords-victory-to-have-assisted-suicide-law-clarified.html.

137 **Debbie's lawyer argued that:** Afua Hirsch, "Debbie Purdy Wins 'Significant Legal Victory' on Assisted Suicide," *Guardian*, July 30, 2009, https://www.theguardian.com/society/2009/jul/30/debbie-purdy-assisted-suicide-legal-victory.

137 **and Britain issued new guidelines:** Sandra Laville, "People Who Assist Suicide Will Face Test of Motives, says DPP," *Guardian*, February 25, 2010, https://www.theguardian.com/society/2010/feb/25/dpp-assisted-suicide-guidelines-starmer-purdy; Director of Public Prosecutions, "Suicide: Policy for Prosecutors in Respect of Cases of Encouraging or Assisting Suicide," Crown Prosecution Service, February 2010, last updated October 2014, https://www.cps.gov.uk/legal-guidance/suicide-policy-prosecutors-respect-cases-encouraging-or-assisting-suicide.

137 **Debbie said that she wanted:** Afua Hirsch, "Victory for Debbie Purdy After Historic Ruling in Right-to-Die Legal Battle," *Guardian*, July 30, 2009, https://www.theguardian.com/society/2009/jul/30/debbie-purdy-assisted-suicide-judgement.

141 **that a proposed aid-in-dying bill had not passed:** Compassion & Choices, "New Mexico," accessed March 2020, https://www.deathwithdignity.org/states/new-mexico/.

141 **The proposed criteria expansion in Oregon:** Elizabeth Hayes, "Oregon Lawmakers Consider Controversial Expansion to Death with Dignity Law," *Portland Business Journal*, March 20, 2019, https://www.bizjournals.com/portland/news/2019/03/20/oregon-lawmakers-consider-controversial-expansion.html; "Oregon House Bill 2217," LegiScan, accessed March 2020, https://legiscan.com/OR/bill/HB2217/2019.

4. MEMORY

145 **while researching online, Brian found:** Final Exit Network, "What We Do," accessed March 2020, https://finalexitnetwork.org/what-we-do/exit-guide-services/.

145 **Brian read that FEN had:** For more on the Hemlock Society and its history, see Faye Girsh, "The Hemlock Story in Brief," Hemlock Society San Diego, 2006, https://www.hemlocksocietysandiego.org/wp-content/uploads/2019/03/brief.pdf; Richard Cote, *In*

Search of Gentle Death: The Fight for Your Right to Die with Dignity (South Carolina: Corinthian Books, 2012); Derek Humphry and Mary Clement, *Freedom to Die: People, Politics and the Right-to-Die Movement* (New York: St. Martin's Griffin, 2000); Derek Humphry, *The Good Euthanasia Guide: Where, What, and Who in Choices in Dying* (Oregon: ERGO, 2004); Derek Humphry, *Good Life, Good Death: The Memoir of a Right to Die Pioneer* (New York: Carrel Books, 2017); Derek Humphry, "Founding the Hemlock Society," interview by Bob Uslander, Dr. Bob Uslander: Integrated MD Care, January 12, 2018, https://integratedmdcare.com/founding-hemlock-sociedy-derek-humphry-ep-8/.

145 **who in 1975 had helped his:** Derek Humphry, *Jean's Way* (Oregon: Norris Lane Press, 2013).

145 **Ideally, Humphry told a *New York Times* reporter:** Andrew H. Malcolm, "Some Elderly Choose Suicide over Lonely, Dependent Life," *New York Times*, September 24, 1984, https://www.nytimes.com/1984/09/24/us/some-elderly-choose-suicide-over-lonely-dependent-life.html.

145 **"They firebomb the houses":** George Howe Colt, *The Enigma of Suicide: A Timely Investigation into the Causes, the Possibility for Prevention and the Paths to Healing* (New York: Simon and Schuster, 1991), 369.

145 **Ten years later, Hemlock claimed:** Girsh, "Hemlock Story in Brief."

146 **At chapter meetings, many held:** For instance, see Randall Beach, "Hemlock Society Attracts Growing Attention," *New York Times*, July 22, 1990; Psyche Pascual, "Right-to-Die Talk Met by Understanding, Protest," *Los Angeles Times*, January 12, 1992.

For more on the relationship between Unitarian Universalists and right-to-die campaigners, see Elaine McCardle, "Choice at the End: In Oregon, Terminally Ill People Have the Right to Seek a Prescription to End Their Lives—Thanks in Large Part to Unitarian Universalists," UU World, April 25, 2016, https://www.uuworld.org/articles/choice-end; Unitarian Universalist Association, "The Right to Die with Dignity: 1988 General Resolution," UUA, 1998, https://www.uua.org/action/statements/right-die-dignity.

146 **In 1991, Humphry offered a direct response:** Derek Humphry, *Final Exit: The Practicalities of Self-Deliverance and Assisted Suicide for the Dying* (California: Hemlock Society USA, 1991).

147 **But then, to pretty much everyone's surprise:** Lawrence K. Altman, "How-To Book on Suicide Is atop Best-Seller List," *New York Times*, August 9, 1991, https://www.nytimes.com/1991/08/09/us/how-to-book-on-suicide-is-atop-best-seller-list.html.

147 **The newspaper called it:** Trip Gabriel, "A Fight to the Death," *New York Times Magazine*, December 8, 1991, https://www.nytimes.com/1991/12/08/magazine/a-fight-to-the-death.html.

147 **Dr. Arthur Caplan, the preeminent bioethicist:** Altman, "How-To Book on Suicide."

147 **and shortly after Ann Wickett, his second ex-wife:** Afterward, Humphry claimed that Ann had long been mentally ill and noted that her cancer was in remission. Gabriel, "Fight to the Death"; Robert Reinhold, "Right-to-Die Group Is Shaken as Leader Leaves His Cancer-Stricken Wife," *New York Times*, February 8, 1990, https://www.nytimes.com/1990/02/08/us/right-to-die-group-is-shaken-as-leader-leaves-his-cancer-stricken-wife.html; Garry Abrams, "A Bitter Legacy: Angry Accusations Abound After the Suicide of Hemlock Society Co-Founder Ann Humphry," *Los Angeles Times*, October 23, 1991, https://www.latimes.com/archives/la-xpm-1991-10-23-vw-283-story.html; "Suicide Note Said to Accuse Author," *Washington Post*, October 27, 1991, https://www.washingtonpost.com/archive/lifestyle/1991/10/28/suicide-note-said-to-accuse-author/f1bcba4e-7cf1-4530-a17f-101523609f60/.

147 **In 1998, the group set up a program**: Girsh, "Hemlock Story in Brief."

147 **Under the program, volunteers were trained to act**: Dr. Dick MacDonald, a physician who was employed by the Hemlock Society and who ran Caring Friends, told me that the organization initially worked with barbiturates. Caring Friends guides would advise Hemlock members on how to procure barbiturates such as Seconal or Nembutal—and would then sit with them while they consumed the drugs. He said that later, under new leadership, Caring Friends gave advice on using other, legally prescribed medications, such as antidepressants.

   MacDonald also explained that the Caring Friends program was financially self-supporting. He said that loved ones often donated to the program after a client's death, "so that within four years or so of having the Caring Friends program there were several million dollars of donations."

148 **In the early 2000s, Hemlock merged**: Derek Humphry, "Farewell to Hemlock: Killed by Its Name," Euthanasia Research & Guidance Organization, February 21, 2005, https://www.assistedsuicide.org/farewell-to-hemlock.html.

149 **Robert had closely studied the subject**: Robert Rivas, "Survey of State Laws Against Assisting in a Suicide," 2017, https://www.scribd.com/document/367153355/Survey-of-State-Laws-Against-Assisting-in-a-Suicide-2017-Update.

149 **As it was, FEN had already been the subject**: Jaime Joyce, "Kill Me Now: The Troubled Life and Complicated Death of Jana Van Voorhis," BuzzFeed, December 27, 2013, https://www.buzzfeed.com/jaimejoyce/kill-me-now-the-troubled-life-and-complicated-death-of-jana; *The Suicide Plan*, season 2, episode 23, produced by Mira Navasky and Karen O'Connor (PBS, 2012), television broadcast; Robbie Brown, "Arrests Draw New Attention to Assisted Suicide," *New York Times*, March 10, 2009, https://www.nytimes.com/2009/03/11/us/11suicide.html; Paul Rubin, "Final Exit Members Going on Trial After 2007 Assisted Suicide of Phoenix Woman," *Phoenix New Times*, March 31, 2011, https://www.phoenixnewtimes.com/news/final-exit-network-members-going-on-trial-after-2007-assisted-suicide-of-phoenix-woman-6448001; "Right-to-Die Group Fined $30K in Minnesota Woman's Suicide," Associated Press, August 24, 2015, https://minnesota.cbslocal.com/2015/08/24/right-to-die-group-heads-for-sentencing-in-womans-suicide/. More collected legal analysis of the Final Exit Network can be found at Professor Thaddeus Pope's *Medical Futility Blog*: Thaddeus Mason Pope, "Final Exit Network," *Medical Futility Blog*, http://medicalfutility.blogspot.com/search?q=final+exit+network.

149 **In 2015, the network received a felony conviction**: "Judge Fines Final Exit Group Convicted of Assisting Minnesota Suicide," Reuters, August 24, 2015, https://www.reuters.com/article/us-usa-minnesota-finalexit/judge-fines-final-exit-group-convicted-of-assisting-minnesota-suicide-idUSKCN0QT25920150824.

149 **It appealed the decision**: *State of Minnesota v. Final Exit Network*, File No. 19HA CR-12-1718 (Dakota County District Court, 2016), https://mn.gov/law-library-stat/archive/ctappub/2016/opa151826-121916.pdf.

149 **Under the state's interpretation, FEN lawyers argued**: *Final Exit Network Inc. v. State of Minnesota*, "Petition for a Writ of Certiorari," 2017, https://www.scotusblog.com/wp-content/uploads/2017/07/16-1479-petition.pdf; *Final Exit Network, Inc., Fran Schindler, and Janet Grossman v. Lori Swanson, in her official capacity as the attorney general of Minnesota et al.*, Case No. 0:18-cv-01025-JNE/SER (US District Court, District of Minnesota, 2018), http://www.thaddeuspope.com/images/Amended_compl_D_Minn_08-2018.pdf.

150 **Barbara Coombs Lee, the president**: "4 Assisted Suicide Group Members Are Arrested,"

Associated Press, February 26, 2009, http://www.nbcnews.com/id/29411514/ns/us_news
-crime_and_courts/t/assisted-suicide-group-members-are-arrested/#.XoDd19NKg0o.

151 **I was reminded of the Jane Collective**: Laura Kaplan, *The Story of Jane: The Legendary
Underground Feminist Abortion Service* (New York: Pantheon Books, 1995); Clyde Haber-
man, "Code Name Jane: The Women Behind a Covert Abortion Network," *New York
Times*, October 14, 2018, Retro Report, https://www.nytimes.com/2018/10/14/us/illegal
-abortion-janes.html.

152 **As it happens, Janet learned**: Ann Neumann, "Going to Extremes," *Harper's*, February 2019,
https://harpers.org/archive/2019/02/going-to-extremes-elderly-assisted-suicide-caregivers/.

153 **She should live as long**: Final Exit Network guides told me that they have dropped clients
with dementia before. One guide recalled a client who seemed confused by what she was
saying—as if, maybe, her husband was coaching her to say it. The guide stopped working
with the client.

154 **Researchers were already warning**: Alzheimer's Association, "Generation Alzheimer's:
The Defining Disease of the Baby Boomers," 2011, https://act.alz.org/site/DocServer
/ALZ_BoomersReport.pdf?docID=521; James R. Knickman and Emily K. Snell, "The
2030 Problem: Caring for Aging Baby Boomers," *Health Services Research* 37, no. 4 (2002):
849–884.

159 **Debra was surprised to learn**: AARP, "Does Medicare Pay for Assisted Living?" accessed
March 2020, https://www.aarp.org/health/medicare-qa-tool/does-medicare-cover-assisted
-living/. Marlo Sollitto, "How to Pay for Assisted Living," AgingCare, accessed March
2020, https://www.agingcare.com/articles/how-to-pay-for-assisted-living-153842.htm.

160 **That meant he was obliged**: Oregon Department of Human Services, "Mandatory Reporting," accessed March 2020, https://www.oregon.gov/DHS/ABUSE/Pages/mandatory
_report.aspx.

161 **"The existential experience of dementia"**: Sallie Tisdale, "Out of Time," *Harper's*, March
2018, https://harpers.org/archive/2018/03/out-of-time/3/.

163 **They might want to leave the house**: One exit guide explained the "discovery plan" this
way: "Generally, the discovery plan is, those present will actually leave the house for two
hours and perform some perfunctory errand, going to lunch, going shopping, going to
a bar or whatever. Then come back and *find* that their family member, their friend, has
deceased while they were gone. There's two reasons for that. First of all, when they're telling the authorities . . . 'Well, we went to lunch and came back and the person was dead,'
that's the truth. We don't want people to be in the position of telling lies. . . . Then the
other thing is that, occasionally, there will be emergency personnel coming into the scene.
If there's two hours, the body will already be cold and it will be clear and no resuscitation
should be attempted."

168 **In 2015, when an Oregon legislator**: Molly Harbarger, "Legislator's Promise to a Dying
Friend: Death with Dignity Amendment to Help ALS, Alzheimer's Patients Fails," *Or-
egonian*, April 30, 2015, https://www.oregonlive.com/politics/2015/04/legislators_promise
_to_a_dying.html; "House Bill 3337," OregonLive, accessed March 2020, https://gov
.oregonlive.com/bill/2015/HB3337/; "Oregon House Bill 2217," LegiScan, accessed March
2020, https://legiscan.com/OR/bill/HB2217/2019.

168 **In Belgium and the Netherlands**: For more on Belgium, see Federal Public Service, "Euthanasia," updated January 27, 2016, accessed March 2020, https://www.health.belgium
.be/en/node/22874; Raphael Cohen-Almagor, "First Do No Harm: Euthanasia of Patients
with Dementia in Belgium," *Journal of Medicine and Philosophy* 41, no. 1 (2016): 74–89;
Raphael Cohen-Almagor, "Euthanasia Policy and Practice in Belgium: Critical Obser-

vations and Suggestions for Improvement," *Issues in Law and Medicine* 24, no. 3 (2009): 187–218; Chris Gastmans, "Euthanasia in Persons with Severe Dementia," in *Euthanasia and Assisted Suicide: Lessons from Belgium*, ed. David Albert Jones et al. (Cambridge: Cambridge University Press, 2017). For more on the Netherlands, see Government of the Netherlands, "Euthanasia, Assisted Suicide and Non-Resuscitation," accessed March 2020, https://www.government.nl/topics/euthanasia/euthanasia-assisted-suicide-and-non -resuscitation-on-request; Dominic R. Mangino et al., "Euthanasia and Assisted Suicide of Persons with Dementia in the Netherlands," *American Journal of Geriatric Psychiatry* 28, no. 4 (2020): 466–477; David Gibbes Miller et al., "Advance Euthanasia Directives: A Contro-versial Case and Its Ethical Implications," *Journal of Medical Ethics* 45, no. 2 (2017): 84–89; Christopher de Bellaigue, "Death on Demand: Has Euthanasia Gone Too Far?" *Guard-ian*, January 18, 2019, https://www.theguardian.com/news/2019/jan/18/death-on-demand -has-euthanasia-gone-too-far-netherlands-assisted-dying; Janene Pieters, "Euthanasia OK'D for Dementia Patients Who Request It When Lucid," *NL Times*, January 7, 2016, https://nltimes.nl/2016/01/07/euthanasia-okd-dementia-patients-request-lucid; Marike E. de Boer, "Advance Directives for Euthanasia in Dementia: Do Law-Based Opportunities Lead to More Euthanasia?" *Health Policy* 98, nos. 2–3 (December 2010): 256–262.

169 **Between 2002 and 2013**: Sigrid Dierickx et al., "Euthanasia for People with Psychiatric Dis-orders or Dementia in Belgium: Analysis of Official Reported Cases," *BMC Psychiatry* 203 (2017).

169 **According to a 2016 report**: Inez D. de Beaufort and Suzanne van de Vathorst, "Dementia and Assisted Suicide and Euthanasia," *Journal of Neurology* 263 (2016): 1463–1467.

169 **In the Netherlands, where euthanasia now accounts for**: "Euthanasia Cases Drop by 7%, Accounting for 4% of Total Deaths in NL," *Dutch News*, April 11, 2019, https://www .dutchnews.nl/news/2019/04/euthanasia-cases-drop-by-7-accounting-for-4-of-total -deaths-in-nl/; Regionale Toetsingscommissies Euthanasie, "The 2018 Annual Report Was Published Today," April 11, 2019, https://www.euthanasiecommissie.nl/actueel /nieuws/2019/april/11/jaarverslag-2018.

170 **According to the Dutch euthanasia review committee's**: Regionale Toetsingscommissies Euthanasie, "Annual Report 2016," April 11, 2019, https://www.euthanasiecommissie.nl /binaries/euthanasiecommissie/documenten/jaarverslagen/2016/april/12/jaarverslag-2016 /RTE_annual_report_2016.pdf.

170 **In fact, many physicians have refused**: Janene Pieters, "Euthanasia Rarely Approved for Advanced Dementia Patients, Despite Lucid Requests," *NL Times*, January 6, 2017, https://nltimes.nl/2017/01/06/euthanasia-rarely-approved-advanced-dementia-patients -despite-lucid-requests; Jaap Schuurmans et al., "Euthanasia Requests in Dementia Cases; What Are Experiences and Needs of Dutch Physicians? A Qualitative Interview Study," *BMC Medical Ethics* 20, no. 66 (2019); Kirsten Evenblij et al., "Factors Associated with Requesting and Receiving Euthanasia: A Nationwide Mortality Follow-Back Study with a Focus on Patients with Psychiatric Disorders, Dementia, or an Accumulation of Health Problems Related to Old Age," *BMC Medicine* 17, no. 39 (2019).

One way around this reticence is the Levenseindekliniek (End of Life Clinic) in the Hague, which was started in 2012 as an independent facility that could help patients whose own doctors wouldn't support them. By 2016, Levenseindekliniek physicians were per-forming around a third of the country's euthanasias involving dementia patients. In 2017, I visited the clinic, which is headquartered in a stately brick home, down the road from the Embassy of Nicaragua. In his office, the clinic's director, Steven Pleiter, confided that his relationship with the Dutch Medical Association was "not smooth." Levenseindek-liniek doctors, he said, had been dismissed as "cowboys," offering euthanasia on the fly.

170 **In 2017, more than two hundred doctors**: "Dutch Doctors Against Euthanasia for Advanced Dementia Patients," *NL Times*, February 10, 2017, https://nltimes.nl/2017/02/10/dutch-doctors-euthanasia-advanced-dementia-patients.

170 **Even Jacob Kohnstamm**: Pieters, "Euthanasia Rarely Approved for Advanced Dementia Patients"; Celeste McGovern, "'Horrible Picture': Dutch Woman Restrained by Family While Being Euthanized," *National Catholic Register*, February 7, 2017, https://www.ncregister.com/daily-news/horrible-picture-dutch-woman-restrained-by-family-while-being-euthanized.

170 **In 2018, 146 dementia patients**: Regionale Toetsingscommissies Euthanasie, "The 2018 Annual Report."

170 **The Dutch Association for Voluntary Ending of Life**: Pieters, "Euthanasia Rarely Approved for Advanced Dementia Patients."

171 **One landmark case, later investigated**: Regionale Toetsingscommissies Euthanasie, "Annual Report 2016," 52–58; Miller et al., "Advance Euthanasia Directives"; "Doctor Reprimanded for 'Overstepping Mark' During Euthanasia on Dementia Patient," *Dutch News*, January 29, 2017, https://www.dutchnews.nl/news/2017/01/doctor-reprimanded-for-overstepping-mark-during-euthanasia-on-dementia-patient/.

172 **"Even if the patient had said"**: Maria Cheng and Mike Corder, "Dutch to Prosecute Doctor Who Euthanized Woman with Dementia," Associated Press, November 9, 2018, https://apnews.com/15805d9d1d4345dab2a657f26697a775.

172 **The physician was initially charged**: "Dutch Euthanasia Case: Doctor Acted in Interest of Patient, Court Rules," BBC News, September 11, 2019, https://www.bbc.com/news/world-europe-49660525.

172 **Dutch doctors continue to debate**: Eva Constance Alida Asscher and Suzanne van de Vathorst, "First Prosecution of a Dutch Doctor Since the Euthanasia Act of 2002: What Does the Verdict Mean?" *Journal of Medical Ethics* 46, no. 2 (2020): 71–75; Gastmans, "Euthanasia in Persons with Severe Dementia."

172 **Those in the business of debating**: Ronald Dworkin, *Life's Dominion: An Argument About Abortion, Euthanasia, and Individual Freedom* (New York: Alfred A. Knopf, 1993).

173 **But some are disturbed**: Cohen-Almagor, "First Do No Harm"; Rebecca Dresser, "Dworkin on Dementia: Elegant Theory, Questionable Policy," *Hastings Center Report* 25, no. 6 (1995): 32–38; C. M. Hertogh et al., "Would We Rather Lose Our Life Than Lose Our Self? Lessons from the Dutch Debate on Euthanasia for Patients with Dementia," *American Journal of Bioethics* 7, no. 4 (2007): 48–56; Eric Rakowski, "The Sanctity of Human Life: Life's Dominion: An Argument About Abortion, Euthanasia, and Individual Freedom, by Ronald Dworkin," *Yale Law Journal* 103, no. 7 (1994): 2014–2118; Paul T. Menzel and Bonnie Steinbock, "Advance Directives, Dementia, and Physician-Assisted Death," *Journal of Law, Medicine and Ethics* 41, no. 2 (2013): 484–500; Norman L. Cantor, "My Plan to Avoid the Ravages of Extreme Dementia," *Bill of Health*, April 16, 2015, https://blog.petrieflom.law.harvard.edu/2015/04/16/my-plan-to-avoid-the-ravages-of-extreme-dementia/; Daniel P. Sulmasy, "An Open Letter to Norman Cantor Regarding Dementia and Physician-Assisted Suicide," *Hastings Center Report* 48, no. 4 (2018); Brian Draper et al., "Early Dementia Diagnosis and the Risk of Suicide and Euthanasia," *Journal of the Alzheimer's Association* 6, no. 1 (2010): 75–82; Margaret P. Battin, "Right Question, but Not Quite the Right Answer: Whether There Is a Third Alternative in Choices About Euthanasia in Alzheimer's Disease," *American Journal of Bioethics* 4, no. 4 (2007): 58–60; Dena S.

Davis, "Alzheimer Disease and Pre-emptive Suicide," *Journal of Medical Ethics* 40, no. 8 (2014): 543–549.

173 In Canada, lawmakers have debated: The Expert Panel Working Group on Advance Requests for MAID, "The State of Knowledge on Advance Requests for Medical Assistance in Dying," 2018, https://cca-reports.ca/wp-content/uploads/2019/02/The-State-of -Knowledge-on-Advance-Requests-for-Medical-Assistance-in-Dying.pdf; Amanda Coletta, "Canada Debates Offering Physician-Assisted Death to Patients Who Aren't Terminally Ill," *Washington Post*, March 29, 2020, https://www.washingtonpost.com/world /the_americas/canada-trudeau-medical-assistance-dying-physician-suicide/2020/03/29 /bd98c4a0-5751-11ea-8efd-0f904bdd8057_story.html; Shannon Proudfoot, "The Impossible Case of Assisted Death for People with Dementia," *Maclean's*, May 20, 2019, https:// www.macleans.ca/society/the-impossible-case-of-assisted-death-for-people-with-dementia/; Shannon Proudfoot, "For People with Dementia, a Fight for the Right to Die," *Maclean's*, May 3, 2019, https://www.macleans.ca/society/for-people-with-dementia-a-fight-for-the -right-to-die/; Marlisa Tiedemann, "Assisted Dying in Canada After Carter v. Canada," Background Paper, Library of Parliament, No. 2019-43-E, November 29, 2019, https://lop .parl.ca/sites/PublicWebsite/default/en_CA/ResearchPublications/201943E; Ipsos, "Eight in Ten (80%) Canadians Support Advance Consent to Physician-Assisted Dying," February 11, 2016, https://www.ipsos.com/en-ca/news-polls/eight-ten-80-canadians-support-advance -consent-physician-assisted-dying.

173 In 2019, Canadian newspapers: "B.C. Man Is One of the First Canadians with Dementia to Die with Medical Assistance," CBC Radio, October 27, 2019, https://www.cbc.ca/radio /thesundayedition/the-sunday-edition-for-october-27-2019-1.5335017/b-c-man-is-one-of -the-first-canadians-with-dementia-to-die-with-medical-assistance-1.5335025.

174 From the start, the Final Exit Network: In the United States, narrower debates around end-of-life care for dementia patients are underway—though they are focused on the withdrawal of treatment rather than active aid in dying. At issue is whether an American adult can specify, in an advance directive, that she wants certain life-prolonging treatments to be withheld or withdrawn, in the event that she is too demented to make the choice herself. The most heated debate concerns spoon-feeding. Can a dementia patient ask, in advance, to *not* be fed—when he loses the ability to feed himself? Effectively, can he ask to be starved? Currently, spoon-feeding is considered "comfort care," something that doctors are required to provide to all patients, regardless of their condition—as opposed to "medical care," like feeding tubes or respirators, which a patient can opt to remove. Patients with dementia often end up being spoon-fed. Even at the point when they are unable to (and sometimes uninterested in) lifting utensils to their lips, they may respond instinctively when a spoon is put before them. Just two dozen states have laws that deal with assisted feeding, and many explicitly prohibit the withdrawal of food and fluids.

In 2017, I read about a woman named Nora Harris, a former librarian and Virginia Woolf scholar with dementia. When she was of sound mind, Harris had written an advance directive asking that no artificial measures be used to prolong her life. Nevertheless, when she lost the ability to communicate and recognize family members, nursing staff began feeding her by hand—and when they raised food to her lips, she obediently opened her mouth to take it in. Her husband, Bill, took the case to court, but a court-appointed lawyer argued that Nora's advance directive was too vaguely worded to be understood and taken literally. The judge agreed. Oregon's long-term care ombudsman also argued that rules around mandatory feeding were necessary, to prevent abuse. The nursing home

NOTES

kept feeding Nora: three state-required meals a day and optional snacks. Lynn Rawlins, the administrator at the care center where Nora lived, said that she had no choice in the matter. "We have to feed them until they stop opening their mouths," she said. "We still have to feed them, even if they choke."

Barak Gaster et al., "Advance Directives for Dementia," *JAMA: Journal of the American Medical Association* 318, no. 22 (2017): 2175–2176; Paul T. Menzel, "Advance Directives, Dementia, and Withholding Food and Water by Mouth," *Hastings Center Report* 44, no. 3 (2014): 23–37; JoNel Aleccia, "Despite Advance Directive, Oregon Dementia Patient Denied Last Wish, Says Spouse," Kaiser Health News, August 25, 2017, https:// www.seattletimes.com/seattle-news/despite-advance-directive-oregon-dementia-patient -denied-last-wish-says-spouse/.

5. MIND

187 **"According to one theory," the website read**: Harvard Medical School, "Depression and Pain," Harvard Health Publishing, updated March 21, 2017, https://www.health.harvard .edu/mind-and-mood/depression-and-pain.

189 **In 2015, Canada's Supreme Court overturned**: Martha Butler and Marlisa Tiedemann, "Carter v. Canada: The Supreme Court of Canada's Decision on Assisted Dying," Background Paper, Library of Parliament, No. 2015-47-E, December 29, 2015, https://lop.parl .ca/sites/PublicWebsite/default/en_CA/ResearchPublications/201547E; *Carter v. Canada (Attorney General)*, 2015 SCC 5 Canada Supreme Court Judgments, No. 35591, https://scc -csc.lexum.com/scc-csc/scc-csc/en/item/14637/index.do.

189 **Lawmakers could be as expansive as**: See, for instance, Canadian Medical Association, "Supporting the Enactment of Bill C-14, *Medical Assistance in Dying*: Submission to the House of Commons Standing Committee on Justice and Human Rights," May 2, 2016, https:// policybase.cma.ca/documents/Briefpdf/BR2016-08.pdf; Canadian Civil Liberties Association, "Submission to the Standing Committee on Justice and Human Rights," May 2016, https://ccla.org/cclanewsite/wp-content/uploads/2018/09/Bill-C-75-CCLA-Submissions.pdf; Laura Wright, "Key Players in the Right-to-Die Decision and Debate," CBC News, April 14, 2016, https://www.cbc.ca/news/politics/doctor-assisted-death-key-players-1.3535912.

190 **Almost immediately, the Parliament and press**: For more on the debate over assisted death and mental illness in Canada, see Canadian Psychiatric Association, "Task Force on Medical Assistance in Dying: 2016 Member Survey Results," 2017, https://www.cpa -apc.org/wp-content/uploads/CPA-MAIDTF-16Surv-Rep-FIN-EN.pdf; Skye Rousseau et al., "A National Survey of Canadian Psychiatrists' Attitudes Toward Medical Assistance in Death," *Canadian Journal of Psychiatry* 62, no. 11 (May 2017): 787–794; Canadian Psychological Association, "Medical Assistance in Dying and End-of-Life Care," May 2018, https://cpa.ca/docs/File/Task_Forces/Medical%20Assistance%20in%20Dying%20and% 20End%20of%20Life%20Care_FINAL.pdf; Canadian Mental Health Association, "Position Paper on Medical Assistance in Dying (MAiD)," August 2017, https://cmha.ca /wp-content/uploads/2017/09/CMHA-Position-Paper-on-Medical-Assistance-in-Dying -FINAL.pdf; Barbara Walker-Renshaw et al., "Carter v. Canada (Attorney General): Will the Supreme Court of Canada's Decision on Physician-Assisted Death Apply to Persons Suffering from Severe Mental Illness?" *Journal of Ethics in Mental Health*, November 2015, https://jemh.ca/issues/v9/documents/JEMH_Open-Volume_Benchmark

_Assisted%20Death-Nov20-2015.pdf; Scott Y. H. Kim and Trudo Lemmens, "Should Assisted Dying for Psychiatric Disorders Be Legalized in Canada?" *CMAJ* 188, no. 14 (October 2016): 337–339; Expert Panel Working Group on MAID Where a Mental Disorder Is the Sole Underlying Medical Condition, "The State of Knowledge on Medical Assistance in Dying Where a Mental Disorder Is the Sole Underlying Medical Condition," Council of Canadian Academies, 2018, https://cca-reports.ca/wp-content/uploads/2018/12/The-State-of-Knowledge-on-Medical-Assistance-in-Dying-Where-a-Mental-Disorder-is-the-Sole-Underlying-Medical-Condition.pdf.

190 **The Federal Special Joint Committee of the House and Senate on Physician-Assisted Dying**: Canadian Parliament, House of Commons Special Joint Committee on Physician-Assisted Dying, "Medical Assistance in Dying: A Patient Centered Approach. Report of the Special Joint Committee on Physician-Assisted Dying," 1st sess., 40th Parliament, February 2016, https://www.parl.ca/DocumentViewer/en/42-1/PDAM/report-1.

190 **They cited reports showing that mental suffering**: J. L. Bernheim et al., "The Potential of Anamnestic Comparative Self-Assessment (ACSA) to Reduce Bias in the Measurement of Subjective Well-Being," *Journal of Happiness Studies* 7, no. 2 (2006): 227–250, cited in Justine Dembo et al., "'For Their Own Good': A Response to Popular Arguments Against Permitting Medical Assistance in Dying (MAID) Where Mental Illness Is the Sole Underlying Condition," *Canadian Journal of Psychiatry* 63, no. 7 (2018): 451–456.

192 **In the famous Sequenced Treatment Alternatives**: A. John Rush et al., "Acute and Longer-Term Outcomes in Depressed Outpatients Requiring One or Several Treatment Steps: A STAR*D Report," *American Journal of Psychiatry* 166, no. 11 (November 2006): 1905–1917.

193 **In 2010, a few years into her residency**: Justine Dembo, "Addressing Treatment Futility and Assisted Suicide in Psychiatry," *Journal of Ethics in Mental Health* 5, no. 1 (2010).

193 **Dembo knew that the vast majority**: Dembo et al., "'For Their Own Good.'"

193 **A central tenet of psychiatry, in fact**: Ibid.; Rousseau et al., "A National Survey"; D. Okai et al., "Mental Capacity in Psychiatric Patients: Systematic Review," *British Journal of Psychiatry* 191 (2007): 291–297; Louis C. Charland and Mark Lachmann, "1.3: Decisional Capacity," Royal College of Physicians and Surgeons of Canada, accessed April 2020, http://www.royalcollege.ca/rcsite/bioethics/cases/section-1/decisional-capacity-e.

194 **But beyond the Toronto conference room**: Scott Y. H. Kim, "Capacity Assessments as a Safeguard for Psychiatric Patients Requesting Euthanasia," *Journal of Ethics in Mental Health* (2006), https://jemh.ca/issues/v9/documents/JEMH_Open-Volume_Commentary_7_Decision_Making_Capacity_to_Consent_To_Medical_Assistance_in_Dying-Kim-Dec%202-2016.pdf; Louis Charland et al., "Decision-Making Capacity to Consent to Medical Assistance in Dying for Persons with Mental Disorders," *Journal of Ethics in Mental Health* (2016).

194 **"How can one distinguish a request"**: Mona Gupta and Christian Desmarais, "A Response to Charland and Colleagues: Science Cannot Resolve the Problems of Capacity Assessment," *Journal of Ethics in Mental Health* (2016), https://jemh.ca/issues/v9/documents/JEMH_Open-Volume_Commentary_1_Science_Cannot_Resolve_Problems_of_Capacity_Assessment_Nov18-2016.pdf.

195 **Broadening assisted death to patients with**: Theo A. Boer, "Does Euthanasia Have a Dampening Effect on Suicide Rates? Recent Experience from the Netherlands," *Journal of Ethics in Mental Health* (2016), https://jemh.ca/issues/v9/documents/JEMH%20article%20Boer%20final%20proof.pdf.

195 **Others condemned the proposal on more practical:** John Maher, "Assisted Death in Canada for Persons with Active Psychiatric Disorders," *Journal of Ethics in Mental Health* (2016), https://jemh.ca/issues/v9/documents/JEMH_Open-Volume-Editorial-Assisted%20 Death%20in%20Canada-May2016.pdf; Center for Addiction and Mental Health, "Policy Advice on Medical Assistance in Dying and Mental Illness," October 2017, https://www .camh.ca/-/media/files/pdfs—public-policy-submissions/camh-position-on-mi-maid -oct2017-pdf.pdf.

196 **"We thus find ourselves in a paradox":** Justine Dembo, "The Ethics of Providing Hope in Psychotherapy," *Journal of Psychiatric Practice* 19, no. 4 (July 2013): 316–322. See also Jocelyn Downie and Justine Dembo, "Medical Assistance in Dying and Mental Illness Under the New Canadian Law," *Journal of Ethics in Mental Health* (2016).

197 **but the wait time to see specialists:** Rachel Loebach and Sasha Ayoubzadeh, "Wait Times for Psychiatric Care in Ontario," *University of Western Ontario Medical Journal* 86, no. 2 (2007): 48–50.

200 **He talked on the phone with an older activist:** Robert Cribb, "Death's Midwife Helps Terminally Ill Canadians End Their Lives," *Toronto Star*, October 21, 2012, https://www .thestar.com/news/gta/2012/10/21/deaths_midwife_helps_terminally_ill_canadians_end _their_lives.html.

201 **A journalist from the *Globe and Mail*:** Adam Maier-Clayton, "As a Person with Mental Illness, Here's Why I Support Medically Assisted Death," *Globe and Mail*, May 8, 2016, https://www.theglobeandmail.com/life/health-and-fitness/health/as-a-person-with -mental-illness-heres-why-i-support-medically-assisted-death/article29912835/.

201 **In the end, legislators had excluded mental illness:** Lawmakers wrote that they had tried to strike "the most appropriate balance between the autonomy of persons who seek medical aid in dying, on the one hand, and the interests of vulnerable persons in need of protection and those of society, on the other." But they also anticipated the disappointment of activists who had been campaigning for a more expansive interpretation of the Supreme Court ruling. Legislators ordered a panel of independent academics to study three categories of patients who had not been included in Bill C-14 but who could possibly be added down the line: "mature minors" under eighteen years old, people with dementia, and people whose primary illness was psychological. Jocelyn Downie and Jennifer A. Chandler, "Interpreting Canada's Medical Assistance in Dying Legislation," IRPP, March 1, 2018, https://irpp.org/research-studies/interpreting-canadas-medical-assistance-in-dying-maid -legislation/.

201 **Dr. Ellen Wiebe, a Vancouver family medicine:** Sheryl Ubelacker, "Doctors Willing to Help Patients Die May Face Emotional Suffering," *Canadian Press*, December 8, 2015, https://www.ctvnews.ca/health/doctors-willing-to-help-patients-die-may-face-emotional -suffering-1.2691083; "Dr. Ellen Wiebe: 'We Should All Have the Right to Die at Our Own Choice,'" *Canadian Press*, March 20, 2016, https://www.macleans.ca/news/canada/dr -ellen-wiebe-we-should-all-have-the-right-to-die-at-our-own-choice/.

203 **"If I kill myself," he told a reporter:** Alex Ballingall, "'I Will Not Live Like This': Legal Challenge to Ottawa's Assisted Dying Law Gains Steam," *Toronto Star*, September 6, 2016, https://www.thestar.com/news/canada/2016/09/06/i-will-not-live-like-this-legal-challenge -to-ottawas-assisted-dying-law-gains-steam.html.

203 **In December 2016, VICE Canada described Adam:** Rachel Browne, "This 27-Year-Old Is Fighting for His Right to Die, Even if It Means Committing a Crime," VICE Canada, December 22, 2016, https://www.vice.com/en_ca/article/bjdwy3/this-27-year-old-is -fighting-for-his-right-to-die-even-if-it-means-committing-a-crime.

204 **But the more news articles and blog posts that appeared**: For instance, the *Toronto Star* quoted Adam as saying: "It would be far more preferable than restraining my hands and jumping off a bridge or a building." Ballingall, "'I Will Not Live Like This'"; Lisa Xing, "'My Life Is a Nightmare': Windsor Man, 27, Wants Legally Assisted Death," CBC News, October 31, 2016, https://www.cbc.ca/news/canada/windsor/assisted-dying-mentally-ill-1.3829839.

204 **When I read Adam's Facebook page**: Johann Wolfgang von Goethe, *The Sorrows of Young Werther* (Germany, 1774).

205 **Today, social scientists still speak of**: S. Stack, "Media Coverage as a Risk Factor in Suicide," *Journal of Epidemiology and Community Health* 57 (2003): 238–240; Thomas Niederkroten-thaler, "Association Between Suicide Reporting in the Media and Suicide: Systematic Review and Meta Analysis," *BMJ* 368 (March 2020), https://www.bmj.com/content/368/bmj.m575.

205 **A 2015 paper in the *Southern Medical Journal***: D. A. Jones and D. Patton, "How Does Legalization of Physician-Assisted Suicide Affect Rates of Suicide?" *Southern Medical Journal* 108, no. 10 (2015): 599–604.

205 **But when Canadian researchers**: Matthew P. Lowe and Jocelyn Downie, "Does Legalization of Medical Assistance in Dying Affect Rates of Non-assisted Suicide?" *Journal of Ethics in Mental Health* (2017), https://jemh.ca/issues/v9/documents/JEMH%20final%20Legislation-iii.pdf.

207 **She kept coming back to a 2015**: Lieve Thienpont et al., "Euthanasia Requests, Procedures and Outcomes for 100 Belgian Patients Suffering from Psychiatric Disorders: A Retrospective Study," *BMJ Open* (2015), https://bmjopen.bmj.com/content/5/7/e007454. See also M. Verhofstadt et al., "When Unbearable Suffering Incites Psychiatric Patients to Request Euthanasia: Qualitative Study," *British Journal of Psychiatry* 211, no. 4 (2017): 238–245.

207 **in Belgium, where since 2002**: Raphael Cohen-Almagor, "Euthanasia Policy and Practice in Belgium: Critical Observations and Suggestions for Improvement," *Issues in Law and Medicine* 24, no. 3 (2009): 187–218; H. R. W. Pasman et al., "Concept of Unbearable Suffering in Context of Ungranted Requests for Euthanasia: Qualitative Interviews with Patients and Physicians," *BMJ* 339 (2009); Sigrid Dierickx et al., "Euthanasia for People with Psychiatric Disorders or Dementia in Belgium: Analysis of Officially Reported Cases," *BMC Psychiatry* 17, no. 203 (2017); David Albert Jones et al., eds., *Euthanasia and Assisted Suicide: Lessons from Belgium* (Cambridge: Cambridge University Press, 2017); Mark S. Komrad, "A Psychiatrist Visits Belgium: The Epicenter of Psychiatric Euthanasia," *Psychiatric Times*, June 21, 2018, https://www.psychiatrictimes.com/couch-crisis/psychiatrist-visits-belgium-epicenter-psychiatric-euthanasia. See also an explanation of euthanasia for mental suffering in the Netherlands: Marije van der Lee, "Depression, Euthanasia, and Assisted Suicide," chap. 18 in *Physician-Assisted Death in Perspective: Assessing the Dutch Experience* (Cambridge: Cambridge University Press, 2012); Scott Y. H. Kim et al., "Euthanasia and Assisted Suicide of Patients with Psychiatric Disorders in the Netherlands 2011 to 2014," *JAMA Psychiatry* 73, no. 4 (2016): 362–368; Hans Pols and Stephanie Oak, "Physician-Assisted Dying and Psychiatry: Recent Developments in the Netherlands," *International Journal of Law and Psychiatry* 36 (2014): 508–514; Kristen Evenblij et al., "Euthanasia and Physician-Assisted Suicide in Patients Suffering from Psychiatric Disorders: A Cross-Sectional Study Exploring the Experiences of Dutch Psychiatrists," *BMC Psychiatry* 19, no. 74 (2019).

208 **By the time the paper was published**: M. Verhofstadt et al., "When Unbearable Suffering Incites Psychiatric Patients to Request Euthanasia," *British Journal of Psychiatry* 211, no. 4 (2017), 238–245, https://pubmed.ncbi.nlm.nih.gov/28970302/.

208 **Other Belgian doctors admitted to euthanizing**: "Belgian Helped to Die After Three Sex

Change Operations," BBC News, October 2, 2013, https://www.bbc.com/news/world -europe-24373107.

208 **Another, because he could not control:** "Belgian Murderer Van Den Bleeken Wins 'Right to Die,'" BBC News, September 15, 2014, https://www.bbc.com/news/world-europe-29209459.

208 **Across the Dutch-speaking region of Flanders:** Charles Collins, "Belgian Ethicist Says Euthanasia Has Become 'Sacralized,'" Crux, July 9, 2018, https://cruxnow.com/interviews /2018/07/belgian-ethicist-says-euthanasia-has-become-sacralized/.

209 **This was Vonkel, the euthanasia nonprofit:** According to Thienpont, by the end of 2018, 1,495 people had visited Vonkel for information and 437 had made euthanasia requests.

210 **Not long after my visit:** Maria Cheng, "What Could Help Me to Die? Doctors Clash over Euthanasia," Associated Press, October 26, 2017, https://apnews.com/4b6877fab2e849269c 659a5854867a7b.

211 **Thienpont told me that because Belgium:** Pablo Nicaise et al., "Mental Health Care De-livery System Reform in Belgium: The Challenge of Achieving Deinstitutionalization Whilst Addressing Fragmentation of Care at the Same Time," *Health Policy* 115, nos. 2–3 (2014): 120–127.

220 **There was no single, decided-upon protocol:** The Canadian Association of MAID Assessors and Providers has since done work in this area. Canadian Association of MAID Assessors and Providers, "Final Report: 2nd Annual Medical Assistance in Dying Conference 2018," December 2018, https://camapcanada.ca/wp-content/uploads/2018/12/MAID2018eng1 .pdf. The Joint Centre for Bioethics at the University of Toronto has also created a ca-pacity assessment tool. Joint Centre for Bioethics, "Aid to Capacity Evaluation (ACE)," accessed April 2020, http://jcb.utoronto.ca/tools/documents/ace.pdf.

220 **She relied heavily on the Appelbaum criteria:** P. S. Appelbaum and T. Grisso, "Assessing Patients' Capacities to Consent to Treatment," *New England Journal of Medicine* 319, no. 25 (1988): 1635–1638.

220 **But elsewhere, some Canadian physicians:** Alec Yarascavitch, "Assisted Dying for Men-tal Disorders: Why Canada's Legal Approach Raises Serious Concerns," *Journal of Eth-ics in Mental Health* (2017), https://jemh.ca/issues/v9/documents/JEMH%20article%20 MAID%20yarascavitch%20final.pdf. See also Samuel N. Doernberg et al., "Capacity Evaluations of Psychiatric Patients Requesting Assisted Death in the Netherlands," *Psy-chosomatics* 57, no. 6 (2016): 556–565; Scott Kim, lecture in *Physician-Assisted Death: Scan-ning the Landscape: Proceedings of a Workshop* (Washington, DC: National Academies of Sciences, Engineering, and Medicine, 2018), 10–12; Lois Snyder Sulmasy et al., "Ethics and the Legalization of Physician-Assisted Suicide: An American College of Physicians Positions Paper," *Annals of Internal Medicine* 167, no. 8 (2017): 576–578.

221 **Opponents noted that in Oregon:** In 2016, for instance, physicians wrote 204 aid-in-dying prescriptions, but just 5 patients were sent for psychological/psychiatric evalua-tion. Public Health Division, Center for Health Statistics, "Oregon Death with Dignity Act: 2016 Summary," Oregon Health Authority, February 10, 2017, https://www.oregon .gov/oha/PH/PROVIDERPARTNERRESOURCES/EVALUATIONRESEARCH /DEATHWITHDIGNITYACT/Documents/year19.pdf. Only Hawaii mandates men-tal health evaluations for medical aid in dying.

221 **More persuasively, skeptics cited:** Linda Ganzini et al., "Prevalence of Depression and Anxiety in Patients Requesting Physicians' Aid in Dying: Cross Sectional Survey," *BMJ* 337 (2008): 1682.

224 **On April 17, Adam's final Facebook post:** Andre Picard, "The Mentally Ill Must Be Part of the Assisted-Dying Debate," *Globe and Mail*, April 17, 2017, https://www

.theglobeandmail.com/opinion/the-mentally-ill-must-be-part-of-the-assisted-dying
-debate/article34721896/.

224 **In another op-ed, published two days later:** Sandra Martin, "Canada's Assisted-Dying
Laws Must Be Open to Those with Mental Illness," *Globe and Mail*, April 19, 2017, https://
www.theglobeandmail.com/life/health-and-fitness/health/canadas-assisted-dying-laws
-must-be-open-to-those-with-mental-illness/article34753182/.

225 **Online, the CBC ran an article about:** Lisa Xing, "After Son's Suicide, Father Pushes for Assisted Dying for Mentally Ill," CBC News, April 21, 2017, https://www.cbc.ca/news/canada
/windsor/adam-maier-claytons-father-takes-on-assisted-dying-advocacy-1.4080553.

6. FREEDOM

227 **Only a handful of people showed up:** "Seomra Spraoi Provides Venue for Assisted Suicide Workshop," Indymedia Ireland, February 18, 2011, http://www.indymedia.ie/article
/98985?condense_comments=true&userlanguage=ga&save_prefs=true.

228 **He had become a kind of celebrity:** For instance, Paul Gallagher, "Euthanasia: Arrival of
UK's First Clinic Offering Advice on Ending Life Condemned as 'Unwelcome and Very
Dangerous,'" *Independent*, October 5, 2014, https://www.independent.co.uk/news/uk
/home-news/arrival-of-euthanasia-advice-clinic-exit-international-in-uk-condemned-as
-unwelcome-and-very-9775803.html; "'Dr. Death' Philip Nitschke Banned from Practicing Medicine in Australia After Helping a Perth Man Commit Suicide," Australian Associated Press, July 23, 2014, https://www.dailymail.co.uk/news/article-2703405/Euthanasia
-campaigner-Nitschke-appeal.html.

229 **One pale woman in a white sweater:** Philip Nitschke and Fiona Stewart, *The Peaceful Pill
Handbook* (Washington: Exit International US, 2010).

229 **Philip had run his first Exit workshop in 1997:** Philip Nitschke and Peter Coris, *Damned
If I Do* (Melbourne: Melbourne University Publishing, 2013); Philip Nitschke, *Killing Me
Softly* (Washington: Exit International US, 2011).

230 **and after Philip became the first person in the world:** "Australian Man First in World to
Die with Legal Euthanasia," Associated Press, September 26, 1996, https://www.nytimes
.com/1996/09/26/world/australian-man-first-in-world-to-die-with-legal-euthanasia.html.

230 **He explained that Australia had later rescinded:** Gareth Griffith, "Euthanasia: An Update"
NSW Parliamentary Library Research Service, Briefing Paper No. 3/2001, March 2001,
https://www.parliament.nsw.gov.au/researchpapers/Documents/euthanasia-an-update
/Euthanasiacorrected.pdf.

231 **Four years later, in 2002:** David Fickling, "Australia Split on Helping Healthy to Die,"
Guardian, November 27, 2002, https://www.theguardian.com/world/2002/nov/27/australia
.davidfickling; "Healthy Woman Thanks Dr. Nitschke, Then Kills Herself," *Sydney Morning Herald*, November 26, 2002, https://www.smh.com.au/national/healthy-woman-thanks
-dr-nitschke-then-kills-herself-20021126-gdfvde.html; *Mademoiselle and the Doctor*, directed
by Janine Hoskin (Australia: iKandy Films, 2004).

232 **In response, pharmaceutical companies released:** Elena Conis, "Valium Had Many An-
cestors," *Los Angeles Times*, February 18, 2008, https://www.latimes.com/archives/la-xpm
-2008-feb-18-he-esoterica18-story.html.

232 **Now pentobarbital was hard to come by:** Sarah E. Boslaugh, ed., *The SAGE Encyclopedia
of Pharmacology and Society* (London: SAGE Publications, 2016), 35.

233 **In 2009, one of Philip's oldest allies:** Andrew Alderson, "Suicide Expert Turns on 'Dr

Death,'" *Telegraph*, May 9, 2009, https://www.telegraph.co.uk/news/health/news/5299634/Suicide-expert-turns-on-Dr-Death.html.

234 **It began in 1988, with an article published in**: Anonymous, "It's Over, Debbie," *JAMA: Journal of the American Medical Association* 259, no. 2 (1988): 272.

234 **Dozens of readers sent letters of protest**: George D. Lundberg, "'It's Over, Debbie' and the Euthanasia Debate," *JAMA: Journal of the American Medical Association* 259, no. 14 (1988): 2142–2143; "It's Almost Over—More Letters on Debbie," *JAMA: Journal of the American Medical Association* 260, no. 6 (1988): 787–789.

235 **"*Murder* is the only word for it"**: Sherwin Nuland, *How We Die: Reflections on Life's Final Chapter* (New York: Knopf, 1994).

235 **The editors of *JAMA***: Lundberg, "'It's Over, Debbie.'"

235 **That same year, an uncelebrated pathologist**: Jack Kevorkian, "The Last Fearsome Taboo: Medical Aspects of Planned Death," *Medicine and Law* 7, no. 1 (1988): 1–14; Detroit Free Press Staff, *The Suicide Machine* (Detroit: Detroit Free Press, 1997); Michael DeCesare, *Death on Demand: Jack Kevorkian and the Right-to-Die Movement* (Baltimore: Rowman and Littlefield, 2015); Neal Nichol and Harry Wylie, *You Don't Know Jack: Between the Dying and the Dead* (USA: World Audience, 2011); "Chronology of Dr. Jack Kevorkian's Life and Assisted Suicide Campaign," *Frontline*, PBS, June 4, 1990, https://www.pbs.org/wgbh/pages/frontline/kevorkian/chronology.html.

235 **Then, in 1990, Kevorkian was featured**: Detroit Free Press Staff, *Suicide Machine*.

235 **"A high school student could do it"**: DeCesare, *Death on Demand*, 51.

235 **According to her husband**: Ron Rosenbaum, "Angel of Death: The Trial of the Suicide Doctor," *Vanity Fair*, May 1990.

235 **In June 1990, Janet took her life**: Lisa Belkin, "Doctor Tells of First Death Using His Suicide Device," *New York Times*, June 6, 1990, https://www.nytimes.com/1990/06/06/us/doctor-tells-of-first-death-using-his-suicide-device.html; James Risen, "Death and the Doctor: Dr. Jack Kevorkian Has Long Taken an Interest in the Dying. But Did He Go Too Far in Assisting a Suicide?" *Los Angeles Times*, June 21, 1990.

236 **Because the state did not have a law**: Isabel Wilkerson, "Inventor of Suicide Machine Arrested on Murder Charge," *New York Times*, December 4, 1990; "Doctor Cleared of Murdering Woman with Suicide Machine," *New York Times*, December 14, 1990; William E. Schmidt, "Prosecutors Drop Criminal Case Against Doctor Involved in Suicide," *New York Times*, December 15, 1990; "Murder Charge Dropped in Suicide Device Case," *Washington Post*, December 13, 1990; Catherine L. Bjorck, "Physician-Assisted Suicide: Whose Life Is It Anyway," *SMU Law Review* 47, no. 2 (1994): 371–397.

236 **But in the end, that charge was dismissed**: The *New York Times* explained, in an article announcing the dismissal of charges: "After a two-day preliminary hearing on the case in Clarkston, Mich., Judge Gerald McNally of Oakland County District Court ruled that the prosecutors had failed to prove that Dr. Kevorkian, 62, had planned and carried out the death of the woman, Janet Adkins. Judge McNally said it was Mrs. Adkins and not Dr. Kevorkian who had caused her death. Noting that Michigan had no specific law against assisting suicide, he called on the State Legislature to address the issue."

236 **In 1991, prosecutors tried again**: Rosenbaum, "Angel of Death."

236 **During the hearing, prosecutors compared**: Ibid.

236 **"We thought patients would be horrified"**: Elisabeth Rosenthal, "In Matters of Life and Death, the Dying Take Control," *New York Times*, August 18, 1991.

237 **Kevorkian built a second suicide machine**: Jack Kevorkian, *Prescription Medicide: The Goodness of Planned Death* (Maryland: Prometheus, 1991); Pamela Warrick, "Suicide's

Partner: Is Jack Kevorkian an Angel of Mercy, or Is He a Killer, as Some Critics Charge? 'Society Is Making Me Dr. Death,' He Says. 'Why Can't They See? I'm Dr. Life!'" *Los Angeles Times*, December 6, 1992, https://www.latimes.com/archives/la-xpm-1992-12-06 -vw-3171-story.html.

237 **By the early nineties, Americans had grown used**: Alexander Morgan Capron, "Looking Back at Withdrawal of Life-Support Law and Policy to See What Lies Ahead for Medical Aid-in-Dying," *Yale Journal of Biology and Medicine* 92, no. 4 (2019): 781–791; Haider Warraich, *Modern Death: How Medicine Changed the End of Life* (New York: St. Martin's Press, 2017); Jessica Nutik Zitter, "How the Rise of Medical Technology Is Worsening Death," *Health Affairs*, November 6, 2017, https://www.healthaffairs.org/do/10.1377 /hblog20171101.612681/full/; Jessica Zitter, "Pricey Technology Is Keeping People Alive Who Don't Want to Live," *Wired*, April 10, 2017, https://www.wired.com/2017/04/pricey -technology-keeping-people-alive-dont-want-live/.

237 **Just a few decades earlier, a majority of deaths**: Atul Gawande, *Being Mortal: Medicine and What Matters in the End* (New York: Metropolitan Books, 2014), 6. Gawande writes, of the United States: "As recently as 1945, most deaths occurred in the home. By the 1980s, just 17 percent did. Those who somehow did die at home likely died too suddenly to make it to the hospital—say, from a massive heart attack, stroke, or violent injury—or were too isolated to get somewhere that could provide help."

237 **There were even new conditions emerging**: Alexander C. White, "Long-Term Mechanical Ventilation: Management Strategies," *Respiratory Care* 57, no. 6 (2012): 446–454.

237 **His objective, he would later explain**: Belkin, "Doctors Tell of First Death."

237 **Kevorkian was a trained pathologist**: George Howe Colt, *The Enigma of Suicide: A Timely Investigation into the Causes, the Possibilities for Prevention and the Paths to Healing* (New York: Touchstone, 1991), 377–384; Isabel Wilkerson, "Physician Fulfills a Goal: Aiding a Person in Suicide," *New York Times*, June 7, 1990, https://www.nytimes.com/1990/06 /07/us/physician-fulfills-a-goal-aiding-a-person-in-suicide.html; Mark Hosenball, "The Real Jack Kevorkian," *Newsweek*, December 5, 1993, https://www.newsweek.com/real -jack-kevorkian-190678; Maura Judkis, "Kevorkian's Macabre Paintings Caught in Auction Dispute," *Washington Post*, October 20, 2011, https://www.washingtonpost.com/blogs /arts-post/post/kevorkians-macabre-paintings-caught-in-auction-dispute/2011/10/20 /gIQAxyOD0L_blog.html.

238 **Before he unveiled the Thanatron**: "Kevorkian Pushes Death Row Organ Giving," Associated Press, October 18, 1993; "Biography," Jack Kevorkian Papers 1911–2017, Bentley Historical Library, accessed April 2020, https://quod.lib.umich.edu/b/bhlead/umich-bhl -2014106?byte=160800215;focusrgn=bioghist;subview=standard;view=reslist.

238 **Once, he left a corpse**: "Body in Auto Is Reported to Be Kevorkian's 26th Assisted Suicide," *New York Times*, November 9, 1995, https://www.nytimes.com/1995/11/09/us/body -in-auto-is-reported-to-be-kevorkian-s-26th-assisted-suicide.html.

238 **Derek Humphry, the founder of the Hemlock Society**: Derek Humphry and Mary Clement, *Freedom to Die: People, Politics and the Right-to-Die Movement* (New York: St. Martin's Griffin, 2000), chap. 9.

238 **"Diane was feeling tired and had a rash"**: Timothy E. Quill, "Death and Dignity—A Case of Individualized Decision Making," *New England Journal of Medicine* 324 (1991): 691–694.

239 **He knew that "pseudo-conversations"**: Timothy E. Quill, *Death and Dignity: Making Choices and Taking Charge* (New York: W. W. Norton, 1993).

239 **"In our discussion"**: Quill, "Death and Dignity."

240 **The _New York Times_ ran an editorial**: "Dealing Death, or Mercy?" _New York Times_, March 17, 1991.

240 **The bioethicist George Annas predicted**: Shari Roan, "Doctor Describes Aiding Cancer Patient's Suicide: Ethics: Many Authorities Support Physician. But He Could Face Charges of Second-Degree Manslaughter," _Los Angeles Times_, March 8, 1991.

240 **"I think these cases are as much an indictment"**: _The Kevorkian Verdict_, directed by Michael Kirk and Michael Sullivan (Boston: PBS, May 14, 1996), television broadcast.

240 **In the eight years following**: Keith Schneider, "Dr. Jack Kevorkian Dies at 83; a Doctor Who Helped End Lives," _New York Times_, June 3, 2011, https://www.nytimes.com/2011/06/04/us/04kevorkian.html.

241 **Some had psychiatric histories and**: According to one paper published in the _Gerontologist_, only 25 percent of Kevorkian's patients were terminally ill and 4 percent had "a history of psychiatric problems." Of 69 patients who were autopsied, 5 had "no anatomical evidence of disease at autopsy." Lori A. Roscoe et al., "A Comparison of Characteristics of Kevorkian Euthanasia Cases and Physician-Assisted Suicides in Oregon," _Gerontologist_ 41, no. 4 (2001): 439–446; Jack Lessenberry, "Specialist Testifies Depression Was Issue in Kevorkian Case," _New York Times_, April 24, 1996.

241 **Kevorkian, for his part, rarely tried to hide**: Ron Devlin and Christian D. Berg, "Long Found 'Not Close to Terminal.' Coroner Says Apparent Assisted Suicide Patient Had 10 Years of Life Left," Morning Call, December 31, 1997, https://www.mcall.com/news/mc-xpm-1997-12-31-3165984-story.html.

241 **In 1993, after Kevorkian was briefly jailed**: "Kevorkian Leaves Jail After 3 Days," _New York Times_, November 9, 1993.

241 **a Harris poll showed that 58 percent of Americans**: Humphry Taylor, "Doctor-Assisted Suicide: Support for Dr. Kevorkian Remains Strong and a 2-to-1 Majority Approves Oregon-Style Assisted Suicide Bill," Harris Poll, January 30, 1995, https://theharrispoll.com/wp-content/uploads/2017/12/Harris-Interactive-Poll-Research-DOCTOR-ASSISTED-SUICIDE-SUPPORT-FOR-DR-KEVORKIAN-R-1995-01.pdf.

241 **It wasn't until 1998 that**: Felicity Barringer, "CBS to Show Kevorkian Video of Man's Death," _New York Times_, November 20, 1998; Arthur Caplan and Joseph Turow, "Taken to Extremes: Newspapers and Kevorkian's Televised Euthanasia Incident," in _Culture Sutures: Medicine and Media_, ed. Lester D. Friedman (Durham, NC: Duke University Press, 2004), 36–54.

241 **When Judge Jessica Cooper delivered**: Edward Walsh, "Kevorkian Sentenced to Prison," _Washington Post_, April 14, 1999.

241 **The same year of Kevorkian's arrest**: Diane E. Meier et al., "A National Survey of Physician-Assisted Suicide and Euthanasia in the United States," _New England Journal of Medicine_ 338 (1998): 1193–1201.

241 **The _Lancet_ medical journal also ran**: "Kevorkian Arrested on Charge of First-Degree Murder," _Lancet_ 352 (1998): 1838.

242 **Underneath the Kevorkian article**: "Australian Doctor Reveals Details of Assisted Suicides," ibid.

242 **A few years later, Philip left**: Nitschke and Coris, _Damned If I Do_; Nitschke, _Killing Me Softly_.

243 **The Netherlands had effectively stopped prosecuting doctors**: Gerrit Van Der Wal and Robert J. M. Dillmann, "Euthanasia in the Netherlands," _BMJ_ 308, no. 6940 (1994): 1346–1349; Judith A. C. Reitjens et al., "Two Decades of Research on Euthanasia from the

Netherlands. What Have We Learnt and What Questions Remain?" *Journal of Bioethical Inquiry* 6 (2009): 271–283.

Furthermore, in 1993, the Dutch Senate passed Bill 22572, which created a legal mechanism for doctors to report assisted deaths and euthanasias to the public prosecutor. David C. Thomasma et al., eds., *Asking to Die: Inside the Dutch Debate About Euthanasia* (New York: Kluwer Academic Publishers, 2000), 11.

243 **but it would take until 2002 for the country to pass a law:** "Dutch Legalise Euthanasia," BBC, April 1, 2002, http://news.bbc.co.uk/2/hi/europe/1904789.stm.

243 **And so, Australia's Northern Territory became:** "Australian Man First in World to Die with Legal Euthanasia," Associated Press, September 26, 1996; Australian Broadcasting Corporation, *The Road to Nowhere*, Four Corners ABC (ABC, 1996), television broadcast.

246 **When he left Bob's house, Philip admitted:** Margaret Simons, "Between Life and Death," *Sydney Morning Herald*, August 31, 2013, https://www.smh.com.au/lifestyle/between-life-and-death-20130826-2skl0.html.

246 **Still, at the press conference announcing:** "The Fight to End a Life," *Sydney Morning Herald*, September 27, 1996, https://www.smh.com.au/national/the-fight-to-end-a-life-19960927-gdfboi.html.

246 **Philip signed his name to a "Declaration":** Dr. Rodney Syme et al., "Melbourne Declaration on Physician-Assisted Dying, Adopted by the 11th International Conference of the World Federation of Right to Die Societies," October 15–18, 1996, http://hrlibrary.umn.edu/instree/melbourne.html.

247 **But then, in March 1997, nine months:** David Kissane et al., "Seven Deaths in Darwin: Case Studies Under the Rights of the Terminally Ill Act, Northern Territory, Australia," *Lancet* 352 (1998): 1097–1102.

247 **That day, Philip had to tell another patient:** Ibid.

247 **So, in 1997, he founded the Voluntary:** Nitschke and Coris, *Damned If I Do*; Nitschke, *Killing Me Softly*.

247 **Philip designed a tiny Nembutal testing strip:** "Nembutal Sampler Kit," Exit International, accessed April 2020, https://exitinternational.net/product/nembutal-sampler-kit/.

249 *The Peaceful Pill Handbook* had: Nitschke and Stewart, *Peaceful Pill Handbook*.

250 **Philip met an elderly couple:** Stephanie Gardiner, "After 60 Years of Life Together, Don and Iris Die Together," *Sydney Morning Herald*, May 3, 2011, https://www.smh.com.au/national/after-60-years-of-life-together-don-and-iris-die-together-20110503-1e646.html; Susan Donaldson James, "Tourists Trek to Mexico for 'Death in a Bottle,'" ABC News, July 31, 2008, https://abcnews.go.com/Health/MindMoodNews/story?id=5481482.

251 **By the time he met Nigel Brayley:** Michael Safi, "Euthanasia Campaigner Dr. Philip Nitschke Suspended by Medical Board," *Guardian*, July 23, 2014, https://www.theguardian.com/world/2014/jul/24/euthanasia-campaigner-dr-philip-nitschke-suspended-by-medical-board; Suzie Keen, "Police Raid Nitschke's Clinic," InDaily, August 1, 2014, https://indaily.com.au/news/2014/08/01/police-raid-nitschkes-clinic/; Helen Davidson, "Philip Nitschke: 'I Wish I Had Responded Differently to Man's Suicide Email,'" *Guardian*, November 12, 2014, https://www.theguardian.com/australia-news/2014/nov/12/philip-nitschke-i-wish-i-had-responded-differently-to-mans-suicide-email; Helen Davidson, "Philip Nitschke Tribunal: A Clinical, Jarring Discussion on Rational Suicide," *Guardian*, November 18, 2014, https://www.theguardian.com/australia-news/2014/nov/18/philip-nitschke-tribunal-hearing-is-there-such-a-thing-as-rational-suicide.

251 **In response, the Medical Board of Australia**: Helen Davidson, "Philip Nitschke Wins Appeal over Medical License Suspension," *Guardian*, July 6, 2015, https://www.theguardian.com/australia-news/2015/jul/06/nitschke-wins-appeal-against-medical-licence-suspension.

253 **In October 2015, Australia's medical board**: Melissa Davey, "Philip Nitschke Banned from Promoting Voluntary Euthanasia as a Doctor," *Guardian*, October 25, 2015, https://www.theguardian.com/australia-news/2015/oct/26/philip-nitschke-banned-from-promoting-voluntary-euthanasia; Philip Nitschke, "Medical Registration Resignation Statement," Exit International, November 27, 2015, https://exitinternational.net/medical-registration-resignation-statement/.

256 **when I saw an article in the *Mirror***: "Fears Grow for Man Who Disappeared After Reportedly Buying 'Euthanasia Drugs' Online," *Mirror*, November 2, 2016, https://www.mirror.co.uk/news/uk-news/fears-grow-man-who-disappeared-9181727.

260 **And so, Philip said, he was starting a new initiative**: Helen Davidson, "Philip Nitschke Launches 'Militant' Campaign for Unrestricted Adult Access to Euthanasia," *Guardian*, December 3, 2016, https://www.theguardian.com/australia-news/2016/dec/04/philip-nitschke-launches-militant-campaign-for-unrestricted-adult-access-to-peaceful-death.

261 **"The guy next door, he has our competitor's book"**: Boudewijn Chabot, *Dignified Dying: Death at Your Bidding* (Netherlands: Boudewijn Chabot, 2014).

262 **Dr. Boudewijn Chabot, a psychiatrist**: Tony Sheldon, "The Doctor Who Prescribed Suicide," *Independent*, June 30, 1994, https://www.independent.co.uk/life-style/the-doctor-who-prescribed-suicide-was-the-dutch-psychiatrist-dr-boudewijn-chabot-right-to-help-a-1425973.html; "Doctor Unpunished for Dutch Suicide," Reuters, June 22, 1994, https://www.nytimes.com/1994/06/22/world/doctor-unpunished-for-dutch-suicide.html; Thomasma et al., *Asking to Die*, 76–82.

262 **By 2016, it accounted for 4 percent**: "Netherlands May Extend Assisted Dying to Those Who Feel 'Life Is Complete,'" Reuters, October 12, 2016, https://www.theguardian.com/world/2016/oct/13/netherlands-may-allow-assisted-dying-for-those-who-feel-life-is-complete.

263 **Even the Dutch Reformed Church tolerated**: Nuland, *How We Die*, chap. 7.

263 **More practically, the machine would reduce**: Adrianne Jeffries, "Silk Road Closure Reportedly Cuts Off Supply of Drug for Assisted Suicide," Verge, October 7, 2013, https://www.theverge.com/2013/10/7/4811920/silk-road-shutdown-cut-off-crucial-source-for-euthanasia-drug-nembutal; "Euthanasia Advocate Philip Nitschke Warns of Online Nembutal Scam," ABC News, September 2, 2014, https://www.abc.net.au/news/2014-09-03/philip-nitschke-warns-of-nembutal-scam/5715408.

265 ***Newsweek*, in its piece, had**: Nicole Goodkind, "Meet the Elon Musk of Assisted Suicide, Whose Machine Lets You Kill Yourself Anywhere," *Newsweek*, December 1, 2017, https://www.newsweek.com/elon-musk-assisted-suicide-machine-727874.

267 **By the time of my visit, some people**: Scott Kim, "How Dutch Law Got a Little Too Comfortable with Euthanasia," *The Atlantic*, June 8, 2019, https://www.theatlantic.com/ideas/archive/2019/06/noa-pothoven-and-dutch-euthanasia-system/591262/; Scott Kim et al., "Euthanasia and Assisted Suicide of Patients with Psychiatric Disorders in the Netherlands 2011–2014," *JAMA Psychiatry* 73, no. 4 (2017): 362–368.

267 **International newspapers like the *Daily Mail***: Sue Reid, "The Woman Killed by Doctors Because She Was Obsessed with Cleaning: Just One of Growing Numbers of Dutch People Given the Right to Euthanasia Because of Mental, Not Terminal, Illness," *Daily Mail*, May 13, 2016, https://www.dailymail.co.uk/news/article-3589929/The-woman-killed-doctors-obsessed-cleaning-Horrifying-Yes-s-just-one-growing-numbers-Dutch-men

-women-given-right-euthanasia-mental-not-terminal-illness.html; Linda Pressly, "The Troubled 29-Year-Old Helped to Die by Dutch Doctors," BBC, August 9, 2018, https:// www.bbc.com/news/stories-45117163; "Euthanasia Clinic Criticized for Helping Woman with Severe Tinnitus to Die," *Dutch News*, January 19, 2015, https://www.dutchnews.nl /news/2015/01/euthanasia-clinic-criticised-for-helping-woman-with-severe-tinnitus-to -die/.

267 **They quoted experts who pointed out, correctly**: Harriet Sherwood, "A Woman's Final Facebook Message Before Euthanasia: 'I'm Ready for My Trip Now,'" *Guardian*, March 17, 2018, https://www.theguardian.com/society/2018/mar/17/assisted-dying-euthanasia -netherlands#maincontent.

268 **In the Netherlands, wrote the psychiatrist**: Kim, "How Dutch Law."

268 **In his 2014 book, *Being Mortal***: Gawande, *Being Mortal*, 245.

268 **In reviewing Gawande's book**: Marcia Angell, "A Better Way Out," *New York Review of Books*, January 8, 2015.

270 **This was the New Technologies in Self-Deliverance**: Russel D. Ogden, "Non–physician Assisted Suicide: The Technological Imperative of the Deathing Counterculture," *Death Studies* 25 (2001): 387–401; Diane Martindale, "A Culture of Death," *Scientific American*, June 1, 2005, https://www.scientificamerican.com/article/a-culture-of-death/.

THE END

273 **According to a 2017 survey by the Kaiser Family Foundation**: Liz Hamel et al., "Views and Experiences with End-of-Life Medical Care in the U.S.," Kaiser Family Foundation, April 27, 2017, https://www.kff.org/report-section/views-and-experiences-with-end-of-life -medical-care-in-the-us-findings/.

273 **In October 2019, leading representatives**: Robin Gomes, "Abrahamic Religions: No to Euthanasia, Assisted Suicide, Yes to Palliative Care," *Vatican News*, October 28, 2019, https://www.vaticannews.va/en/vatican-city/news/2019-10/abrahamic-religions-life -euthanasia-suicide-palliative.html; Tom Blackwell, "Catholics Could Be Denied Last Rites, Funerals If They Undergo Doctor-Assisted Suicide: Canadian Bishop," *National Post*, March 6, 2016, https://nationalpost.com/news/religion/catholics-could-be-denied -last-rites-funerals-if-they-undergo-doctor-assisted-suicide-canadian-bishop-says; "Swiss Bishop to Priests: No Last Rites for Patients Seeking Assisted Suicide," Catholic News Service, December 8, 2016, https://www.ncronline.org/news/world/swiss-bishop-priests -no-last-rites-patients-seeking-assisted-suicide.

277 **"It could not be otherwise"**: Andrew Coyne, "On Assisted Suicide, the Slope Is Proving Every Bit as Slippery as Feared," *Globe and Mail*, January 17, 2020, https://www .theglobeandmail.com/opinion/article-on-assisted-suicide-the-slope-is-proving-every-bit -as-slippery-as/.

277 **In January 2020, three Belgian doctors**: "Belgian Doctors Go on Trial for Murder for Helping Woman End Life," Reuters, January 14, 2020, https://www.theguardian.com /world/2020/jan/14/belgian-doctors-go-on-trial-for-for-helping-woman-end-life; "Belgian Euthanasia: Three Doctors Accused in Unprecedented Trial," BBC, January 14, 2020, https://www.bbc.com/news/world-europe-51103687; Bruno Waterfield, "Tine Nys: Belgian Euthanasia Doctor Was Only 'Half-Trained,'" *The Times*, January 21, 2020, https://www.thetimes.co.uk/article/tine-nys-belgium-euthanasia-doctor-was-only-half -trained-0wjmnc00l.

277   **But just a month after the trial began**: Elian Peltier, "Belgium Acquits Three Doctors in Landmark Euthanasia Case," *New York Times*, January 31, 2020, https://www.nytimes.com/2020/01/31/world/europe/doctors-belgium-euthanasia.html.

277   **According to an Associated Press report**: Raf Casert, "Belgian Court Acquits 3 Doctors in Euthanasia Case," Associated Press, January 31, 2020, https://apnews.com/bd4a489924bac998ef0af3f3e446f3b7.

278   **In Britain, a former Supreme Court justice**: Owen Bowcott, "Ex–Supreme Court Justice Defends Those Who Break Assisted Dying Law," *Guardian*, April 17, 2019, https://www.theguardian.com/society/2019/apr/17/ex-supreme-court-jonathan-sumption-defends-break-assisted-dying-law.

279   **Then, a few months later, French media**: "French Police Seize Illegal Euthanasia Drugs in Raids," *Le Monde*, October 16, 2019, https://www.lemonde.fr/police-justice/article/2019/10/15/un-trafic-de-barbituriques-demantele-en-france_6015639_1653578.html. A spokesperson from the US Department of Homeland Security told me that her office was not involved in the investigation. A spokesperson from US Customs and Border Protection referred me to the Food and Drug Administration, whose spokesperson told me in an email that he had no information to provide. A spokesperson for the Department of Justice told me in an email that "due to ongoing litigation, we're unable to comment on this issue."

280   **Already, stories have appeared**: Bradford Richardson, "Insurance Companies Denied Treatment to Patients, Offered to Pay for Assisted Suicide, Doctor Claims," *Washington Times*, May 31, 2017, https://www.washingtontimes.com/news/2017/may/31/insurance-companies-denied-treatment-to-patients-o/; Andrea Peyser, "Terminally Ill Mom Denied Treatment Coverage—but Gets Suicide Drug Approved," *New York Post*, October 24, 2016, https://nypost.com/2016/10/24/terminally-ill-mom-denied-treatment-coverage-but-gets-suicide-drugs-approved/.

280   **"In this profit-driven economic climate"**: Helena Berger, "Assisted Suicide Laws Are Creating a 'Duty-to-Die' Medical Culture," The Hill, December 17, 2017, https://thehill.com/opinion/civil-rights/365326-how-assisted-suicide-laws-are-creating-a-duty-to-die-medical-culture.

280   **when the country's population is aging**: US Department of Health and Human Services, Administration on Aging, "A Profile of Older Americans: 2009," accessed April 2020, https://acl.gov/sites/default/files/Aging%20and%20Disability%20in%20America/2009profile_508.pdf; "A Profile of Older Americans: Older People Projected to Outnumber Children for the First Time in U.S. History," US Census, March 13, 2018, https://www.census.gov/newsroom/press-releases/2018/cb18-41-population-projections.html; James R. Knickman and Emily K. Snell, "The 2030 Problem: Caring for Aging Baby Boomers," *Health Services Research* 37, no. 4 (2002): 849–884.

280   **In 2010, the number of people**: Loraine A. West et al., "65+ in the United States," United States Census Bureau, June 2014, https://www.census.gov/content/dam/Census/library/publications/2014/demo/p23-212.pdf.

280   **Already, in 2017, Americans spent more than**: Centers for Medicare Services, "National Health Expenditures 2018," accessed April 2020, https://www.cms.gov/Research-Statistics-Data-and-Systems/Statistics-Trends-and-Reports/NationalHealthExpendData/NHE-Fact-Sheet; Karen E. Joynt Maddox et al., "US Health Policy—2020 and Beyond," *JAMA: Journal of the American Medical Association* 321, no. 17 (2019): 1670–1672; OECD, "Health Expenditure," 2018, accessed April 2020, https://www.oecd.org/els/health-systems/health-expenditure.htm.

280   **Up to a quarter of all Medicare spending**: Juliette Cubanski et al., "Medicare Spending

at the End of Life: A Snapshot of Beneficiaries Who Died in 2014 and the Cost of Their
Care," Kaiser Family Foundation, July 14, 2016, https://www.kff.org/medicare/issue-brief
/medicare-spending-at-the-end-of-life/; Matthew A. Davis et al., "Patterns of Healthcare
Spending in the Last Year of Life," *Health Affairs* 35, no. 7 (July 1, 2016); Ian Duncan et
al., "Medicare Cost at End of Life," *American Journal of Hospice and Palliative Care* 36, no.
8 (2019): 705–710.

281 **According to the 2017 Kaiser Family Foundation study**: Hamel et al., "Views and Experiences."

281 **National death phobia is so institutionalized that, in 2009**: Paula Span, "A Quiet End to
the 'Death Panels' Debate," *New York Times*, November 20, 2015, https://www.nytimes
.com/2015/11/24/health/end-of-death-panels-myth-brings-new-end-of-life-challenges
.html; JoNel Aleccia, "Docs Bill Medicare for End-of-Life Advice as 'Death Panel' Fears
Reemerge," Kaiser Health News, February 15, 2017, https://khn.org/news/docs-bill
-medicare-for-end-of-life-advice-as-death-panel-fears-reemerge/.

281 **In 2013, three years after the passage of the Affordable Care Act**: "Kaiser Health Tracking
Poll: March 2013," Kaiser Family Foundation, March 20, 2013, https://www.kff.org/health
-reform/poll-finding/march-2013-tracking-poll/. See also Olga Khazan, "27% of Surgeons
Still Think Obamacare Has Death Panels," *The Atlantic*, December 19, 2013, https://www
.theatlantic.com/health/archive/2013/12/27-of-surgeons-still-think-obamacare-has-death
-panels/282534/.

281 **"Rallying a party base against death"**: Jill Lepore, "The Politics of Death," *New Yorker*,
November 22, 2009.

281 **A study in the *Journal of Medical Ethics***: Margaret Battin et al., "Legal Physician-Assisted
Dying in Oregon and the Netherlands: Evidence Concerning the Impact on Patients in
'Vulnerable' Groups," *Journal of Medical Ethics* 33, no. 10 (2007): 591–597.

282 **hospice utilization in the state**: Death with Dignity National Center, "The Impact of Death
with Dignity on Healthcare," December 7, 2018, https://www.deathwithdignity.org/news
/2018/12/impact-of-death-with-dignity-on-healthcare/; National Hospice and Palliative
Care Organization, "NHPCO Facts and Figures, 2018 Edition," revised July 2, 2018, https://
39k5cm1a9u1968hg74aj3x51-wpengine.netdna-ssl.com/wp-content/uploads/2019/07/2018
_NHPCO_Facts_Figures.pdf; Linda Ganzini et al., "Oregon Physicians' Attitudes About
and Experiences with End-of-Life Care Since Passage of the Oregon Death with Dignity
Act," *JAMA: Journal of the American Medical Association* 285, no. 18 (2001): 2363–2369; Margaret Pabst Battin and Timothy Quill, eds., *The Case for Physician-Assisted Dying: The Right
to Excellent End-of-Life Care and Patient Choice* (Baltimore: Johns Hopkins University Press,
2004), 176–180; Timothy E. Quill and Franklin G. Miller, eds., *Palliative Care and Ethics*
(Oxford: Oxford University Press, 2014), 242–277.